AF717536

Holystic Medicine
The Patron Saints of Medicine

The Hagiography of Health and Illness

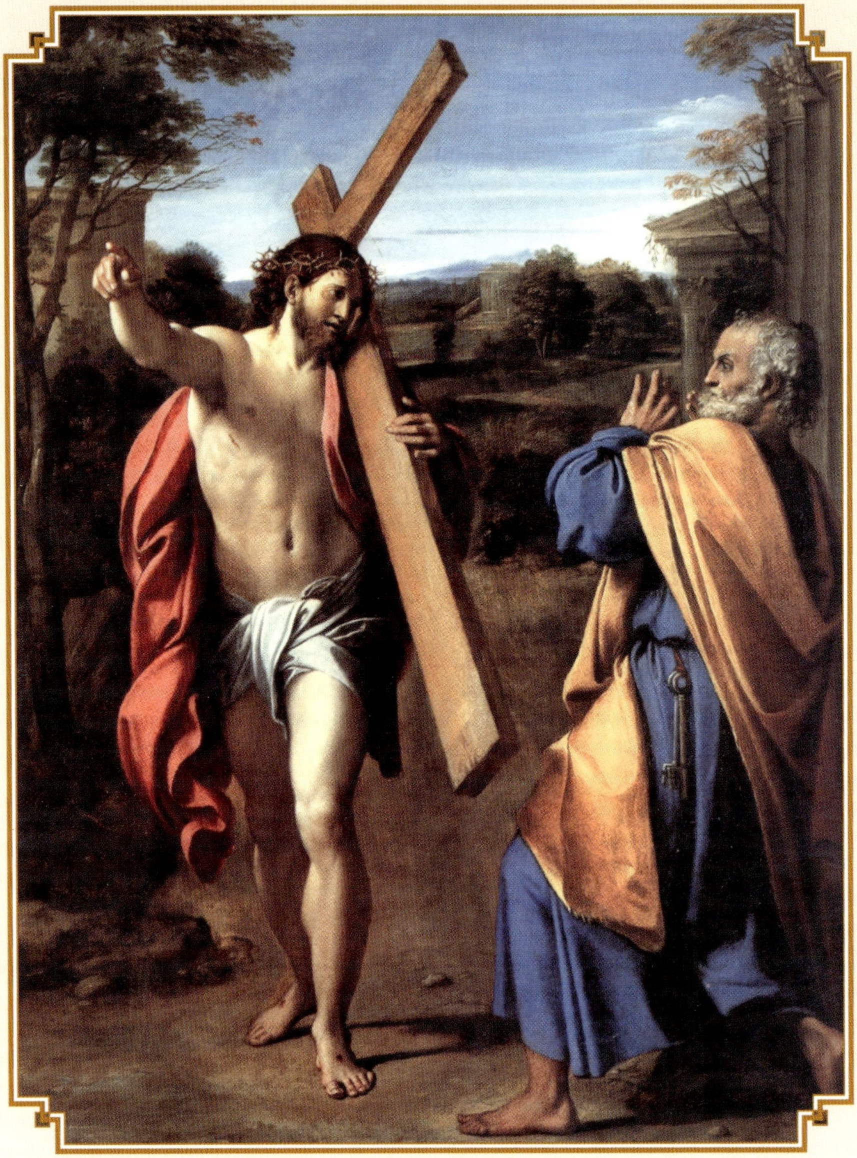

Christ Appearing to Saint Peter on the Appian Way (Domine, Quo Vadis?),
Annibale Carracci, 1601-1602. National Gallery, London, UK.

Holystic Medicine

The Patron Saints of Medicine

The Hagiography of Health and Illness

SEYMOUR I. SCHWARTZ, MD
Distinguished Alumni Professor
Department of Surgery
University of Rochester School of Medicine and Dentistry
Rochester, New York

CHRISTOPHER HOOLIHAN, MLS
Rare Books and Manuscripts Librarian
Edward G. Miner Library
University of Rochester Medical Center
Rochester, New York

Quality Medical Publishing, Inc.
ST. LOUIS, MISSOURI
2012

Copyright © 2012 by Quality Medical Publishing, Inc.

All rights reserved. No part of this publication may be reproduced, stored in a retrieval system, or transmitted in any form or by any means, electronic, mechanical, photocopying, recording, or otherwise, without prior permission of the publisher.

Printed in the United States of America

The publishers have made every effort to trace the copyright holders for borrowed material. If they have inadvertently overlooked any, they will be pleased to make the necessary arrangements at the first opportunity.

BOOK DESIGN Diane Beasley
COVER DESIGN Amanda Yarberry Behr

Quality Medical Publishing, Inc.
2248 Welsch Industrial Court
St. Louis, Missouri 63146
Telephone: 1-800-348-7808
Web site: *http://www.qmp.com*

LIBRARY OF CONGRESS CATALOGING-IN-PUBLICATION DATA

Schwartz, Seymour I., 1928-
Holystic medicine--the patron saints of medicine : the hagiography of health and illness / Seymour I. Schwartz, Christopher Hoolihan.
p. ; cm.
Includes bibliographical references.
ISBN 978-1-57626-348-8 (hardcover)
I. Hoolihan, Christopher. II. Title.
[DNLM: 1. Saints--Biography. 2. History of Medicine. 3. Religion and Medicine. WZ 150]

610.92'2--dc23

2011043645

Seymour I. Schwartz is the Distinguished Alumni Professor of Surgery at the University of Rochester School of Medicine and Dentistry, Rochester, New York, where he spent his entire academic career and was chair of the Department of Surgery. He edited seven editions of the popular surgical textbook, *Principles of Surgery,* and two editions of *Maingot's Abdominal Operations.* He authored seven additional surgical books. He was the editor-in-chief of *Yearbook of Surgery* for 21 years and the *Journal of the American College of Surgeons* for 7 years. Dr. Schwartz served as president of the American College of Surgeons, the American Surgical Association, and the Society of Clinical Surgery. He also authored seven books on American cartography and history; the latest is *Gifted Hands: America's Most Significant Contributions to Surgery.* He is a member of the Institute of Medicine and the American Philosophical Society.

Christopher Hoolihan is the Rare Books and Manuscripts Librarian at the Edward G. Miner Library, University of Rochester Medical Center, Rochester, New York. He is the compiler of the three-volume annotated catalog of the Edward G. Miner, MD, Collection of American Popular Medicine and the author of articles on the history of medical publishing and nineteenth century medical book illustration.

Preface

It is improbable and anachronistic that the idea of this first compendium of saints whose patronage pertains specifically to medical issues emanates from an academic surgeon dedicated to the dissemination of scientific knowledge. But, over my five decades of lecturing and writing about surgery, I have purposefully included reference to the patron saints of infirmities, diseases, symptoms, physically and physiologically disadvantaged individuals, and the persons who address and care for the afflicted in those narratives. Admittedly, the inclusion was generally planned to offer an allegory for embellishment, to romanticize and thereby maintain interest.

My use of the patron saints of medicine personally began with Saint Agatha and her patronage for breast disease. Incorporated within the legend of Saint Agatha is a description of the first bilateral mastectomy, the first immediate mammary reconstruction, and a sequence of events that can be used to emphasize that death associated with breast disease is not the result of the local lesion but rather of the systemic consequences. Exposing my audiences to saints continued during lectures on organ transplantation, which were often initiated with a representation of Saints Cosmas and Damian caring for a Caucasian with a successfully transplanted black leg from an exhumed Moor. Similarly, trauma lectures frequently were introduced with a painting of Saint Sebastian skewered with arrows.

I did not include what many regard to be myths as part of a scientific dialog to indicate acceptance of the concept that cure can result from invoking saints. Rather, I assembled references to the saints and their medical patronage to help appreciate the fact that there was a time when science did not dominate the practice of medicine. It was a time when those who were afflicted with illness, those who were unable to procreate, and those who feared becoming victims of devastating diseases or plagues were unaware of the pathologic processes responsible for their distress, and, as in other adverse circumstances, looked to the heavens for help. There remain some for whom these practices have continued into the present. A segment of society continues to apply prayers to prevent, cure, and palliate ailments—thus the invocation of patron saints of medicine, which was a pervasive and integral part of a distant heritage, persists.

This volume is offered as a compilation of relationships and tales mainly from the distant past. Although those relationships and tales continue to form the bases of beliefs for some, most readers should regard them as being of interest, perhaps intriguing, and potentially entertaining. The book is structured to provide factual biographic as well as legendary information. The narrative is meant to provide neither support nor disputation.

Seymour I. Schwartz

Acknowledgments

Throughout the project, the graphic artistry of Gianna Nixon-Saldinger has been integral to the optimal presentation of the illustrations and tables. Her total involvement in the project has raised her to a saintly esteem in our thoughts. Coincidentally, while writing the acknowledgment after completing the manuscript, we became aware of Saint Gianna Berreta Molla (1922-1962), who was an Italian pediatrician, wife, and mother known to have refused an abortion and a hysterectomy during her fourth pregnancy despite knowing that she was at risk. In 1962, she delivered her child by Caesarian section but died of peritonitis and sepsis. She was canonized by John Paul II in 2004. Her feast day is April 28, and she provides patronage for mothers, preborn children, and the pro-life movement.

Reverend Daniel Condon, Chancellor and Diocesan Director, Legal Services, of the Roman Catholic Diocese of Rochester, kindly reviewed the manuscript to ensure that there were no transgressions. Past President Nicholas J. Healy of Ave Maria University and Reverend George Heyman of St. Bernard's School of Theology and Ministry also reviewed the manuscript and illustrations to define potential sites for publication and distribution.

This publication is a rekindling of a relationship between myself and publisher Karen Berger after a hiatus of two decades. Both of the works we have done together have benefited enormously from her eye for elegance and insistence on perfection.

Contents

A

1 Abraham of Saint Cirgues . . . 2
2 Achatius . . . 3
3 Adamo of Fermo . . . 5
4 Adelard . . . 6
5 Adrian of Nicomedia . . . 8
6 Aedh Mac Bricc . . . 9
7 Aemilianus . . . 10
8 Agapitus . . . 11
9 Agatha . . . 12
10 Agrippina of Mineo . . . 14
11 Alban of Mainz . . . 15
12 Albana . . . 16
13 Albert of Trapani . . . 17
14 Albertinus . . . 18
15 Albinus of Angers . . . 19
16 Aldegonde . . . 20
17 Alderic . . . 21
18 Alena . . . 22
19 Alexander . . . 23
20 Aloysius Gonzaga . . . 24
21 Alphonsus Maria de Liguori . . . 26
22 Amable . . . 28
23 Amalburga of Maubeuge . . . 29
24 Amalburga of Munsterbilzsen . . . 30
25 Amo . . . 31
26 Anastasius the Persian . . . 32
27 Andrew the Apostle . . . 33
28 Andrew Avellino . . . 35
29 Anianus . . . 36
30 Anne . . . 37
31 Annemund . . . 38
32 Anno . . . 39
33 Ansbert . . . 40
34 Anthony della Chiesa . . . 41
35 Anthony the Great . . . 42
36 Anthony of Padua . . . 44
37 Aphrodisius . . . 46
38 Apollinaris of Ravenna . . . 47

39 *Apollonia* 48
40 *Apronia* 49
41 *Arnould* 50
42 *Arnulf of Soissons* 52
43 *Asclepius of Limoges* 53
44 *Asperenus* 54
45 *Athanasius* 55
46 *Aurelianus of Limoges* 57
47 *Austriclinianus* 58
48 *Avertan* 58
49 *Avertinus* 59
50 *Aybert* 60

B

51 *Balbina* 62
52 *Baldus* 63
53 *Balsamia* 64
54 *Balthasar* 65
55 *Barbara* 66
56 *Bartholomew* 68
57 *Basil the Great* 70
58 *Baudelius* 72
59 *Bavo* 73
60 *Beatus* 74
61 *Benedict the Moor* 75
62 *Benedict of Nursia* 76
63 *Bernard of Rodez* 78
64 *Bernardino of Siena* 79
65 *Bernulph of Utrecht* 81
66 *Bertha* 82
67 *Berthaldus of Reims* 83
68 *Berthilon* 84
69 *Bertilia* 85
70 *Beuve* 86
71 *Bibiana* 87
72 *Blase* 88
73 *Boetianus* 90
74 *Bonitus* 91
75 *Bonosa* 92
76 *Bruno of Cologne* 93
77 *Burchard* 94

C

78 *Cadoc of Llancarfan* 96
79 *Caesarius of Nazianzen* 98
80 *Calogeros* 99
81 *Camillus of Lellis* 100
82 *Candida* 102
83 *Caprasius* 103
84 *Casilda of Toledo* 104
85 *Casimir* 105
86 *Castorius* 106
87 *Catald of Taranto* 107

88 *Catherine of Alexandria* 108
89 *Catherine of Siena* 109
90 *Catherine of Vadstena* 111
91 *Ceranus* 112
92 *César de Bus* 113
93 *Cessator* 114
94 *Charalampos* 115
95 *Charitina* 116
96 *Charles Borromeo* 117
97 *Charles the Good* 119
98 *Christine of Saint Trond* 120
99 *Christopher* 121
100 *Chrysolius* 123
101 *Clare of Assisi* 124
102 *Clarus of Albi* 126
103 *Clarus of Vexin* 127
104 *Claude of Besançon* 128
105 *Clodoald* 129
106 *Clotilda* 130
107 *Colette* 131
108 *Colman of Stockerau* 132
109 *Columba of Sens* 133
110 *Columban* 134
111 *Conrad of Piacenza* 135
112 *Consortia* 136
113 *Cornelius* 137
114 *Cosmas and Damian* 138
115 *Crescentia* 140
116 *Cunégonde* 141
117 *Cunera* 142
118 *Cuthbert of Lindisfarne* 143
119 *Cyriacus* 144

D

120 *Dalmatius Moner* 146
121 *Damasus* 147
122 *Daniel of Padua* 148
123 *Danio* 149
124 *Defendens* 150
125 *Denis* 151
126 *Deodatus* 152
127 *Desideratus* 153
128 *Desiderius of Langres* 154
129 *Desiderius of Vienne* 155
130 *Dinoaldus* 156
131 *Dizaint* 157
132 *Dominic of Silos* 158
133 *Dominic of Sora* 159
134 *Domitian of Maestricht* 160
135 *Donanus* 161
136 *Donatus* 162
137 *Drogo* 163
138 *Dulcidius of Agen* 164
139 *Dymphna* 165

E

140 *Ebrulf* 168
141 *Edmund the Martyr* 169
142 *Edward the Confessor* 171
143 *Eligius* 173
144 *Elizabeth of Hungary* 175
145 *Emerentiana* 176
146 *Emilien* 177
147 *Engelmund* 178
148 *Engratia* 179
149 *Enimia* 180
150 *Erasmus* 181
151 *Ethelburga* 182
152 *Etheldreda* 183
153 *Eugenia* 184
154 *Eulalia of Barcelona* 185
155 *Eustace* 186
156 *Eutropius* 187
157 *Exsuperius* 188
158 *Ezekiel Moreno y Diaz* 189

F

159 *Faith* 192
160 *Fara* 193
161 *Félix of Bourges* 194
162 *Félix of Nantes* 195
163 *Felix of Nola* 196
164 *Felix of Split* 197
165 *Ferreolus* 198
166 *Fiacre* 199
167 *Fidelis of Spello* 202
168 *Firminus* 203
169 *Flamina* 204
170 *Flavitus* 205
171 *Florentius* 206
172 *Forannan* 207
173 *Fortunatus of Fano* 208
174 *Fourteen Holy Helpers* 208
175 *Fraimbaud* 210
176 *Framechildis* 211
177 *Franca of Piacenza* 212
178 *Francis of Paola* 213
179 *Francis de Sales* 214
180 *Francis Xavier* 216
181 *Fredegand* 218
182 *Friard* 219
183 *Frisius* 220
184 *Fursey* 221

G

185 *Gall of Clermont* 224
186 *Gaucherius* 225
187 *Gebhard of Konstanz* 226
188 *Gebuinus of Lyon* 227

189 *Genevieve* 228
190 *Gengulf* 230
191 *Gens* 231
192 *George* 232
193 *Gerald of Mayo* 234
194 *Gerard of Brogne* 235
195 *Gerard of Lunel* 236
196 *Gerard Majella* 237
197 *Gereon* 238
198 *Germanus of Auxerre* 239
199 *Germanus of Montfort* 241
200 *Germanus of Paris* 242
201 *Germanus of Scotland* 243
202 *Germer* 244
203 *Gertrude of Nivelles* 245
204 *Gervasius of Milan* 247
205 *Gibrian* 248
206 *Gilbert of Meaux* 249
207 *Gilbert of Neufontaines* 250
208 *Gildas* 251
209 *Giles* 252
210 *Gislenus* 253
211 *Giuseppe Moscati* 254
212 *Gobrianus* 255
213 *Godeberta* 256
214 *Godehard* 257
215 *Godeleva* 258
216 *Godfrey of Le Mans* 260
217 *Godo* 261
218 *Gratus* 262
219 *Gregory of Armenia* 263
220 *Gregory the Great* 264
221 *Gregory of Utrecht* 266
222 *Guenole* 267
223 *Guibert* 268
224 *Guimerra* 269
225 *Gummarus* 270
226 *Gunsaldus* 271
227 *Gurloes* 272
228 *Guy of Anderlecht* 273

H

229 *Haberilla* 276
230 *Hadeloga* 277
231 *Hartman of Brixen* 278
232 *Henry II* 279
233 *Hervé* 280
234 *Hidulf* 281
235 *Hildegund* 282
236 *Hildevert* 283
237 *Hiltrude* 284
238 *Honoratus of Toulouse* 285
239 *Honorina of Conflans* 286
240 *Hubert of Liège* 287
241 *Hugh of Cluny* 288
242 *Hugh of Grenoble* 290
243 *Hyacinth* 292

I

244 *Ida of Nivelle* ... 294
245 *Ignatius of Antioch* ... 295
246 *Inventus* ... 296
247 *Isberga* ... 297

J

248 *James the Greater* ... 300
249 *Jean François Régis* ... 301
250 *Jeanne Françoise de Chantal* ... 302
251 *Joachim of Siena* ... 304
252 *Job* ... 305
253 *John of Arras* ... 307
254 *John the Baptist* ... 308
255 *John Chrysostom* ... 309
256 *John of God* ... 311
257 *John the Great Sinner* ... 313
258 *John Licci* ... 315
259 *John of Ortica* ... 316
260 *Joseph* ... 317
261 *Josse* ... 319
262 *Julia of Troyes* ... 320
263 *Julian of Alexandria* ... 321
264 *Julian of Brioude* ... 322
265 *Julian the Hospitaler* ... 323
266 *Juliana of Collalto* ... 325
267 *Juliana Falconieri* ... 326
268 *Juliana of Nicomedia* ... 327

K

269 *Kilian* ... 330

L

270 *Lambert of Maastricht* ... 332
271 *Landericus* ... 333
272 *Lando* ... 334
273 *Lawrence* ... 335
274 *Lazarus of Bethany* ... 336
275 *Lazarus the Poor Man* ... 338
276 *Leander* ... 339
277 *Leo of Rouen* ... 341
278 *Leobonus* ... 342
279 *Leocadia* ... 343
280 *Leodegar* ... 344
281 *Leonard of Noblac* ... 346
282 *Leonard of Vandoeuvre* ... 348
283 *Leontius* ... 349
284 *Léothade* ... 350
285 *Leudomer* ... 351
286 *Leutfridus* ... 352
287 *Libaria* ... 353
288 *Liborius of Le Mans* ... 354
289 *Licinius* ... 355

290 *Loup of Chalon* 356
291 *Loup of Limoges* 357
292 *Loup of Lyon* 358
293 *Loup of Sens* 359
294 *Loup of Troyes* 360
295 *Lubin of Chartres* 361
296 *Lucian of Beauvais* 363
297 *Lucius of Cavargna* 364
298 *Lucy of Syracuse* 365
299 *Ludan* 367
300 *Luglius and Luglianus* 368
301 *Luke the Evangelist* 369
302 *Lutgardis* 371

M

303 *Macarius of Antioch* 374
304 *Macra* 375
305 *Madelbertha* 376
306 *Maginus of Tarragona* 376
307 *Magnobodus* 377
308 *Magnus of Füssen* 378
309 *Malo* 379
310 *Mamas* 380
311 *Manechildis* 381
312 *Marciana* 382
313 *Marculf* 383
314 *Margaret of Antioch* 384
315 *Margaret Mary Alacoque* 385
316 *Marguerite d'Youville* 386
317 *Marianus* 388
318 *Martha of Bethany* 389
319 *Martial of Limoges* 391
320 *Martin of Tours* 392
321 *Marus* 394
322 *Mary of Egypt* 395
323 *Mary of Oignies* 397
324 *Mathias the Apostle* 398
325 *Maturinus* 399
326 *Matrona of Capua* 400
327 *Maudez* 401
328 *Maurice* 402
329 *Maurus* 403
330 *Maximilian Kolbe* 404
331 *Maximinus of Besançon* 406
332 *Mazerand* 407
333 *Medard* 408
334 *Medicus* 409
335 *Méen* 410
336 *Mennas* 411
337 *Menoux* 412
338 *Meriadoc* 413
339 *Michael the Archangel* 414
340 *Millefort* 415
341 *Molagga* 416
342 *Mommolinus* 417
343 *Mucius* 418

N

344 *Namphanius* . . . 420
345 *Nepotianus* . . . 421
346 *Nicasius* . . . 422
347 *Nicholas of Bari* . . . 423
348 *Nomadia* . . . 424
349 *Norbert* . . . 425
350 *Notburga* . . . 427

O

351 *Odile* . . . 430
352 *Omer* . . . 431
353 *Onenna* . . . 432
354 *Orana* . . . 433
355 *Ortarius* . . . 434
356 *Osmund* . . . 435
357 *Oswald of Northumbria* . . . 436
358 *Otto of Bamberg* . . . 438
359 *Ouen of Rouen* . . . 439

P

360 *Pacificus* . . . 442
361 *Pancras of Rome* . . . 443
362 *Pantaleon* . . . 444
363 *Patroclus* . . . 446
364 *Paul of Narbonne* . . . 447
365 *Paulina do Coração Agonizante de Jesus* . . . 448
366 *Peregrine Laziosi* . . . 450
367 *Peter of Alcántara* . . . 451
368 *Peter the Apostle* . . . 452
369 *Peter Chrysologus* . . . 454
370 *Peter Damian* . . . 455
371 *Peter Thomas* . . . 456
372 *Peter of Verona* . . . 458
373 *Petronilla* . . . 459
374 *Phaletrus* . . . 460
375 *Pharaildis* . . . 461
376 *Philip Benizi* . . . 462
377 *Philip Neri* . . . 463
378 *Philomena* . . . 465
379 *Piat* . . . 466
380 *Pirminus* . . . 467
381 *Placido of Recanati* . . . 468
382 *Polycarp* . . . 469
383 *Porcarius* . . . 470
384 *Portianus* . . . 471
385 *Praejectus of Clermont* . . . 472
386 *Priscus* . . . 473
387 *Psalmodius* . . . 474

Q

388 *Quintianus* 476
389 *Quintinus* 477
390 *Quirinus* 478
391 *Quiteria* 480

R

392 *Radegunde* 482
393 *Raphael* 483
394 *Ratho* 484
395 *Raymond Nonnatus* 485
396 *Raymond of Toulouse* 486
397 *Regina of Alise* 487
398 *Reginald* 488
399 *Regulus* 489
400 *Reineldis* 490
401 *Remaclus* 491
402 *Remigius* 492
403 *Rene Goupil* 493
404 *Richarius* 495
405 *Rigobert* 496
406 *Rita of Cascia* 497
407 *Roch* 499
408 *Roland of Chèzery* 501
409 *Roland de'Medici* 502
410 *Rolande* 503
411 *Romanus of Rouen* 504
412 *Rosalia* 505
413 *Rose of Lima* 506

S

414 *Sabina* 510
415 *Salvator of Horta* 511
416 *Saturninus of Toulouse* 512
417 *Scholastica* 513
418 *Sebastian* 514
419 *Senan of Saint-Pol-de-Léon* 516
420 *Serenicus and Serenus* 517
421 *Servatius* 518
422 *Severinus of Noricum* 519
423 *Servulus* 520
424 *Severus of Agde* 521
425 *Sigismund of Burgundy* 522
426 *Simplicianus* 523
427 *Stanislaus Kostka* 524
428 *Stapinus* 526
429 *Sulpicius Pius* 527
430 *Sulpicius Severus* 528
431 *Swithbert* 529
432 *Symphorian* 530
433 *Syre* 531

T

434 *Tanche* 534
435 *Taracus* 535
436 *Teresa and Sanchia of Portugal* 536
437 *Teresa of Ávila* 538
438 *Thaumast* 540
439 *Theobald of Provence* 541
440 *Theodard* 542
441 *Theodoric of Mont d'Or* 543
442 *Theodulph* 544
443 *Thérèse de Lisieux* 545
444 *Tiburtius* 546
445 *Tillo* 547
446 *Timothy* 548
447 *Trophimus of Arles* 549
448 *Turibius* 550

U

449 *Ubaldo of Gubbio* 552
450 *Udaut* 553
451 *Ulrich of Augsburg* 554
452 *Ursicinus* 555
453 *Ursmar* 556
454 *Ursus of Aosta* 557

V

455 *Valentine of Passau* 560
456 *Valentine of Rome* 561
457 *Vaury* 562
458 *Vedastus* 563
459 *Venantius of Camerino* 564
460 *Venantius of Tours* 565
461 *Ventura of Castello* 566
462 *Veranus* 567
463 *Veronus* 568
464 *Victor of Campbon* 569
465 *Victurnianus* 570
466 *Vincent de Paul* 571
467 *Vincent Ferrer* 573
468 *Vitalis of Salzburg* 575
469 *Vitus* 576
470 *Vulganius* 578

W

471 *Walaricus* ... 580
472 *Walburga* ... 581
473 *Walfroy* ... 582
474 *Walstan* ... 583
475 *Walter of Poitiers* ... 584
476 *Walter of Pontoise* ... 585
477 *Werenfrid* ... 586
478 *William Firmatus* ... 587
479 *William Tempier* ... 588
480 *Willibrord* ... 589
481 *Wolfgang* ... 591

Z

482 *Zenaide* ... 594
483 *Zenobius* ... 595
484 *Zoilus* ... 596
485 *Zosimus* ... 597

References ... 599
Calendar of Saints ... 603
Index of Medical Conditions ... 615
Index of Medical Specialties ... 625
Illustrations ... 627

Introduction

The saints will aid if men will call;
For the blue sky bends over all!

– Samuel Taylor Coleridge
The Rime of the Ancient Mariner

The presence of medical issues has been recorded throughout the ages. Illnesses, diseases, disorders, and bodily injuries were documented by oral histories and written words from the earliest of times to the present. The dramatic epidemics that have affected society over the ages have been recounted. Contemporaneous methods of maintaining health and managing medical adversities have been integral to that documentation.

Over the years, the care of individuals and the populace has been increasingly based on scientific solutions. As practiced today, medicine is essentially a product of the analysis of evidence that is the consequence of translating facts frequently defined or confirmed in the laboratory or by clinical trials. But the so-called rational approach is hardly new; the oldest extant scientific document, the Edwin Smith Papyrus, a manuscript copy of a work originally written about 4000 years ago, details the logical treatment of traumatized patients and is implicitly based on experience.

During the era of the building of the pyramids, disease management was frequently based on empiricism. As time passed, some methods of treatment became established, occasionally falling into disrepute later. Alongside the generally accepted empirical therapies and those based on previous experience, intervention by a higher power was often invoked. Initially, pagan gods, represented by idols or items of nature, were propitiated to effect cures or to prevent disease or physical disaster. The shaman or medicine man, in addition to administering herbs and potions, interceded between the affected one and a higher healing power.

As Christianity spread and became an expansive influence over Western civilization, a new avenue of support became available. As written in James 5:15, "The prayer of faith will save the sick." First it was the Holy Spirit, and then He was joined by those worthy of His special love—the saints. The word *saint* derives from the Latin word "sanctus," meaning "consecrated." "Saint" appeared in its current form initially in the French language and was adopted into the English language. Perhaps it is not by chance that the French word for health, "sante," is strikingly similar.

The saints were regarded as distributors of special gifts, often related to an individual's health. At the same time that belief in the Holy Spirit and saints of the Catholic Church were becoming more widespread, scientific knowledge acquired in the past was lost to Western Europe and lay sequestered among non-Christian Arabic societies. During these so-called Dark Ages and Middle Ages, which preceded the Renaissance and the reintroduction of reason, a reliance on prayer and beseeching higher powers to ameliorate individual and societal illnesses became more pervasive. Prayer filled the void when knowledge was nonexistent. Also, at that time, and extending into the early part of the Renaissance, the Church, by fiat, disallowed priests and monks to treat wounds and illnesses with other than prayer. A series of edicts passed between 1130 and 1247 precluded monks and priests from treating illness by other than relics, prayer, and exhortation.

In the first millennium and a half of the Common Era, the Catholic Church initially recognized the veneration of human beings who were martyred in the cause of their faith and who had performed supernatural deeds (miracles). Those individuals and their names or relics were often invoked to effect cures of medical ailments. Thus there came into being within Christianity a group of patron saints who were considered to be individually capable of altering the course of specific medical afflictions.

Evidence of the solicitation of the services of doctors and saints during the Middle Ages is provided in the *Rubáiyát* written by Omar Khayyám in the early twelfth century and translated by Edward Fitzgerald in the second half of the nineteenth century:

Myself when young did eagerly frequent
Doctor and Saint, and heard great argument
About it and about: but evermore
Came out by the same door where in I came.

A saint is an individual who demonstrated Christian perfection during life and is regarded to be "a person with God." A basic tenet of Catholicism is that God makes the saint; the Church merely identifies him or her. Canonization is the act by which the Christian Church declares that a deceased individual is recognized to be a saint, is worthy of a universal cult (a formal following), and that his or her name merits inclusion on a canon, or ecclesiastically accepted exclusive list. Originally, individuals were recognized as saints without a formal process.

The Roman Canon of the Mass contains only the names of saints who were martyred, and that of the Virgin Mary and Saint Joseph. The list was initially constituted by individuals who were martyred by giving their lives for the cause of Christianity. Priority as the first martyr is generally assigned to the convert, Saint Stephen, who is referred to in Luke's account in the Acts of the Apostles.

In the first four centuries of the Common Era, martyrdom was the result of Roman persecution of Christians. The memorial day for each saint was established by the date of death, because it was believed that the saint was reborn at death into life everlasting and continued to carry out miracles of intercession as "a friend of God." Some time around the fourth century, the list of saints was expanded to include individuals who were categorized as "confessors," namely those who evidenced their faith by exceptional words and deeds, and who died peacefully after a life of virtue and holiness. They were missionaries, pastors, caretakers of the poor and the sick, and defenders of the faith.

In earlier ages, veneration or acclimation was regional and confined to a local appreciative audience that related to each specific saint. As such, from the fifth to the tenth century, veneration was under the aegis of local bishops, who determined whether a martyr had truly died for his or her faith in Christ and whether worship of that martyr was permissible for a particular disease. Toward the end of the first millennium, the Holy See became more involved and authoritative. The canonization of Saint Ulrich (Udalric), Bishop of Augsburg, by Pope John XV in 993 is the first example of a papal canonization of a saint from outside Rome. Gradually, rules for canonization began to evolve. In 1234, Pope Gregory IX issued "Decretals" (Pontifical Laws) that established the absolute jurisdiction of the pontiff over all causes of saints and made the laws binding on the Universal Church. From that point, only the pope had the power to canonize.

In October 1517, the Reformation (of Catholicism) was catalyzed by the publication of Martin Luther's 95 theses against indulgences. The cornerstone of the Reformation was "justification by faith alone," and the ultimate authority of the Scripture itself, which disallowed interpretation by the pope. For Protestants, the pope lost his authority, and the saints lost any right of domain. The most common artistic expression before the Reformation consisted of portraits or representations of patron saints. These gave way to secular subjects. For non-Catholics, the feast days that celebrated the saints' deaths were erased and the calendar was sanitized of their presence.

Meanwhile, within Catholicism, in 1588, Pope Sixtus V moved forward with the process of sanctification by creating the Congregation for the Causes of Saints, which was charged with preparing for canonization and authenticating relics. In 1634, Pope Urban VII published a Bull reserving for the Holy See the exclusive right of beatification and canonization. The papacy gained full control, and canonical procedures were defined. In 1670, the Congregation Committee of Cardinals was established as a refinement of Pope Sixtus V's initiative to distribute the central administration of the Church among the cardinals. Saints who were canonized before that date are referred to as "precongregational." In the seventeenth century, local calendars indicating the saints' memorial days were fused into a universal calendar for the entire Roman Catholic Church.

Although the process for making saints remains one of the Church's greatest enigmas, according to Woodward, matched only by the Mass, definitive rules for canonization have been established. In 1917, the formal procedures were modified and incorporated in the Code of Canon Law. Before that time, 50 years had to have elapsed before the process of canonization could be initiated. Since then, at least 5 years must have elapsed from the time of death of the candidate, but the pope can waive that limitation, as has occurred recently in the instances of Mother Teresa and Pope John Paul II.

In September 1997, the Holy See press office made public an update on canonical procedure for causes of beatification and canonization. The document indicates that the process is defined in the Apostolic Constitution "Divinus Perfectionis Magister," promulgated by Pope John Paul II on January 25, 1983.

Usually the bishop of the diocese in which the subject under consideration died initiates the process of beatification in response to or stimulated by a promoter group ("Actor Causae") consisting of members of the diocese. The stimulus for recognizing the subject is either martyrdom or "holiness or holy virtue." Also, the subject cannot have been the object of a public cult during his or her life. The bishop forms a diocesan tribunal to consider the subject's virtues and gather pertinent documents. At that point, the individual being considered is assigned the title "Servant of God," and is called "Venerable." Before beatification, the local bishop often examines the corpse, but in the Roman Catholic Church an uncorrupted body (one that has not decomposed) is not a sign of sanctity.

After the diocesan investigation concludes that beatification may be appropriate, the local assessment and the supporting documents are forwarded to the Congregation for the Causes of Saints, made up of cardinals and bishops. The postulator, who resides in Rome, oversees preparation of a summary of the documentation, or "Positio," which is reviewed by eight or nine theologians. In 1983, Pope John Paul II significantly changed a process that had been initiated in the fourteenth century by the Avignon popes, abolishing the time-honored argument between an advocate, who defended the appropriateness of beatification of a given subject against a Promoter of the Faith or "Devil's Advocate," who argued against the beatification.

If most of the theologians, based on historiographic evidence, favor beatification, the Congregation for the Causes of Saints formally initiates a consideration of the issue. A favorable judgment by that group is followed by presentation of the cause to the Holy Father, whose approval results in the authorization for the Congregation to draft a decree that is read to the public.

In the case of beatification of a confessor, the theological consultants assess the holiness and heroic virtue of the candidate. Holiness is evidenced by a two-tiered set of virtues: the three supernatural virtues of faith, hope, and charity (the love of God and neighbors) and the four cardinal moral virtues of prudence, justice, fortitude, and temperance.

The issue of the role of miracles in the processes of beatification and canonization has been in flux. *Thaumatology,* a word that derives from Greek, meaning "wonder or marvel," is the consideration of miracles. In the past, many miracles had medical implications; now virtually all miracles are medical cures. In 1948, a medical panel of experts, known as "Consulta Medica," was constituted to determine whether a reported miracle was in any way scientifically explicable. The Consulta Medica is drawn from a panel of 60 Roman physicians, all Roman Catholic, generally professors or hospital administrators. With the advent of more extensive extirpations, more effective radiation therapy, and more successful chemotherapy directed at leukemia and other cancers, it became imperative to determine whether a medical therapeutic explanation was in any way a possibility. The Consulta Medica issues a finding as to whether the cure is inexplicable, after which a group of theologians determine whether it is truly a miracle.

In the past, for beatification of confessors, two miracles "of the first class" must have had eyewitnesses in the ordinary and Apostolic processes; that is, those conducted within the Holy See. Three eyewitnesses were required if they were not found in Apostolic processes. Four witnesses were needed if there was hearsay testimony. Today one miracle is required for the beatification of nonmartyrs. Once the miracle is affirmed, the Holy Father may issue approval for beatification, which conveys the title "Blessed." The papal declaration of beatification is not regarded as infallible.

The beatification of martyrs, defined as innocent victims who died for the Faith at the hand of a tyrant opposed to the Faith, previously required one authenticated miracle, but now requires none. For the canonization of confessors or martyrs, an affirmed miracle that occurred after beatification is required, but this requirement can be abolished by the pope. The process is complete when the pope issues a Bull of Canonization in which he commends the public veneration of the saint and the addition of the saint's memorial day to the Church's calendar. A declaration of sainthood is not an "ex cathedra" papal pronouncement, and therefore its infallibility is a point of argument.

More than 10,000 Christian saints have been identified by Church authorities; the overwhelming majority are precongregational. Between January 22, 1588, when Pope Sixtus V created the Sacred Congregation of Rites to deal with the causes of saints, and 1978, when Pope John Paul II was elevated to the papacy, a total of 302 canonizations were issued by the 23 popes of the Holy See. During John Paul II's pontificate, extending up to the Holy See press office report of December 28, 2005, there were 1138 beatifications and 482 canonizations. The 1988 issue of *Index ac Status Causarum* (Index on the Status of Causes) listed 1369 active causes. In 2011, John Paul II was beatified, and the miracle ascribed to him was the cure of Parkinson's disease in an individual.

In the Eastern Orthodox Church, the equivalent of canonization is termed *Glorification.* There is no formal service of beatification. Glorification is considered to be an act of God and grows from the consensus of the Church. After the evidence of saintliness grows, as manifest by verifiable miracles, a Glorification may be performed by any bishop, the name of the saint is inscribed in the calendar of saints, and a memorial day is assigned for a celebratory feast.

Anglicans have a calendar of saints, but, since the Reformation, only King Charles I has been canonized in the Church of England. Some Lutherans have a calendar of saints, but most Protestants reject canonization and prayer requests to the dead.

Hagiography, which derives from the Greek word "hagio," meaning "holy or sacred," and "graphy," meaning "writing," is the study of the lives of saints, and generally refers to an analysis of the lives of individuals who have been canonized by the Roman Catholic Church. The formalized study has a long history, dating as far back as the Roman Empire in the fourth century.

The *Golden Legend,* by Jacobus de Voraigne (ca. 1230-1298), a collection of the legendary lives of the major saints of the medieval Church, with an emphasis on miracles, was one of the most popular religious works of the Middle Ages and was one of the earliest books printed. A Latin edition was printed about 1469, and a French edition was printed at Lyon in 1473. Before 1500, about two editions appeared each year, including those printed in German, Czech, French, Italian, and three English editions by William Caxton, who introduced the movable-type printing press into England.

The idea of *Acta Sanctorum,* a compilation of the lives of saints recognized by the Catholic Church, was conceived by the Dutch Jesuit Heribert Rosweyde (1569-1665). It was continued by Jean Boland (1596-1665) and Godfrey Henschen (1601-1681) in Antwerp, where the first two volumes were published in 1643. Henschen devoted his life to the project, and by the time of his death, 24 volumes had been published. As of 1988, 62 volumes had been published.

The association of Jesuit scholars who participated in the project of hagiography became known as the Bollandists. When the Society of Jesus was suppressed by Pope Clement XIV in 1773, the Bollandists moved to Brussels, where, after the reestablishment of the Society of Jesus in Belgium, a new Societé des Bollandistes was created under the patronage of the Belgian government, and, by 1867, a collection of 61 volumes was published in Paris. In 1882, a quarterly review on hagiography, *Analecta Bollandiana,* was initiated and continues to this day.

The most comprehensive work on saints is *Bibliotheca Sanctorum,* which includes more than 10,000 entries. Only a small portion of the saints in this work were canonized by popes. Several other compilations of names of saints have been published in English, French, Italian, Spanish, and German. Included on the lists of saints are those who have been recognized formally by the Holy See and others who have been recognized only regionally.

Included among the large cadre of universally and locally recognized saints is a group that has been formally considered for their patronage of various illnesses. Some of these saints have been associated with more than one illness. Many illnesses and infirmities have the patronage of several saints. Most saints invoked for medical conditions also have been assigned patronage for trades unrelated to medicine, and for countries and cities.

In some cases, the legend associated with a saint offers an explanation for their patronage, but, in most instances, the life and legend of the saint do not explain the patronage for the specific illness or disorder, and the patronage is based on alleged cures associated with invocation of that saint's name or powers attributed to that saint's relics.

Among the patron saints of medicine, particularly those for whom an association between their lives and specific patronage is apparent, fascinating legends have appeared. In some instances, the purported events have been very dramatic. The tales of Saints Agatha, Anthony of Padua, Blase, Cosmas and Damian, Edward the Confessor, Fiacre, Leodegar, Lucy, Peregrine, and Sebastian are examples of intriguing legends that formed the bases for patronage.

The spectrum of diseases and disorders for which saints have been invoked is a reflection of personal and societal concerns. In the early days of Christianity, which were characterized by widespread persecution by the Romans, torture was pervasive. Decapitation was commonplace, and the invocation of a saint who had lost his or her head to the blade for the cure of severe headache is an obvious association. Similarly, saints who were martyred by being wounded with thorns, nails, and arrows, and those who sustained fractures and dislocations of their limbs, often on the rack, were invoked for the cure of injuries or ailments with symptoms and signs similar to those caused by the various types of personal injury they had sustained.

Also, in the early days of Christianity, and extending through the Middle Ages and into the Renaissance, there was a focus on procreation, because of the need for large families to provide the labor force for an agricultural economy and to compensate for a high infant mortality. At the other end of the societal spectrum, for the nobility, the production of an heir was a dominant issue. Therefore, for the rich and the poor alike, saints were often called on to ensure fertility, a normal pregnancy, and, in an era during which there was no anesthesia or obstetrical expertise, an uncomplicated labor.

Throughout this period, infant mortality was almost an anticipated event. Infections prevailed before any appreciation of bacterial or viral causes. Epidemics were prevalent, including plague and pestilence. Rabies and tuberculosis (phthisis) were rampant. Leprosy and scrofula were commonplace, blindness was more common, and the diet contributed to gout and urinary calculi.

The dramatic elements of all of those conditions in an age devoid of scientific medical care provided fertile soil for intercession by a higher, presumably all-powerful, force. For the Christian world, the saints provided such a force.

Jonathan Swift wrote: "Physicians ought not to give their judgment of religion, for the same reason that butchers are not admitted to be jurors on life and death" (*Thoughts on Various Subjects,* 1703). Rudolph Virchow, the father of modern pathology, stated: "There can be no scientific dispute with respect to faith, for science and faith exclude one another" (*Disease, Life, and Man,* 1958). By contrast, the Nobel laureate Francis Collins recently presented evidence for belief in his 2006 *The Language of God.*

This book in no way addresses the issue of belief. It is a reference work, a compilation of the lives of those saints who have been canonized because of their impact on the health of individuals and society. An extensive search of the English, French, Italian, German, and Spanish literature has uncovered more than 400 names of saints related to illness or health.

For each of the individuals canonized, we have listed the memorial day (usually the date of death) and the patronage and the saint's life and legend, as can be uncovered. Factual biography is combined with the legendary information that provided the basis for patronage. In addition, for each specific disease or disorder, the list of patron saints who have been invoked is provided, as well as a calendar of memorial days.

Holystic Medicine
The Patron Saints of Medicine

The Hagiography of Health and Illness

A

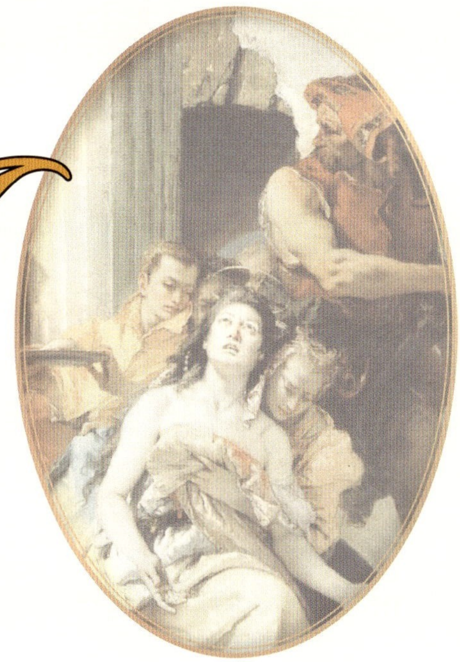

1

Abraham of Saint Cirgues

MEMORIAL DAY **June 15**

PATRONAGE **Fever, children's diseases**

LIFE & LEGEND

Abraham, whose name is derived from Hebrew, meaning "father of many nations," was born on the banks of the Euphrates river. As a young man he decided to visit the monasteries that were then flourishing in the Egyptian wilderness. During the course of his journey, Abraham was taken captive by pagan Arabs. After 5 years of hardship, he was delivered from captivity by an angel. His subsequent wanderings ended near Clermont-Ferrand, in south-central France, where he established a monastery in the vicinity of the church dedicated to Saint Cirgues. Abraham was given the gift of miraculous healing, which he was particularly wont to bestow during the feast of Saint Cirgues. Abraham lived to an old age, dying ca. 480, and was buried in the monastery he founded. Reports circulated of miraculous healing of fever at his tomb, and thus Abraham came to be invoked for the remission of fever. Du Broc de Segange notes the presence of a spring near the church of Saint Cirgues that was known as late as the seventeenth century as "le fon de Saint Abraham."

Infants were immersed in its waters for relief from "une maladie douloureuse et cachée, dont les cris de ces petits êtres souffrants ne sont que indice [a painful and hidden illness of which the cries of the little suffering children indicate its seriousness]."

REFERENCES 16, 36

2

Achatius (Acatius, Agathius)

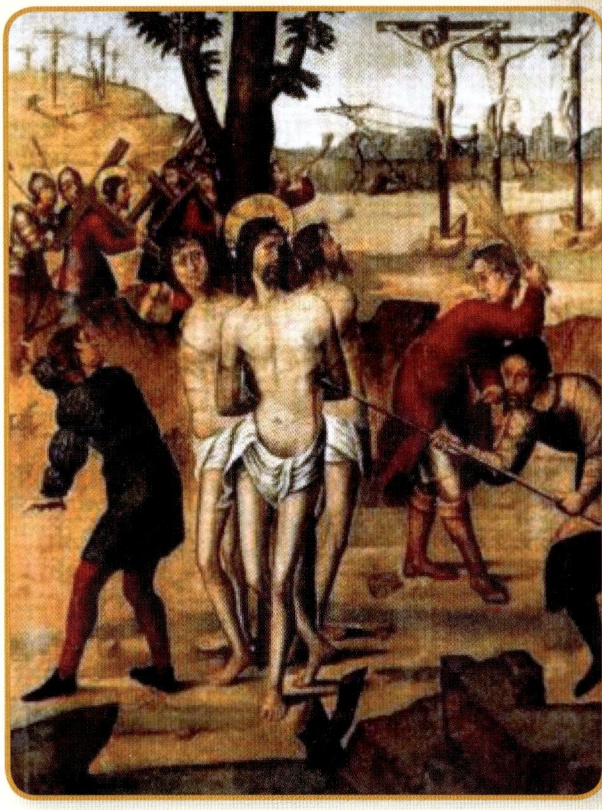

MEMORIAL DAY **May 8**

PATRONAGE **Headache, soldiers, several Italian towns**

LIFE & LEGEND

The name Achatius is derived from Hebrew, meaning "holding." Achatius was a Cappadocian centurion in the imperial army of Byzantium. He was prominent in Christian circles and was arrested because of his faith. He refused to worship pagan gods, was tortured with thorns piercing his head (accounting for his headache patronage), and was put to death ca. 303. He is one of the Fourteen Holy Helpers, who are the patron saints of daily life.

The first extensive narrative of the story of Saint Achatius appears in the *Catalogus Sanctorum* of Petrus de Natalibus, which was compiled between 1370 and 1400 and was first printed at Vincenza in 1493. According to that legend, Achatius was a primicerius under Emperors Hadrian and Antoninus. Achatius was sent to lead a force as part of the Theban Legion, and to engage a much larger enemy. An angel appeared to Achatius and his men, telling them that they would gain victory through Christ, and they all embraced Christianity.

After they were victorious, the troops climbed to the top of Mount Ararat, where angels descended from heaven and instructed them in their new faith. The enemy regrouped and expanded their ranks, resulting in the ultimate defeat of the recently converted Christians. The Christians refused to recant their new faith and were tortured. They were stoned, but the stones miraculously rebounded from them. They also were able to walk over a series of spikes. Following these failed torture attempts, the Christians were crowned with thorns and pierced with lances. At the order of King Sapor, they were led to Mount Ararat, where they were crucified.

Achatius is occasionally confused with a bishop of Armenia and also with an officer under the command of the Emperors Hadrian and Antoninus, both with the same name. The bishop Achatius and the commander Achatius were also martyred after being tortured by being flogged with thorns.

Constantine the Great built a church to honor Achatius, whose relics were moved to a spring near a monastery at Squillace in the heel of Italy, where miracles were reported. A relic of his arm was taken to Guardavalle and also to Cuenca and Avila in Spain.

REFERENCES 39, 42

3

Adamo of Fermo

MEMORIAL DAY **May 16**

PATRONAGE **Epilepsy**

LIFE & LEGEND

A native of Fermo, located in the Marche northeast of Ascoli Piceno, Italy, Adamo's name is derived from Hebrew, meaning "man, earth." He entered the monastery of San Savino in the nearby hills of Vissiano, and was later elected abbot of San Savino. Some years after his death, ca. 1210, the remains of Adamo were removed to Fermo's cathedral, Santa Maria Assunta, in Cielo. Numerous miracles were reported to have occurred at his tomb.

REFERENCES 14, 16, 36

4

Adelard (Adalard, Adelhad, Adalardus, Alard)

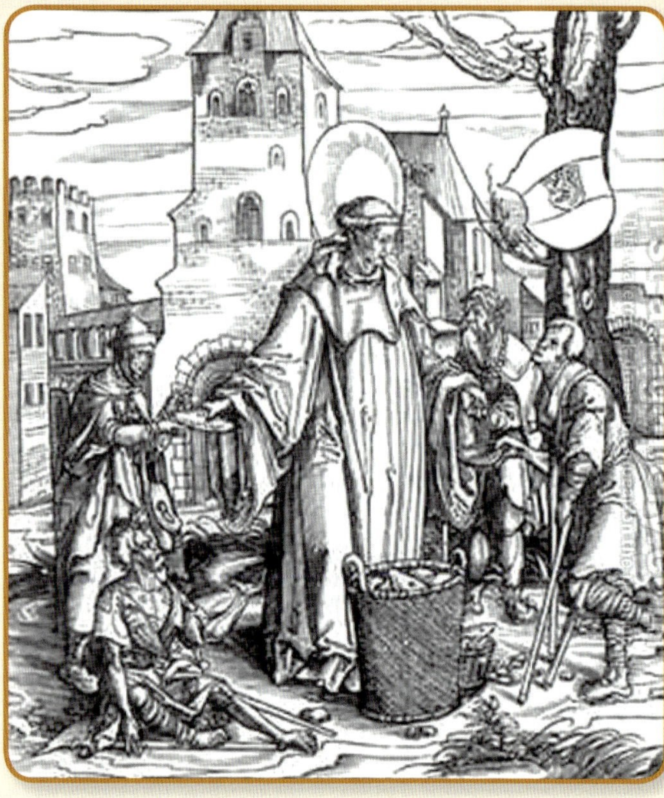

MEMORIAL DAY **January 2**

PATRONAGE **Fever, typhoid, typhus, paralysis, deafness, contagious diseases, measles, muteness, gardeners**

LIFE & LEGEND

Adelard's name has a Germanic derivation, meaning "noble and brave." He was the grandson of Charles Martel, the Frankish king famous for his victory at Tours in 732. Adelard was also the nephew of Pepin the Short, the king of the Franks, and the first cousin of Charlemagne. Adelard was born ca. 752 and was educated at the Palatine School at the court of Charlemagne. He grew up in the French court, where he was made count of the palace at a young age.

In 773, Adelard left the court to enter a Benedictine monastery in Corbie, Picardy. He initially served as a gardener at the monastery, but he moved to Monte Cassino to gain greater seclusion for meditation. He was ordered by Charlemagne to return to Corbie where he was elected abbot. At the same time, Charlemagne made him prime minister to the king of Italy, who was Charlemagne's son, Pepin. Adelard tutored Pepin's son, Bernard, who later became king of Naples.

Because it was thought that he sympathized with Bernard in Bernard's revolt against Emperor Louis the Debonair (Charlemagne's successor) in 817, Adelard was exiled to the island of Heri (Noirmoutier today). After 7 years, Emperor Louis realized that he had made a mistake and appointed Adelard to be one of his chief advisors.

In 822, Adelard and his brother, Wala, founded the New Corbie monastery in Saxony. Adelard died at the Corbie monastery in Picardy, France, on January 2, 827. He was canonized by Pope John XIX in 1026, and he is honored by many churches and towns in France and along the lower Rhine.

REFERENCES 13, 15, 45

5

Adrian of Nicomedia

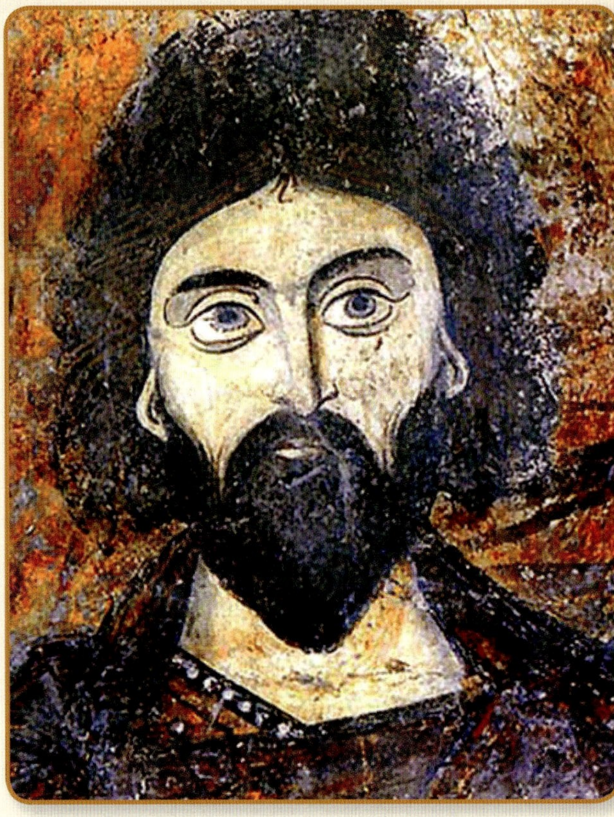

MEMORIAL DAY **September 8**

PATRONAGE **Plague, infertility**

LIFE & LEGEND

Adrian, a name derived from Latin "Hadrian," meaning "from Hadria," is said to have been an officer in the imperial court at Nicomedia when he was converted to Christianity after witnessing the piety and courage of a group of recently arrested Christians. He himself was then arrested and imprisoned. After refusing to apostatize, Adrian was executed ca. 304 by having his limbs broken and his hands and feet cut off. His young wife, Natalia, previously a Christian, was witness to her husband's martyrdom and managed to hide one of his severed hands in her garments. She died soon after at Argyropolis, where the relics of Adrian and the others martyred at Nicomedia were buried. It is unclear why he is invoked in times of plague, but, according to Fossyeux, Adrian "is invoked against the plague during the mass against epidemic, according to a twelfth-century writing in the Bibliotheque d'Amiens, and also against sudden death, as noted in the fifteenth century in the Bibliotheque de l'Ecole de Medecine de Montpellier."

REFERENCES 6, 25, 36

6

Aedh Mac Bricc

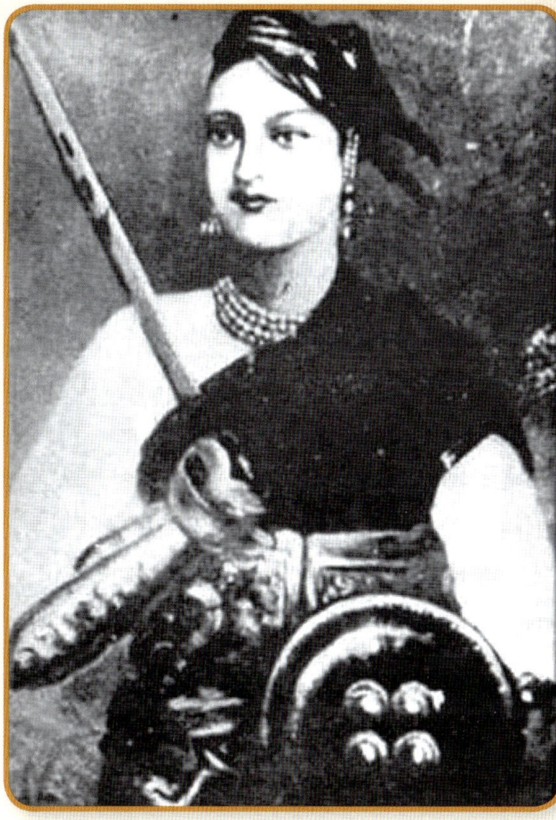

MEMORIAL DAY **November 10**

PATRONAGE **Headache, plague**

LIFE & LEGEND

When his brothers withheld his patrimony after the death of their father, Aedh responded by carrying off a girl from their household. Saint Illathan, bishop of Rathlithen in Offaly, Ireland, persuaded Aedh to renounce his patrimony and return the girl. Aedh remained with Illathan, who blessed him and convinced him to establish a monastery in the diocese at Cill-air in Westmeath, Ireland. Aedh later became a bishop. Many miracles are attributed to Aedh during his lifetime, including the healing of Saint Brigid, who came to Aedh for relief from her chronic headaches.

REFERENCES 6, 14, 36

7

Aemilianus

MEMORIAL DAY **December 6**

PATRONAGE **Pharmacists**

LIFE & LEGEND

Among those martyred ca. 484 during the persecution of orthodox Christians in northern Africa by the Vandal king, Huneric, an Arian, were the physician Aemilianus, whose name is derived from Latin, meaning "rival" or "emulating," and his wife Dativa. Late in the Middle Ages the cult of Aemilianus (Emiliano) was popular in Naples. In the fourteenth century he was chosen as a patron saint by the pharmacists of Naples, and he remains a patron saint of pharmacists.

REFERENCES 36, 46, 50

8

Agapitus

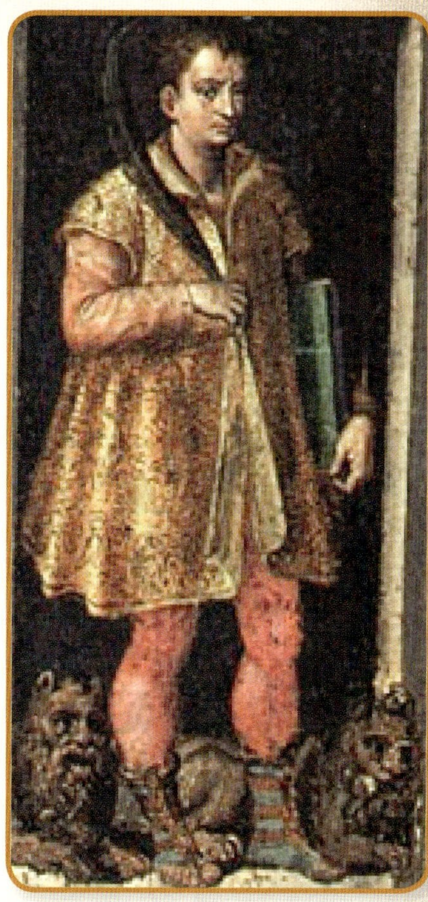

MEMORIAL DAY **April 18 (formerly August 18)**

PATRONAGE **Colic, pregnant women, tooth disorders, infant dentition**

LIFE & LEGEND

Agapitus' name is derived from Greek, meaning "beloved." Agapitus became caught up in the persecutions of the Christians in Antioch. As a 15-year-old, he was brought before the governor representing the Emperor Aurelian and professed his faith. Because he refused to recant, Agapitus was tortured and thrown to wild animals in the arena. He was protected by divine intervention, and the animals refused to attack him. Ultimately he was beheaded ca. 267 at Palestrina, where he was buried. His relics, which are located at Palestrina and at Besançon, have been successfully invoked to cure colic and tooth disorders and to ameliorate the discomfort of pregnant women. Because the story of his life has been questioned, his sainthood was limited to local status in 1969.

REFERENCE 9

9

Agatha

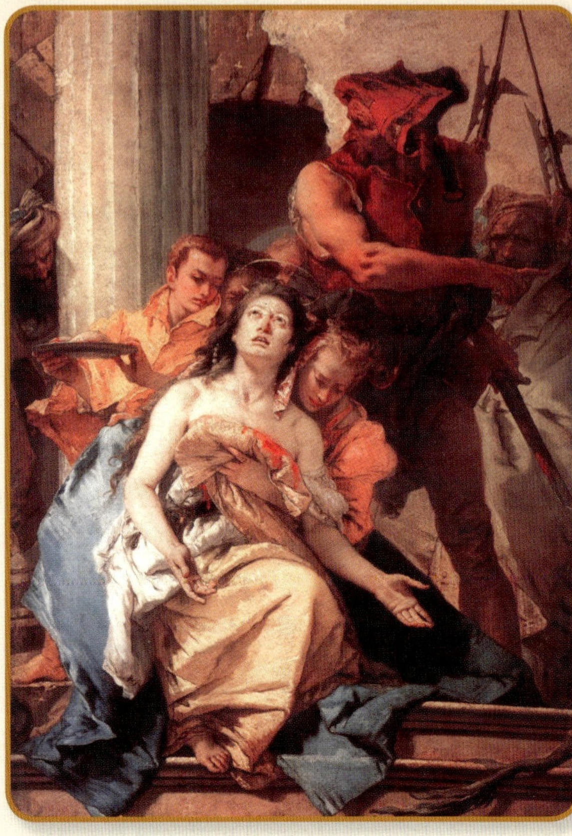

MEMORIAL DAY **February 5**

PATRONAGE **Breasts (breast cancer patients), sterility, nurses, wet nurses, torture victims, natural disasters, volcanic eruptions, fire and lightning, bell-founders (because of the shape of amputated breasts), Catania (Sicily), Palermo (Sicily), Zamarramala (Spain), Mount Etna, Malta**

LIFE & LEGEND

Agatha, whose name is derived from the Greek word for "good," is one of the most highly venerated virgin martyrs of Christian antiquity. Although her martyrdom is authenticated, there is no reliable source for her life or her death. Both the cities of Catania and Palermo in Sicily claim the honor of her birth. According to the Latin Acts, she was born into a distinguished family and was a beautiful young lady, who was consecrated to God from her early years. It is agreed by all sources that her martyrdom took place at Catania in the year 251.

During the third consulship of the Roman Decius, at a time of broad, sweeping persecution, the senator Quintianus had lustful desires for her. When she refused his advances, he committed her to the charge of Aphrodisia, the equivalent of a modern madam, who was to expose her to sexual assaults and prostitution. Agatha's steadfast refusal to adapt to that pathway, and her firm commitment to remain a servant of Jesus Christ, led Quintianus to torture her. This was highlighted by the removal of her breasts using pincers, which is the genesis of her distinctive iconography.

The apostle Saint Peter comforted her in a vision, and, according to some legends, reconstituted her breasts overnight. According to one version, Quintianus then had her rolled naked over burning coals, but she suffered no pain and survived that torture. She then died peacefully in her sleep in her jail cell. Another version indicates that she was saved from the planned fiery exposure by an earthquake and that she died peacefully before her sentence could be imposed.

Within the legend is the earliest chronicled report of the modern surgical procedure of bilateral mastectomy and, also, immediate reconstruction. In addition, the legend is an allegory for the medical truism that death related to breast cancer is the result of systemic involvement and not local disease.

About the year 500, Pope Symmachus built a church in Rome on the Aurelian Way in honor of Saint Agatha, but the structure has fallen into decay. Her relics are distributed in many places, including the Monastery of Saint Stephen on the Isle of Capri and in Constantinople. It is claimed that eruptions from Mount Etna have been averted on several occasions by the citizens of Catania who took the veil of Saint Agatha out of her tomb and carried it in procession. Also, her intercession allegedly preserved the island of Malta from the Turkish invasion in 1551. Saint Agatha continues to be invoked against eruptions of Mount Etna. In some places, bread, known as Agatha bread, and water are blessed during mass on her feast day after the Consecration.

REFERENCES 6, 9

10

Agrippina of Mineo

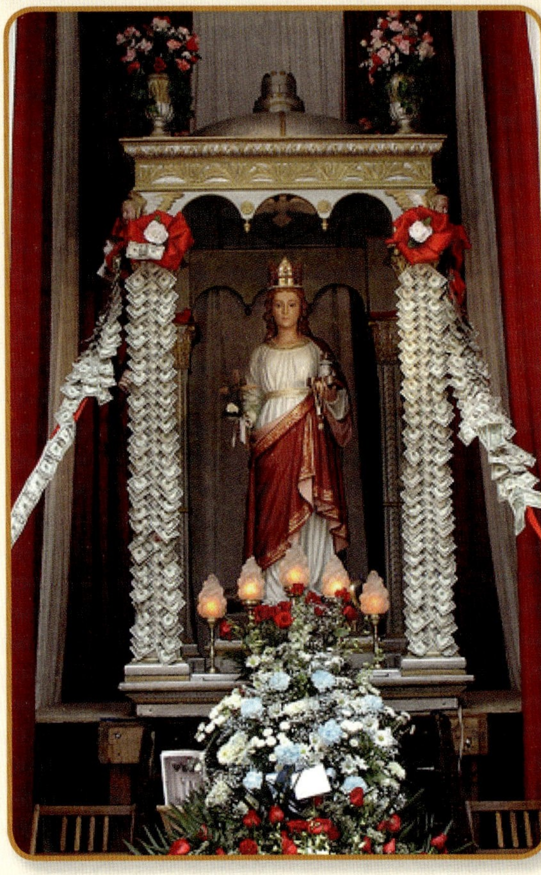

MEMORIAL DAY **June 23**

PATRONAGE **Leprosy, infections, thunderstorms, evil spirits**

LIFE & LEGEND

Agrippina is derived from Latin, meaning "feet first," suggesting a breech delivery. Agrippina, who died in 262, was venerated as a virgin martyr, but the Catholic Church has removed her from the Roman Catholic Calendar. She was born of Roman nobility and was martyred by being beheaded or scourged during either the Valerian or Diocletian persecution.

Her body was taken to Mineo, Sicily, by her three sisters, also devout Christians, named Bassa, Paula, and Agathonica. The story of their journey is replete with miracles. Pleasant fragrances accompanied her body, which was venerated along the way; the weight of her corpse was miraculously light, and clouds protected the sisters throughout the voyage. Her gravesite became a popular pilgrimage destination and is noted for curing infections, particularly leprosy, and other miracles. Some of her relics were translated to Constantinople. For the past 94 years, people in the North End of Boston have had a 3-day festival celebrating the saint.

REFERENCE 14

11

Alban of Mainz

MEMORIAL DAY **June 21**

PATRONAGE **Hernia, epilepsy, kidney stones, sore throat, urinary tract disorders**

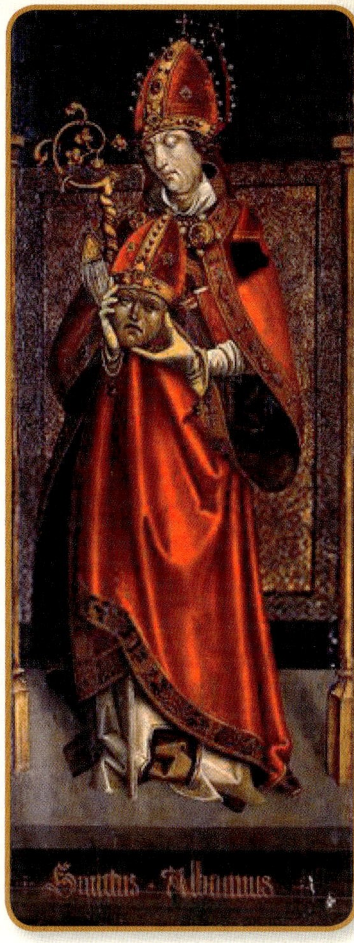

LIFE & LEGEND

The name Alban is derived from a geographic location, perhaps Albania in this case. There are two Saint Albans—one was a Christian martyr who was killed in the third or fourth century in Britain, whereas Saint Alban of Mainz lived 100 years later. He was born in either Greece or Albania and fled with Saint Ursus from Naxos, Greece, to Naples, Italy, to escape persecution. Ursus and Alban were sent by Saint Ambrose of Milan to evangelize Gaul and Germany. Ursus was killed on the way, and Alban continued to Mainz, where he became famous as a preacher who converted many pagans.

Alban helped Aureus of Mainz regain his bishopric, from which he had been deposed by a local antagonist faction. During an attack by Vandals ca. 406, both Aureus and Alban were killed. Alban was beheaded while praying, and, according to legend, carried his head in his hands to the place where he wished to be buried. A church built at his gravesite became a large Benedictine monastery, which continues to bear his name today. His patronage for throat diseases relates to his beheading. There are reports that his name also has been invoked for epilepsy and a variety of disorders of the urinary tract.

REFERENCES 6, 36

12

Albana

MEMORIAL DAY **March 31**

PATRONAGE **Hydrops, epilepsy**

LIFE & LEGEND

Albana lived during the thirteenth century and was the founder of the priory of Leigneu-en-Forez near Montbrison in central France. Pilgrims visited her tomb, especially on her feast day, to drink waters from a fountain outside the cloisters that was dedicated to her memory. The waters were reported to cure hydrops and epilepsy. In 1846, Albana's remains were transferred from her original tomb to the sacristy of the church.

REFERENCES 16, 36

13

Albert of Trapani

MEMORIAL DAY **August 7**

PATRONAGE **Fever, yellow fever, jaundice, throat ulcers, infertility**

LIFE & LEGEND

A native of the city of Trapani, this Carmelite priest is also known as Albert of Sicily. After being ordained to the priesthood, Albert, whose name is derived from French, meaning "noble" or "famous," was sent to Messina, where he was well known as a mendicant preacher and a worker of miracles. In 1296, he became superior of the Carmelite order in Sicily. During the final years of his life, Albert lived as a hermit near Messina. Although never formally canonized, Albert's cult was approved in 1476.

REFERENCES 6, 14, 16, 36

14

Albertinus

MEMORIAL DAY **August 31**

PATRONAGE **Hernia**

LIFE & LEGEND

Also known as Albertinus of Montone, the place of his birth, Albertinus became a monk in the Camaldolese monastery of Santa Croce at Fonte Avellana in the Marches near the Umbrian border in Italy. He was elected prior general of this congregation in 1270 but later declined his election as bishop of Osimo (near Ancona) so that he could continue a life of solitude until his death in 1294.

REFERENCES 14, 36, 46

15

Albinus (Aubin) of Angers

MEMORIAL DAY **March 1**

PATRONAGE **Sick children, kidney diseases**

LIFE & LEGEND

A native of Vannes in Brittany, Albinus, whose name is derived from Latin, meaning "white," entered the monastery of Tincillac (Cincillac) as a young man. He was elected abbot at age 35. In 529, Albinus was appointed bishop of Angers, where he was noted for his piety, preaching, assistance to the poor, and ransoming of slaves from barbarians. Albinus performed many miracles during his lifetime, and many were attributed to him after his death ca. 550. In one instance he is said to have brought a dead child back to life—thus his patronage of sick children.

REFERENCES 6, 14, 16, 36

16
Aldegonde

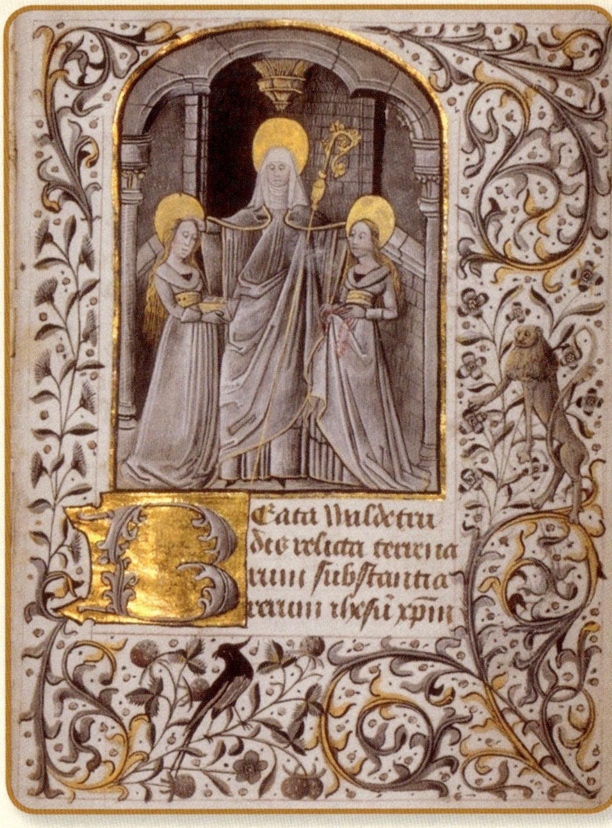

MEMORIAL DAY **January 30**

PATRONAGE **Cancer, wounds, eye diseases, fever, headache, breast diseases, children's diseases, scabies, ulcers**

LIFE & LEGEND

Aldegonde's name is derived from a Germanic term meaning "noble warrior." She was born in France in 639 at the time of King Dagobert and is honored as a Frankish virgin and abbess who died of breast cancer in 684. She was related to the Merovingian royal family; her father and mother were later canonized as Saint Walbert and Saint Bertilia. Aldegonde had been promised in marriage to an Anglo-Saxon prince, but she fled and allegedly walked across the waters of the Sambre River. It is said that the prince chased her into the forest, full of rage and with the intent of ravishing her, but he could never find her. At Maubeuge, on the banks of that river, she built a small nunnery that later became an abbey of Benedictine nuns. Her relics are enshrined at the church in Maubeuge. In art, she is shown as a Benedictine abbess, crowned, with a dove and veil near her.

REFERENCE 33

17

Alderic (Elric)

MEMORIAL DAY **February 6**

PATRONAGE **Fever, asthma**

LIFE & LEGEND

Alderic belonged to the royal family of France. Following the example of Saint Richard, king of England, and Saint Adelard, the father of Charlemagne, Alderic renounced the dignities of this world to embrace the hermetic life. He secretly left France and became a swineherd for the monastery at Fussenich, where his royal background remained unknown. One day, overcome in the wilderness with fever, Alderic was refused water by a young woman returning from a spring. Too ill to go to the source himself, Alderic prayed. In response, an angel descended to where Alderic stood and commanded him to strike the earth with his staff. Immediately a spring of pure, sweet water issued from the earth. He died ca. 1200. Miraculous cures were associated with those waters as late as the seventeenth century, particularly in cases of fever and asthma.

REFERENCES 16, 36

18

Alena

MEMORIAL DAY **June 17**

PATRONAGE **Eye diseases, tooth diseases**

LIFE & LEGEND

Alena's name is derived from Gaelic, meaning "rock." Alena's father, Evolde, was lord of Dielbeek (near Brussels) and a pagan. When her father discovered that she had secretly been instructed in the Christian faith and had been baptized (an event stemming from Evolde's accidental acquaintance with a party of Christians in Foret), he ordered that she be kept under strict guard. Alena was nonetheless able to elude her father's men and attend services near the chateau at Foret. One day in 640, an arm was found on the altar of the chapel at Foret. When Alena herself did not appear, her Christian friends set out in search of her, eventually finding her body in the woods. Evolde's orders had apparently been misunderstood, and, in the course of capturing the young woman, one of her arms had been severed—an injury from which she must have died soon after. After Alena's burial near the small church, a series of miraculous cures made her gravesite a place of pilgrimage. Notable among these was the restoration of sight to one of the local nobility. The reason of her patronage of those afflicted with tooth diseases remains unknown. After the martyrdom of his daughter, Evolde acknowledged his responsibility for her unintended death. Both he and his wife were subsequently instructed and baptized as Christians.

REFERENCES 16, 36, 46

19

Alexander

MEMORIAL DAY **July 11**

PATRONAGE **Hemorrhage, hemorrhoids, headache, infertility, childbirth**

LIFE & LEGEND

Alexander, whose name is derived from Greek, meaning "defending men," was one of the seven martyred sons of Saint Felicity, who was martyred at Rome in 165, presumably with her sons. The cult of Felicity flourished in late classical Rome. She was commonly depicted with seven male figures—her sons. Although there is scant documentary evidence regarding the martyred Alexander, he has been ascribed patronage for the above-listed medical disorders. The fact that he was beheaded speaks to the issues of headache and hemorrhage. The patronage for infertility probably related to his mother's fecundity.

REFERENCES 14, 36, 46

20

Aloysius Gonzaga

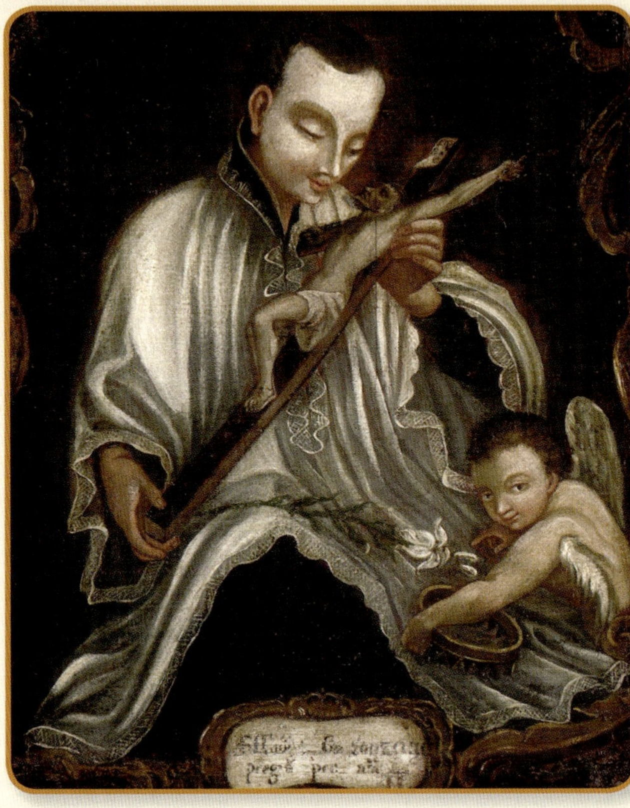

MEMORIAL DAY **June 21**

PATRONAGE **AIDS, plague, sore eyes, youth**

LIFE & LEGEND

Aloysius was born into a wealthy noble family at Castiglione delle Silviere in northern Italy on March 8, 1568, and named Luigi Gonzaga. It was assumed that, as the eldest son, he would follow in his father's footsteps, and he started military training. At age 8, he was sent to Florence to serve as a page at the court of Grand Duke Francesco I de'Medici. Aloysius became ill with a kidney disease that compromised his activities throughout his life. He developed an interest in devoting himself to a religious life. When he returned home, he met Cardinal Borromeo, who gave Aloysius his first communion in 1580.

Aloysius became ascetic and sought to enter the Jesuit order. The family moved to Spain to assist Empress Mary of Austria. There he served as a page for the Infante Don Diego. In 1584, the family returned to Italy, where Aloysius gave up his right of inheritance and was accepted into the Jesuit order. In 1588, he began to prepare for the priesthood and received the lower ordinations. In 1590, he had a vision in which the Archangel Gabriel indicated that he would die within a year.

The following year the plague broke out in Rome, and Aloysius attended patients in the hospital. He became infected but initially recovered. After he had another vision that he would die on a specific day, despite apparent good health, he suddenly died. He was buried in the Church of the Annunciation in Rome. His remains were removed to Saint Ignazio, where they remain in an elegant urn in the Lancelotti Chapel. His head was translocated to the basilica that bears his name in the city of his birth. He was canonized by Pope Benedict XIII in 1726 and declared patron saint of young students 3 years later. In 1926, Pope Pius XI named him patron of Christian youth.

REFERENCES 6, 9, 45

21

Alphonsus Maria de Liguori

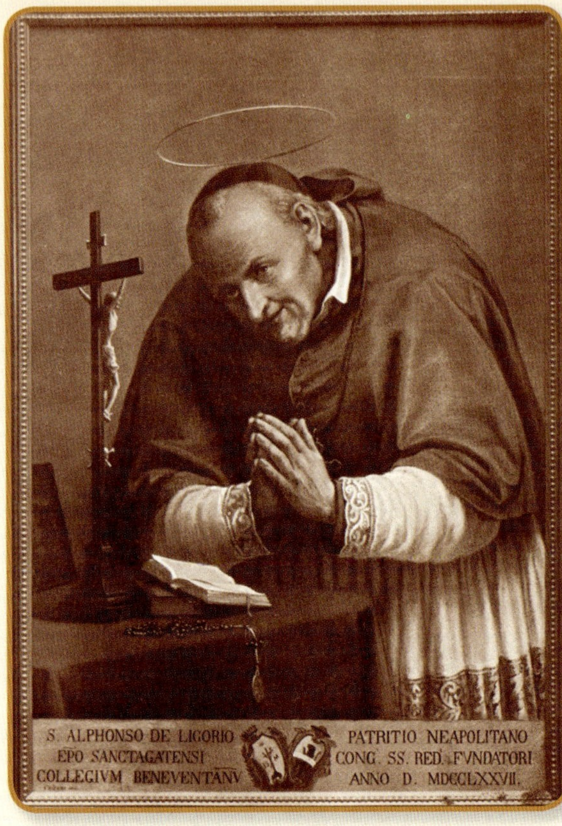
S. ALPHONSO DE LIGORIO
EPO SANCTAGATENSI
COLLEGIVM BENEVENTANV
PATRITIO NEAPOLITANO
CONG. SS. RED. FVNDATORI
ANNO D. MDCCLXXVII.

MEMORIAL DAY **August 1**

PATRONAGE **Arthritis, confessors, moralists, theologians, scrupulosity**

LIFE & LEGEND

The name Alphonsus has a Germanic origin, meaning "ready, prompt, and noble." Alphonsus was one of the eighteenth century's greatest missionaries of the Church. He was born into an impoverished noble family on September 27, 1696, near Naples, Italy. He was a child prodigy—as evidenced by his completion of a doctorate in law from the University of Naples when he was only 16. By the time he was 27, he had risen to a position of leadership at the Neapolitan bar.

In 1723, while performing an act of charity at the Hospital for Incurables, Alphonsus had an epiphany, accompanied by mysterious lights and the calling of an inner voice to give himself unto God. He immediately left law and became a novitiate to the Fathers of the Oratory. He was ordained at age 30 and initially conducted missions and preached in the vicinity of Naples.

He was the founder and de facto head of a group of nuns known as the "Congregation of the Most Holy Redeemer." In 1762, he was appointed by Pope Clement XIII bishop of Saint Agatha of Goths, which was on the road between Naples and Capua. He is most notable for his writings as a moral theologian, but his true prominence is that of a missionary.

He was afflicted with rheumatic arthritis and rheumatic fever, which left him partially paralyzed and with a bent neck that is notable in his later portraits and iconography. He was ill frequently during his later years and received the sacraments of the dying on eight separate occasions. He died at age 91 in Nocera di Pagani near Naples. He was canonized by Pope Gregory XVI in 1839 and declared a Doctor of the Church in 1871 because of the additions he made to theologic thought.

REFERENCES 9, 45

22
Amable

MEMORIAL DAY **June 11**

PATRONAGE **Snakebites, mental illness**

LIFE & LEGEND

Amable, a native of Riom (Puy-de-Dome), lived during the fifth century. He was assigned to the church in his native village after his ordination to the priesthood. Later he was called to serve in the cathedral at Clermont, probably by Saint Sidonius Apollinaris. Little has been written about his life, but it is believed by some that Amable was buried at Riom in the church of Saint Benigne that he himself had built. Other sources maintain that he was buried at Clermont and that his remains were transferred to Riom in the tenth century. In either case, numerous miracles occurred at the tomb of Amable, most notably the cure of those bitten by venomous animals. In the seventh century, the church that Amable had constructed was enlarged and took his name.

REFERENCE 16

23

Amalburga (Amelia) of Maubeuge

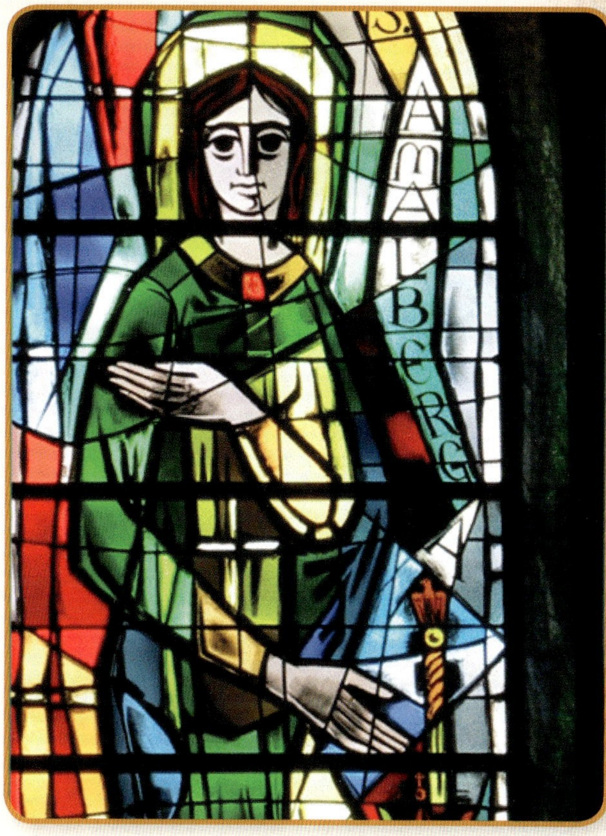

MEMORIAL DAY **July 10**

PATRONAGE **Bruises, arm pain, fever, wounds, Ghent (Belgium)**

LIFE & LEGEND

The name Amalburga has a Germanic origin, meaning "work" or "effort." She was born during the first half of the seventh century and married Count Witger, Duke of Lothargina and Count of Brabant. She was the mother of Saint Emebert, Saint Reineldis, Saint Pharaldis, and Saint Gudula, all of whom she personally educated. After the youngest of her children reached adulthood, Amalburga and her husband joined Benedictine monasteries, he at Lobbes and she at Maubeuge, where they respectively remained for the rest of their lives. Legend indicates that she crossed a lake on the back of a giant sturgeon, accounting for her being represented with a fish. She died in 690 and was buried with her husband at the Lobbes monastery. Her relics were placed in Saint Peter's abbey church in Ghent, accounting for patronage of that city.

REFERENCES 6, 9, 36

24

Amalburga of Munsterbilzsen

MEMORIAL DAY **July 10**

PATRONAGE **Broken arms, fever**

LIFE & LEGEND

There were two women with the same name who lived at about the same time and were supposedly canonized. According to a story not given much credit, one Amalburga was a beautiful young woman whom King Pepin desired to marry to his son Charles (Charlemagne). She refused, fled, and was pursued. On one occasion her arm was broken in the church where she had taken refuge. Whether this story is true or not, Amalburga was indeed a nun at Munsterbilzsen in Belgium. She died ca. 770. She is the patron saint of those with broken arms, and, according to Kerler, is invoked in cases of fever. The two Amalburgas share the same memorial day.

REFERENCES 6, 36

25

Amo

MEMORIAL DAY **October 23**

PATRONAGE **Fever**

LIFE & LEGEND

Amo, the second bishop of Toul in the northeast of France (Meurthe-et-Moselle), lived during the fourth century and is invoked by those suffering from fever.

REFERENCES 16, 36

26

Anastasius the Persian

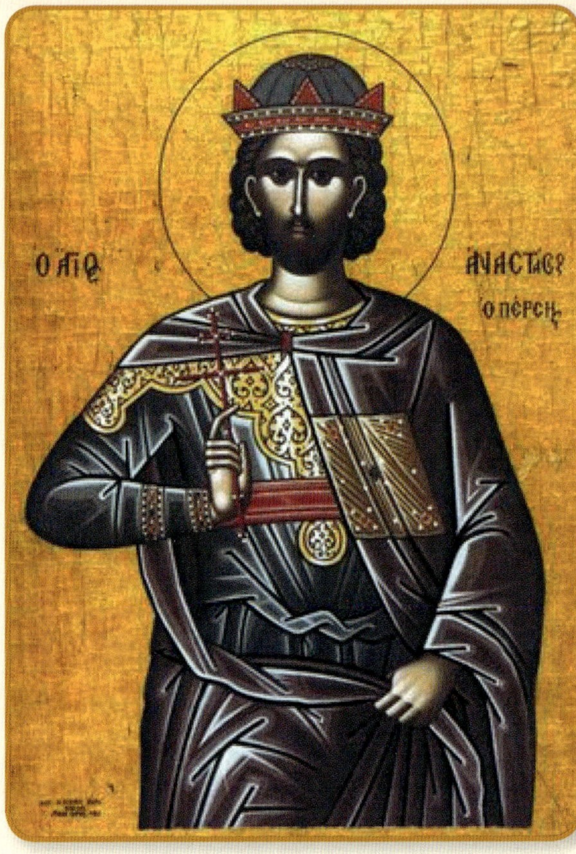

MEMORIAL DAY January 22

PATRONAGE Headache

LIFE & LEGEND

Among the trophies brought back to Persia by King Chosroes after his capture of Jerusalem in 614 were fragments of the cross of Christ. On hearing news of this cross, a young Persian soldier named Magundat became curious about the Christian religion. He became so impressed by the teachings of this religion that he left the army and lodged with a Persian Christian in Hierapolis in Asia Minor. He eventually went to Jerusalem, where he was baptized with the name Anastasius, which is derived from Greek, meaning "resurrection," and assumed the monastic habit in 621.

After a time, Anastasius traveled to Caesarea, which was then under Persian rule. He was arrested by the Persian governor, Marzabanes, for converting to Christianity. Anastasius was sentenced to hard labor, beaten, and tortured for repeatedly refusing to renounce his adopted faith. When Chosroes was informed of the situation, he allowed Anastasius to renounce Christ privately in his presence, but to remain a Christian in his heart if he chose, or return to royal service. After refusing this compromise, Anastasius was returned to Persia, where he again refused the entreaties and threats of the king's representatives. In 628, with more than 60 other Christians, Anastasius was strangled on the banks of the Euphrates. His head was then severed, accounting for his patronage.

REFERENCES 6, 14, 16, 36

27

Andrew (Andreas, Endres) the Apostle

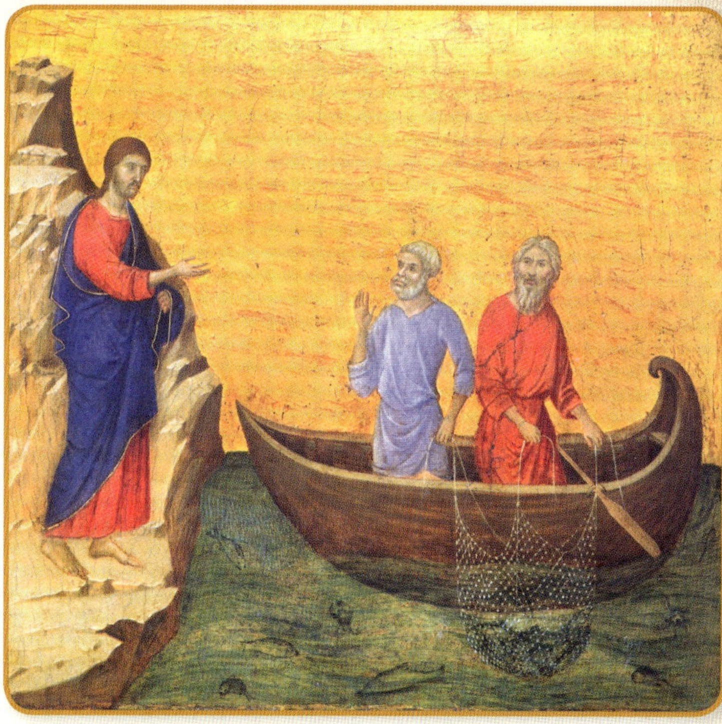

MEMORIAL DAY **November 30**

PATRONAGE **Gout, sore throat, infertility, unmarried women, fishermen, fish dealers, singers, Scotland, Russia, Greece, Malta, Prussia, Amalfi**

LIFE & LEGEND

Andrew, whose name is derived from Greek, meaning "manhood" or "valor," was born in Bethsaida on the shore of the Sea of Galilee. He was the younger brother of Simon Peter, and, like him, was a fisherman. He was a disciple of John the Baptist and is known as the first Apostle. He introduced Jesus to Peter and was a follower of Jesus before and after the crucifixion. Andrew was chosen to be one of the Twelve, was present at the Last Supper, and is always considered to be one of the first four.

He is said to have preached in Cappadocia, Galatia, Bithynia, the Scythian deserts, Byzantium, Thrace, Macedonia, Thessaly, and Achasia. During the reign of Nero, he was ordered to be crucified at Patrae in Achasia by the Roman Governor Aegas. It was specified that, to increase his suffering, he should be bound, not nailed, to a saltire (X-shaped) cross. He died on November 30, AD 60.

His relics were moved from Patras to Constantinople by the Emperor Constantine in 345. At that occasion, Saint Regulus was purportedly instructed by an angel to stop at Fife on the coast of Scotland, where he established the settlement of Saint Andrew. In the seventh century, Saint Wilfrid installed some of Saint Andrew's relics at the settlement. In the thirteenth century, when Constantinople fell to the French, the relics were moved to the cathedral at Amalfi, where some still remain. Following Robert Bruce's victory at the Battle of Bannockburn in 1314, Saint Andrew was named the Patron Saint of Scotland, and at the end of that century, the saltire cross became the national flag. The head of the saint was given to Pope Pius II in 1461. Most of the relics, including the small finger and part of the top of the cranium, were kept in the Vatican until they were sent back to the church of Saint Andrew in Patras by Pope Paul VI in 1964.

REFERENCES 9, 33, 42

28

Andrew Avellino

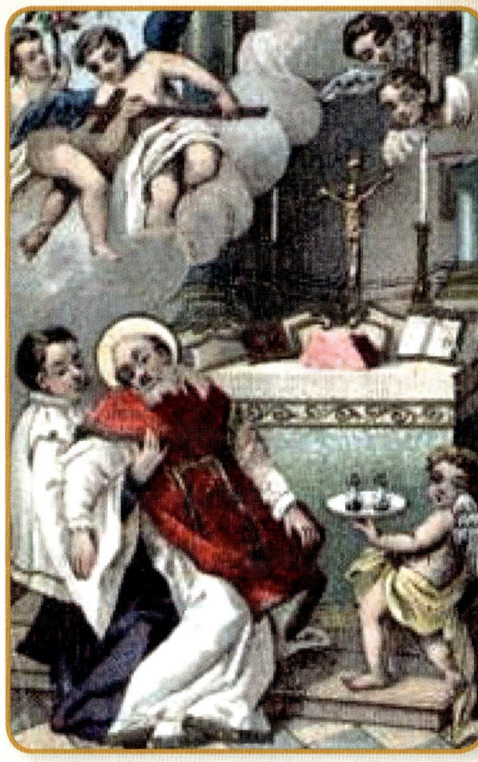

MEMORIAL DAY **November 10**

PATRONAGE **Stroke, sudden death, apoplexy**

LIFE & LEGEND

Andrew Avellino was born in 1521 in the town of Castronuovo, Sicily (now named Castronuovo di Sant Andrea). His baptismal name was Lancelotto. Andrew was well schooled, first at Venice, where he studied humanities and philosophy, and then at Naples, where he obtained the degree of Doctor of Laws. He was ordained as a priest when he was 26 years old, and he became the lawyer to the ecclesiastic court of Naples.

In that capacity, while pleading a case for a friend, he knowingly lied. When he subsequently noted the passage in the Bible, "The mouth that belieth killeth the soul," he renounced the legal profession and devoted himself to a spiritual life. In the course of carrying out an assignment by the archbishop of Naples to reform a scandalous convent, he was assaulted and severely wounded. He was taken to the monastery of the Theatines to recuperate, and entered that order. At that time he took the name of Andrew the Apostle.

He was elected superior of the Order of Theatines, and he established many new houses of the order throughout Italy, including in Milan and Piacenza. On November 10, 1608, he suffered a massive stroke while conducting a mass and died. His remains were enshrined in the church of Saint Paul in Naples. He was beatified by Pope Urban VIII and canonized by Pope Clement XI in 1712.

REFERENCES 9, 41, 44

29

Anianus

MEMORIAL DAY **November 17**

PATRONAGE **Sick children**

LIFE & LEGEND

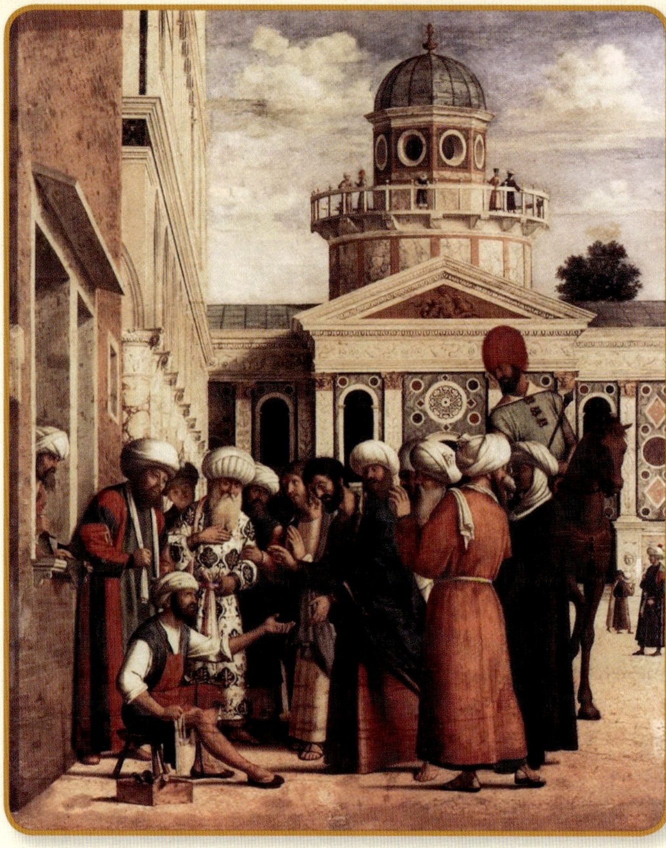

A native of Vienne, Anianus lived for many years as a hermit near his native city. He later succeeded Saint Evurtius as bishop of Orleans. When Attila and his Huns threatened Orleans in 451, Anianus helped organize its defense, and summoned the aid of the Roman general, Aetius. Although the city was taken, the late-arriving Roman army drove the Huns back across the Seine without their captives or booty. After his death, ca. 453, sick children were taken to the tomb of Anianus to be healed of their illnesses. Kerler records the instance of a dead child being brought back to life at the tomb.

REFERENCES 6, 14, 36

30

Anne (Anna)

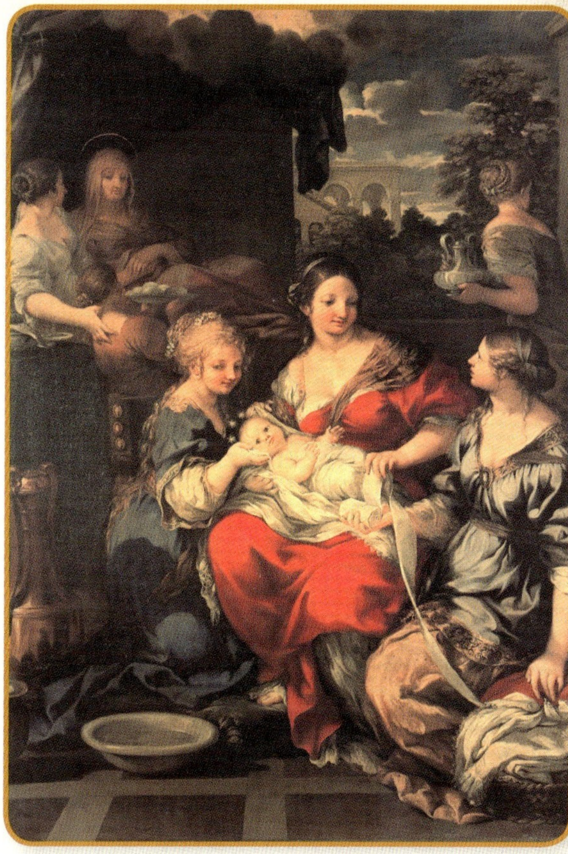

MEMORIAL DAY **July 26**

PATRONAGE **Sterility, pregnancy, childbirth, mothers, grandparents, carpenters, lace makers, miners, poverty, seamstresses, stablemen, Canada, France, Quebec**

LIFE & LEGEND

Anne, whose name is a variant of Hannah and means "grace," was the mother of the Virgin Mary. According to the Gospel of James, she and her husband, Joachim, who were childless for many years, were visited by an angel, and they were told that she would conceive a child. In the fourth century, and later in the fifteenth century, the concept that Mary was born of Anne by virginal birth was accepted. However, this belief was condemned by the Church in 1677.

The relics of Saint Anne were brought from the Holy Land to Constantinople in 710 and kept in the church of Saint Sophia until 1333. The head of Saint Anne was included among the relics at Mainz up to 1510 when it was stolen. She is generally depicted in a red robe with a green mantel, often with a book in hand.

REFERENCE 9

31
Annemund

MEMORIAL DAY **September 28**

PATRONAGE **Epilepsy**

LIFE & LEGEND

Born into a prominent Gallo-Roman family (his father was prefect at Lyons), Annemund was trained at the court of Dagobert I and was an adviser to Clovis II. He was later appointed bishop of Lyons and was befriended (and tonsured) by Saint Wilfrid of York during the latter's stay in Lyons while on journeys to and from Rome. Annemund was murdered at Macon in 658 during the disturbances that followed the death of Clovis II. Wilfrid was present at the execution and offered to die with his friend, but as a foreigner he was allowed to return home. Kerler cites a document of the thirteenth century that refers to Annemund as a patron saint of epileptics.

REFERENCES 6, 14, 16, 36

32

Anno

MEMORIAL DAY **December 4**

PATRONAGE **Gout**

LIFE & LEGEND

The son of an impoverished Swabian nobleman, Anno was educated at the Episcopal school at Bamberg, which he later headed. His many accomplishments brought Anno to the attention of the emperor, Henry III, who made him one of his chaplains. In 1056, Anno was promoted to archbishop of Cologne and chancellor of the empire. He was deeply involved in the politics of his age, including the difficult regency of the son of Henry III, the competing papacies of Alexander III and Cadalus of Parma, and the unpopular appointment of his nephew Conrad as bishop of Trier, which resulted in the latter's murder. In spite of his rather unedifying involvement in the political and ecclesiastic controversies of his age, Anno founded or reformed monasteries, built churches, and distributed large sums to the poor. In his later years, he retired to the abbey at Sieburg, where he lived his final year in repentance. Butler maintains that "it is for the virtue of his private life that he is numbered among the saints."

REFERENCES 6, 14, 36, 46

33
Ansbert

MEMORIAL DAY **February 9**

PATRONAGE **Fever**

LIFE & LEGEND

When Ansbert, whose name is derived from German, meaning "Godly bright," entered a marriage arranged by his father, a prominent nobleman at court, with the daughter of Count de Renty, chancellor to the king, he and his bride, Angadrisma, agreed that marriage was not their true calling and that each would pursue the monastic life. Ansbert entered the abbey at Fontenelle, where he was ordained a priest and later became abbot. When Ouen, the archbishop of Rouen, died, Ansbert succeeded him on the Episcopal throne in 684. During the ceremonies, in which the remains of Saint Ouen were transferred to the abbey that later bore his name, Ansbert was miraculously cured of a fever. This led to his patronage. Ansbert was later deposed from the episcopate on the basis of false accusations maintained by Pepin, mayor of the palace. He retired to the monastery of Hautmont in Hainault, where he died ca. 695.

REFERENCES 6, 16, 36

34

Anthony della Chiesa

MEMORIAL DAY **May 2**

PATRONAGE **Fever**

LIFE & LEGEND

Anthony was born in 1394. Much against the wishes of his father, the Marchese della Chiesa, Anthony entered the Ordine dei Padri Predicatori at Vercelli, near his home town of San Germano. His life was a model of prayer and austerity, and Anthony attained a great reputation as a preacher and director of souls. He successively headed the order's monasteries at Como, Savona, Florence, Bologna, and Genoa, and he was noted as an active opponent of the antipope Felix V and the practice of usury. Both du Broc de Segange and Kerler maintain that Anthony was made archbishop of Florence by Pope Eugenius IV, a dignity not mentioned in Butler or other sources. According to du Broc de Segange, Anthony died of a fever in the thirteenth year of his episcopate in 1459. Subsequently, miraculous cures of fevers have been attributed to invocation of his sainthood.

REFERENCES 6, 14, 16, 36, 46

35

Anthony the Great (Anthony the Abbot)

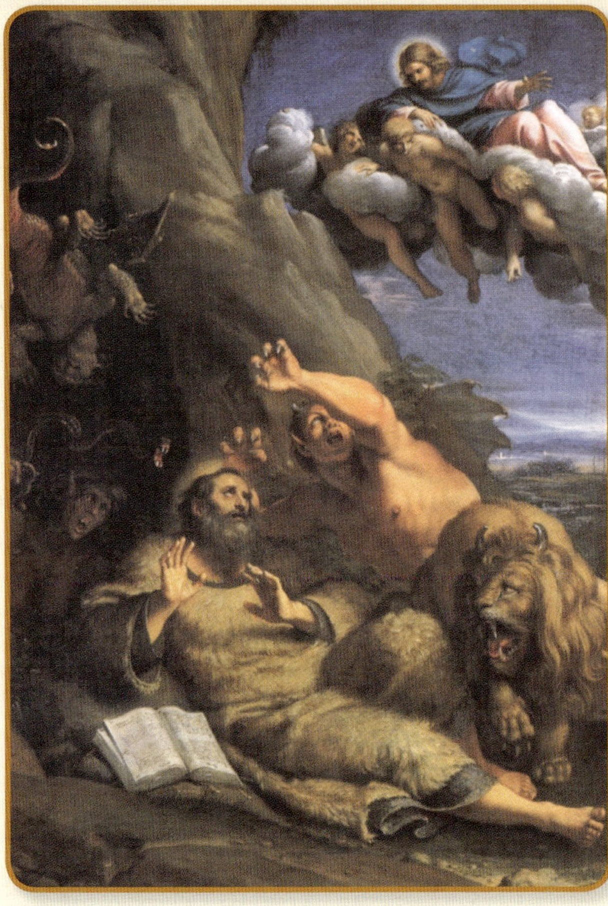

MEMORIAL DAY **January 17**

PATRONAGE **Amputees, eczema, epilepsy, ergotism, erysipelas, skin diseases and rashes, shingles (herpes zoster), herpes, basket makers, brush makers, butchers, domestic animals, monks, swineherds, gravediggers**

LIFE & LEGEND

The name Anthony is derived from Latin, meaning "inestimable." Anthony was born to wealthy parents near Heracleus, Egypt, ca. 251. He dispensed his wealth to the needy and adopted a harsh, anchoritic lifestyle in the desert. As such, he and Saint Paul the Hermit are considered to be the fathers of Christian monasticism. Anthony founded two monasteries on the shores of the Nile, one at Pispir and the other at Arsinoe. The monks at those monasteries supported themselves by making baskets and brushes.

Anthony was noted for his successful treatment of skin disease with pork fat; hence his patronage of skin diseases, pigs, and swineherds. Saint Anthony's Fire, or ignis sacer (holy fire), was the name applied to ergotism, caused by eating grain products contaminated with the fungus *Claviceps pupurea,* which manifested as painful seizures and dry gangrene of the fingers and toes. It was given its name because monks of the Order of Saint Anthony were successful at treating the disorder in the Middle Ages. In Italy and Malta, shingles is also known as Saint Anthony's Fire. Anthony buried Paul the Hermit, which accounts for his patronage of gravediggers. Anthony died at about age 105 at Mount Colzim, Egypt. All that we know of him comes from a biography written by Saint Athanasius.

REFERENCES 6, 9

36

Anthony of Padua (Anthony of Lisbon)

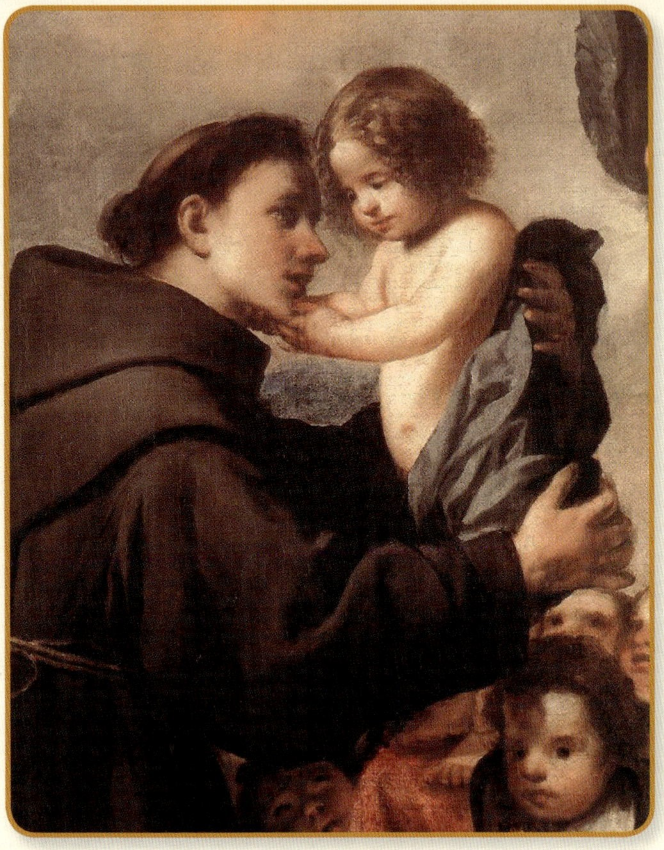

MEMORIAL DAY **June 13**

PATRONAGE **Pregnant women, sterility, childbirth, fever, starvation, [limb replantation],* animals, lost articles, mariners, oppressed and poor people, swineherds, travelers, American Indians, Brazil, Lisbon, Portugal, Padua (Italy), Anzio (Italy)**

LIFE & LEGEND

Anthony of Padua, who is one of the most celebrated and beloved of the saints, was born as Fernando de Bulhoes to a wealthy family in Lisbon in 1195. He initially was ordained as an Augustinian, but in 1220 he became a Franciscan and took the name Anthony in honor of Saint Anthony the Great (Abbot). This change of order resulted from his witnessing the conveyance to his church of the bodies of the first Franciscan martyrs who died that year in Morocco. Anthony left for Morocco but took ill shortly after arrival and, on his return, was shipwrecked at Sicily.

*Proposed patronage

When he was assigned to a rural hospice near Bologna, he was called on to provide a homily, which made a great impression. This led to his commission to preach throughout Lombardy and part of France, and it was as a preacher that Anthony's reputation was established. In 1230, he was released from all other duties and took up residence in Padua, where he composed his sermons on the saints. His convincing oratory earned him the title "hammer of the heretics." He is remembered for the quotation, "Actions speak louder than words; let your words teach and your actions speak."

One of the miracles ascribed to him took place at Padua, where a young man, repentant at having kicked his mother, cut off his foot. Saint Anthony miraculously rejoined the foot to the leg—the first reported replantation. Among his other miracles were rendering poisoned food innocuous by making the sign of the cross, and also preaching a sermon to fish. An apparition of the infant Jesus is said to have visited Anthony, thus accounting for his usual iconographic depiction holding the infant. Anthony died in Padua on June 13, 1231, and was canonized 352 days later, the second most rapid canonization in history. His relics are in the Basilica of Saint Anthony in Padua. He was proclaimed a Doctor of the Church in 1946 by Pope Pius XII.

REFERENCES 9, 42, 45

37

Aphrodisius

MEMORIAL DAY **April 28**

PATRONAGE **Epilepsy**

LIFE & LEGEND

Aphrodisius was a Jewish prefect or priest who lived during the first century in Heliopolis. He recognized the virgin prophesied in Isaiah when he saw the idols in the temples crumble at the passage of Mary, Jesus, and Joseph during their flight from Herod's persecution. According to this same legend, Aphrodisius provided the family shelter during their years of exile. Another legend claims that Aphrodisius learned of the miracles of Jesus from Alexandrian Jews returning from Jerusalem, and that he himself went to Palestine and became one of Jesus' disciples. Different legends maintain that he was present at the Pentecost and received the Holy Spirit, or that after the death of Jesus he went to Antioch, where he was baptized by Saint Peter.

What is of greater historical certainty is that Aphrodisius traveled to Rome and that he accompanied Saint Sergius Paulus into Gaul to evangelize the pagans. He is said to have lived for many years as a hermit in a cave, and later in life he became the first bishop of Beziers. Aphrodisius was arrested and beheaded for his faith ca. 60 to 65. After his execution, he is said to have risen, picked up his severed head, and carried it to the cave where he used to live. The earliest Christians in the region built a chapel on this site, where Charlemagne later erected a church in his honor. The name of Aphrodisius is invoked in cases of epilepsy in children.

REFERENCES 16, 36

38

Apollinaris of Ravenna

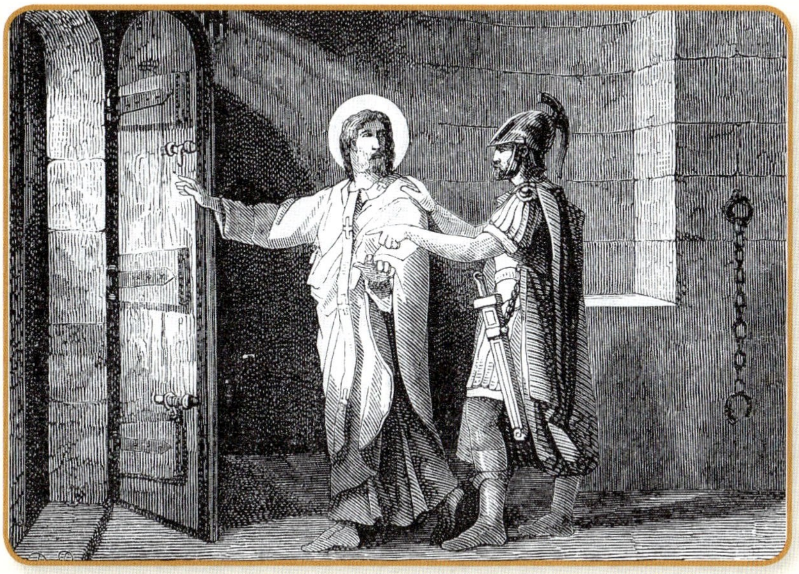

MEMORIAL DAY **July 23**

PATRONAGE **Urinary stones, calculi, Ravenna**

LIFE & LEGEND

A native of Antioch and reputedly a disciple of Peter, Apollinaris, whose name refers to the Greek god Apollo, was the first bishop of Ravenna during the first century. He was noted not only for his zeal in trying to convert the citizens of this important Adriatic port, but also for the miraculous cures he worked there and elsewhere in Emilia Romagna. On four different occasions Apollinaris was arrested, tortured, and expelled from the city for his missionary activity. On the fourth occasion, consequent to Vespasian's banishment of Christians, Apollinaris hid in the suburb of Classis, where one day he was recognized by a mob, beaten, and left for dead. The magnificent basilica erected in his honor in Ravenna, the city of his patronage, was consecrated in 549.

REFERENCES 14, 36, 46

39

Apollonia

MEMORIAL DAY **February 9**

PATRONAGE **Toothache, dentistry**

LIFE & LEGEND

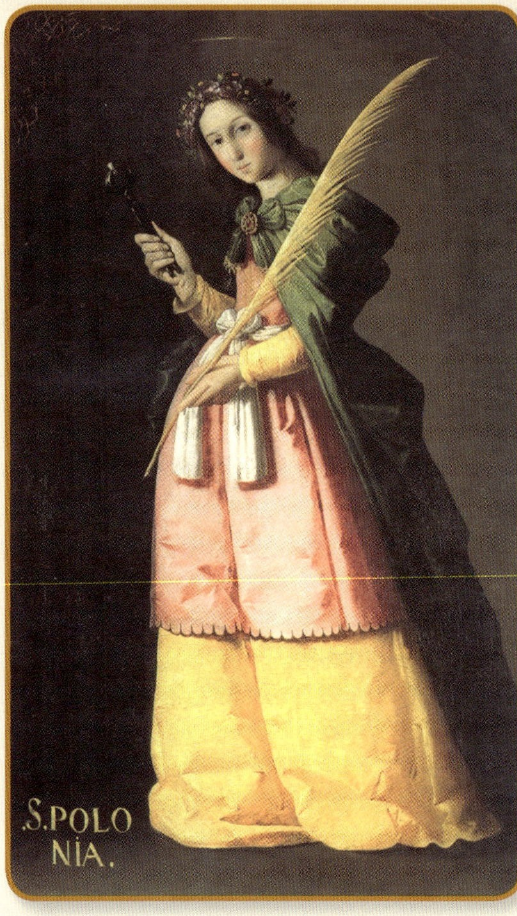

Apollonia's name is derived from the Greek god Apollo, and nothing is known about her birth or early life. During an uprising against the Christians in Alexandria before the persecution of Decius, she was one of a group of virgin martyrs who were seized in 249. Her torture included having her teeth violently removed or broken, accounting for her patronage. She was threatened with being burned alive if she did not renounce her religion, at which point she ran into the flames and died. She is designated as one of the Fourteen Holy Helpers. Her relics were preserved in the former church of Saint Apollonia in Rome. Her relics are currently at the Basilica de Santa Maria in Trastavere, Italy, and at churches in Antwerp, Brussels, Liege, Porto, and Cologne.

REFERENCES 6, 9, 42, 45

40

Apronia (Evronie)

MEMORIAL DAY **July 15**

PATRONAGE **Labor**

LIFE & LEGEND

Apronia was the sister of Saint Evre, the seventh bishop of Toul. She lived in that city under her brother's spiritual direction. After the death of Evre, Apronia returned to Troyes, the city of her birth, where she died ca. 450. After her death, the remains of the saintly woman were returned to Toul.

REFERENCES 16, 36

41

Arnould (Arnulphus)

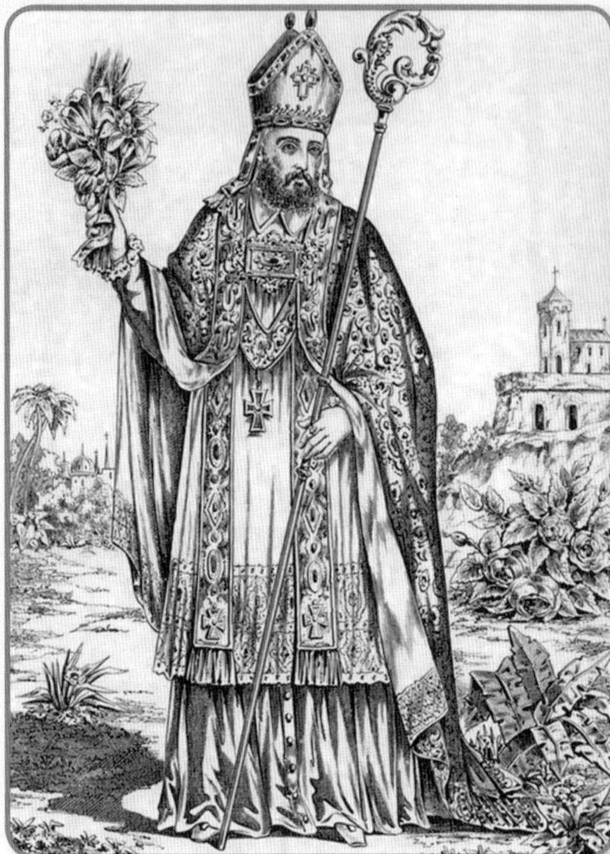

MEMORIAL DAY **January 29**

PATRONAGE **Fever, neck disorders, throat disorders**

LIFE & LEGEND

Born during the eighth century into a noble family of Cysoing near Lille, France, Arnould, whose name is derived from German, meaning "powerful eagle," was sent at an early age to learn the profession of arms under the tutelage of a kinsman. He quickly perfected all the accomplishments and virtues of a chevalier, including piety and generosity to the poor. His character earned Arnould the spite of enemies, who, on at least two occasions, falsely accused him of misdeeds. When he was accused of stealing treasure from his lord, Arnould was not only exonerated but adopted by the nobleman in question. One day when he was riding in the countryside with this same nobleman, Arnould observed in the distance a party of armed men whom he recognized as enemies of the aged chevalier. Arnould gave his lord his own horse, which was faster. His lord escaped, but Arnould was captured. After much maltreatment, Arnould's captors wrapped a cord around his neck, suspended him from a tree, and gradually strangled him by placing their feet on his shoulders.

Arnould was buried at Cysoing, where miraculous cures were almost immediately reported to take place at his tomb—particularly among those suffering from fevers and maladies of the neck. Those afflicted with the latter were able to wrap around their necks the same cord with which Arnould had been martyred. According to du Broc de Segange, it was also once common for those who had been cured of fever or a neck disorder to make a votive offering at his tomb in the form of a silver cord.

REFERENCE 16

42

Arnulf (Arnoul) of Soissons

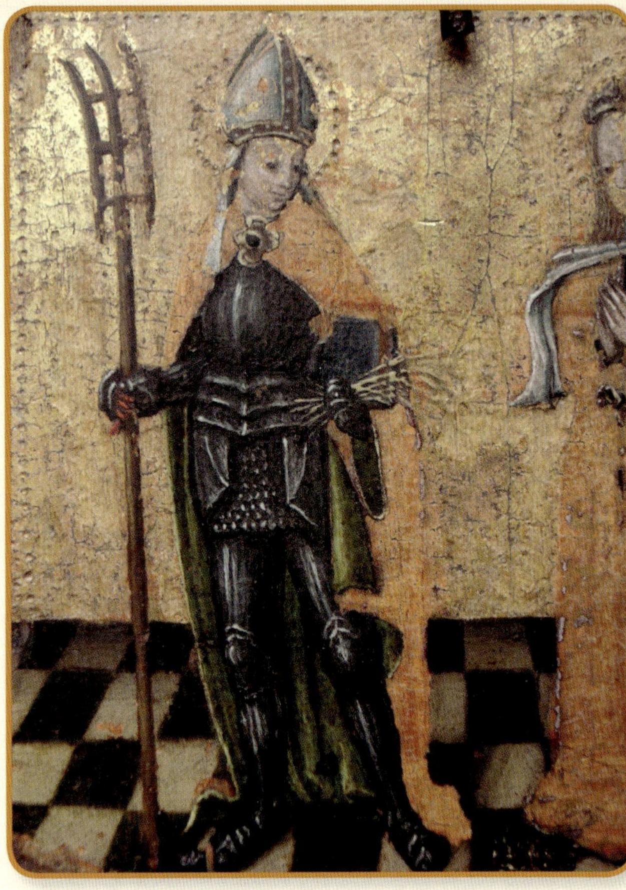

MEMORIAL DAY **August 15**

PATRONAGE **Pregnancy**

LIFE & LEGEND

Born in Flanders, ca. 1040, Arnulf, whose name is derived from German, meaning "eagle and wolf," distinguished himself as a soldier in the armies of kings Robert and Henri I of France. He later became a monk in the monastery of Saint Medard at Soissons, and eventually he assumed the life of a recluse within his cell. Even in this state, his holiness did not remain hidden from the eyes of men. Arnulf was called from his life of constant prayer and repentance to be made bishop of Soissons in 1081. After being driven from his see by a usurper, Arnulf resigned the episcopacy and founded a monastery at Oudenbourg in Flanders. According to Kerler, Arnulf prophesied the birth of a boy to the consort of King Philip of France, and he thus became a patron saint of pregnant women. Arnulf died ca. 1087.

REFERENCES 6, 14, 36

43

Asclepius (Asclipe) of Limoges

MEMORIAL DAY **December 23**

PATRONAGE **Hemorrhage**

LIFE & LEGEND

Asclepius was bishop of Limoges and founder of the Benedictine monastery in that city during the eighth century. He received support from Charlemagne for the restoration of the Benedictine convent at Bourges, of which one of the daughters of Charlemagne is said to have been abbess.

REFERENCES 16, 36

44

Asperenus

MEMORIAL DAY **August 3**

PATRONAGE **Headache**

LIFE & LEGEND

Asperenus was the first bishop of Naples during the first century. He converted to Christianity after being cured of an illness by Saint Peter, who later consecrated him as bishop.

REFERENCES 14, 36, 46

45

Athanasius

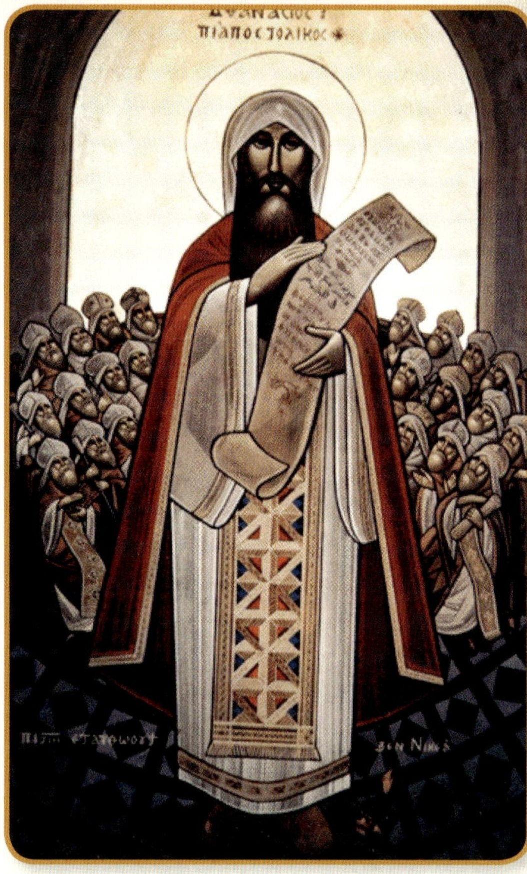

MEMORIAL DAY **May 2**

PATRONAGE **Headache**

LIFE & LEGEND

Born of Christian parents in Alexandria, Athanasius, whose name is derived from Greek, meaning "immortal," was educated in traditional classical literature, theology, and scriptural studies. He developed a lifelong association with the monks and hermits of the Egyptian desert, including Saint Anthony, whose life he chronicled. Athanasius was ordained a deacon in 318 and accompanied Bishop Alexander of Alexandria to the council held at Nicaea that excommunicated the heretic Arius. This marked the beginning of Athanasius' lifelong struggle against Arianism, which insisted that Jesus was not of the substance of God, but only the best of created beings.

In 327, Athanasius succeeded Alexander as bishop of Alexandria. Although Arianism had been condemned at Nicaea nearly a decade earlier, Athanasius still had to contend with the revival of this quickly spreading heresy throughout Egypt and the Mediterranean. When Emperor Constantine directed Athanasius to readmit Arius to full communion, he refused. Athanasius was subsequently compelled to defend himself before the emperor for various charges brought against him by his enemies among the Arians and their allies the Meletians. When cleared of the charges, he was then accused of the murder of a Meletian bishop, who was actually in hiding.

More charges were added, and, in 336, Athanasius was banished by the emperor to the city of Trier in Gaul. Recalled to his see in 338 by a son of the recently deceased Constantine, Athanasius was denounced on charges of sedition and was again deposed. He fled to Rome, where he was cleared of the calumnies by a synod, but he was not able to return to his see until the death of the Arian usurper in 345. With the murder of Constans, the co-emperor, Athanasius lost his imperial protector. Constans' brother, Constantius, an Arian sympathizer, assumed control of both the eastern and western halves of the empire and took advantage of the situation to suppress the popular and influential Athanasius once and for all. Athanasius was condemned by Arian-dominated councils at Arles and Milan and was forced to find refuge in the monasteries of the Egyptian desert.

As a champion of Christian orthodoxy, Athanasius was unable to return to Alexandria until Julian the Apostate assumed the imperial throne in 361. Shortly thereafter, Athanasius was forced to once again seek safety in the Egyptian desert because of his opposition to Julian's intention to reimpose paganism throughout the empire. When Julian died suddenly in 363, Athanasius returned briefly from exile, only to flee again when Emperor Valens banished all orthodox bishops in 365. The emperor reversed his position 4 months later, and Athanasius returned to Alexander after 17 years' intermittent exile to secure the victory of orthodoxy promulgated at the Council of Constantinople in 381. Given the unceasing struggles in which he was engaged, it is small wonder that Athanasius, who died in 373, is the patron saint of those suffering from headaches.

REFERENCES 6, 14, 16, 36

46

Aurelianus of Limoges

MEMORIAL DAY **May 8**

PATRONAGE **Ear diseases, deafness, lightning**

LIFE & LEGEND

According to a legend that emerged in the tenth century, Saint Martial had been a disciple of Jesus and was later sent by Saint Peter to evangelize in the province of Gaul. Du Broc de Segange accepts this story, including the account of two pagan priests who were killed by lightning when they tried to interfere with the proselytizing mission of Martial and his companions. One of these two priests was Aurelianus, who, after being brought back to life by the prayers of Martial, converted to Christianity and succeeded him as bishop of Limoges. This legend stands in contrast to most accounts, which place Martial in France ca. 250. The relics of Aurelianus are enshrined in the church that bears his name in Limoges. For obvious reasons, his name is invoked as a protection against lightning. Aurelianus is also the patron of those suffering from ear diseases and deafness—possibly because his name has mutated in some places to Aureille ("oreille" is "ear" in French).

REFERENCES 16, 36

47

Austriclinianus

MEMORIAL DAY **October 15**

PATRONAGE **Fever, gout**

LIFE & LEGEND

Austriclinianus is supposed to have been one of the companions of Saint Martial in the evangelization of Gaul during the third century.

REFERENCES 16, 36

48

Avertan (Averrano)

MEMORIAL DAY **February 25**

PATRONAGE **Plague**

LIFE & LEGEND

Avertan was born in Limoges during the fourteenth century. He entered the Carmelite monastery in his native city, where he led the life of a contemplative monk. He became seriously ill in Lucca while traveling to Rome to visit the city's holy sites. He died in Lucca and was later invoked by its citizens for relief during the plague.

REFERENCES 16, 31, 36

49

Avertinus

MEMORIAL DAY **May 5**

PATRONAGE **Headache, epilepsy, mental disorders, vertigo, difficult children**

LIFE & LEGEND

Born in England, Avertinus was a canon of Saint Gilbert and was ordained to the diaconate by Thomas of Canterbury (Thomas Becket), whom he attended through all his troubles. Avertinus accompanied Thomas to the city of Tours, where they attended the council that deposed Antipope Victor in 1163. After their return to England, Thomas was murdered. Avertinus again crossed the Channel and sought a life of solitude and prayer in the forest of Cange, near Saint Pierre de Vencay. Even in the wilderness, his holiness attracted those who sought his prayers, counsel, and miraculous cures. Avertinus died ca. 1180. His tomb was visited by those seeking relief from headache well into the modern period. Fletcher maintains that Avertinus is also the patron saint of those suffering from epilepsy and mental disorders and that the saint was invoked in the management of difficult children (the old French word "avertineux" refers to such individuals).

REFERENCES 6, 14, 16, 24, 36

50

Aybert

MEMORIAL DAY April 7

PATRONAGE Fever

LIFE & LEGEND

A native of Espeen, near Tournay, Aybert was inclined from his earliest years to a life of ascetic austerity. He was received as disciple by one of the monks in the monastery of Saint Crespin, where he shared the life of a recluse with his spiritual father. Both men accompanied their abbot on a journey to Rome where the abbot had to attend to monastery business. On their return to Hainault, Aybert joined the monastic brotherhood on a permanent basis. He remained there for 25 years before withdrawing into the wilderness, where he died in 1140. Water from a well that bears his name at the abbey of Saint Crespin was noted for its power to heal those sick with fever.

REFERENCES 16, 36

B

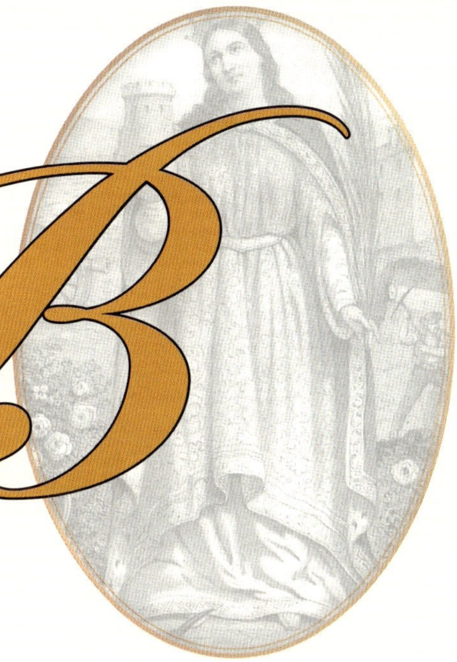

51
Balbina

MEMORIAL DAY **March 31**

PATRONAGE **Scrofula, goiter**

LIFE & LEGEND

Balbina, whose name is derived from Latin, meaning "stuttering," was the daughter of the martyred Roman tribune Quirinus. She and her father were both baptized by Pope Alexander I. They were both martyred at Rome during the reign of Emperor Hadrian, ca. 130, and they were both buried along the Appian Way. Balbina is supposed to have been cured of scrofula by Pope Alexander; hence her patronage of those suffering from enlargement and degeneration of the lymph nodes in the neck. Kerler maintains that Balbina is also the patron saint of those with goiter.

REFERENCES 6, 14, 16, 36, 46

52
Baldus

MEMORIAL DAYS **September 15, October 29**

PATRONAGE **Gout, colic, toothache**

LIFE & LEGEND

The standard account of Baldus' life comes from a manuscript of the fourteenth century in which the saint is described as a native of Spain or Portugal. During his adolescence, Baldus had a premonition that he would one day murder his mother and father. To prevent this, he left home and settled in another region, where he married. Because they were anxious to see their son again, Baldus' parents traced him to his new place of residence. They were met at the door by their daughter-in-law, who received them hospitably and allowed the weary travelers to rest in the bed that she and her husband usually occupied. She then went out to find her husband, who returned in her absence. Baldus saw two figures in his bed and assumed that his wife was betraying him with another man. Overcome by jealousy, Baldus took up an ax and killed the sleeping couple, his parents.

When Baldus realized what he had done, he abandoned his wife and home and assumed a nomadic existence that took him on pilgrimages to the Holy Sepulchre in Jerusalem, to the tombs of the apostles in Rome, and to other holy sites before he finally crossed the Alps and settled near Sens (Gaul). Baldus was received there by Bishop Artemius, to whom Baldus confided his tragic story. As penance,

Artemius gave Baldus his own staff and commanded him to plant it on a nearby hill and to water the staff from the river below. Baldus accepted this penance gladly, carrying bucket after bucket of water to the top of the hill. In response to his penitence and obedience, the staff eventually put out roots, branches, and fruit. Baldus built himself a cell on this hilltop, where he died ca. 620. A church was eventually constructed there in his name. Cures took place at that site related to the diseases for which he was assigned patronage.

REFERENCES 36, 46

53 Balsamia

MEMORIAL DAYS **October 25, November 16**

PATRONAGE **Pregnant women, labor**

LIFE & LEGEND

Perhaps of Italian origin, Balsamia emigrated during the fifth century to Reims in Gaul, where she was employed as a wet nurse. She is notable for having served as wet nurse to Saint Remigius. For this reason, she is also known in France as Sainte Nourrice (French for "wet nurse"). Balsamia is also said to have been the mother of Saint Celsinus (Soussin).

REFERENCES 16, 18, 36, 46

54
Balthasar

MEMORIAL DAY **July 23**

PATRONAGE **Epilepsy, travelers**

LIFE & LEGEND

Balthasar, which means "God or Lord protect the king" in Phoenician, was one of the three wisemen (Magi) who journeyed from the East to worship the infant Jesus. They came first to Jerusalem, where they inquired of Herod, "Where is he who has been born King of the Jews? For we have seen his star in the East, and have come to worship him" (Matthew 2:2). Disturbed by this threatening portent, Herod inquired of the chief priests and scribes where the Christ was to be born. Their answer was Bethlehem of Judea, where Herod sent the three visitors to locate the child and bring back word of him. When the Magi saw the star over Bethlehem, they entered the house and saw the child with Mary his mother. They immediately fell down and worshipped Him. "Then, opening their treasures, they offered him gifts, gold and frankincense and myrrh" (2:11). The last we hear of the Magi is news of their departure: "And being warned in a dream not to return to Herod, they departed to their own country by another way" (2:12).

By the eighth century, the Magi had acquired names: Balthasar, Caspar, and Melchior. The supposed relics of all three were deposited in the Cologne cathedral in 1164, having come to Germany from Milan and before that from Constantinople. The Magi are commonly venerated as patron saints of travelers. Balthasar is the only one of the three with a medical connection, but the reasons for his patronage of epilepsy are unknown.

REFERENCES 6, 36

55
Barbara

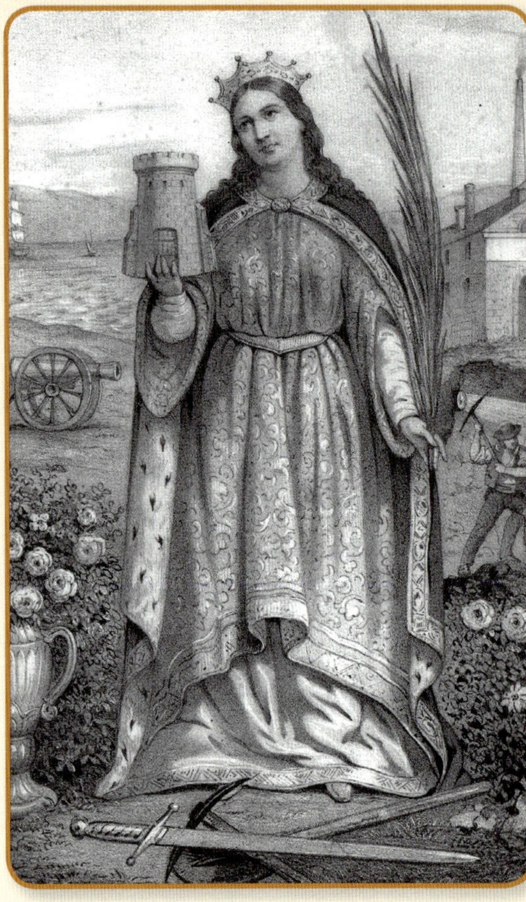

MEMORIAL DAY **December 4**

PATRONAGE **Sudden and violent death, plague, fever, lightning, fire, artillery, miners, firefighters, stonemasons, mathematicians**

LIFE & LEGEND

Barbara's name means "foreign" and has the same derivation as "barbarian." She was born in the latter half of the third century in Nicomedia, the daughter of a wealthy man named Dioscorus. Because she destroyed the images of the pagan gods in her home, her father shut her in a tower, which he planned to contain two windows. Barbara had a third window inserted as a symbol of the Holy Trinity, and she devoted herself to Christianity. Her father attempted to remove her from the tower, but her prayers opened the wall, allowing her escape. She hid in the mountains, where a shepherd betrayed her. He was transformed into marble, and his herd was transformed into grasshoppers.

Dioscorus brought Barbara before Prefect Marcianus in Rome, where she was commanded to renounce her faith. She refused, and after she survived multiple tortures, she was eventually beheaded by her father, who was immediately struck by lightning and killed.

Saint Barbara is one of the Fourteen Holy Helpers. Her name was dropped from the list for universal veneration by Pope Paul VI in 1969 because of the lack of factual material about her. She is still venerated by the Eastern Orthodox Church, where she is known as Great Martyr Barbara. Her relics were translocated from Constantinople to Kiev in the twelfth century, where they are now preserved at Saint Vladimir's Cathedral.

REFERENCES 6, 9, 14, 36, 46

56

Bartholomew

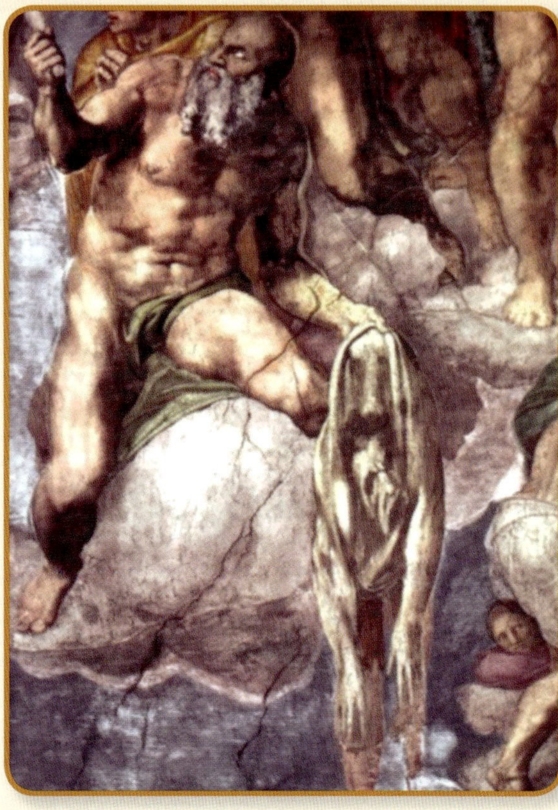

MEMORIAL DAY **August 24**

PATRONAGE **Dermatology, plastic surgery, neurologic diseases, skin diseases, twitching, bookbinders, butchers, cobblers, cheese merchants, leather workers, tanners, trappers, Armenia**

LIFE & LEGEND

Bartholomew, actually Nathaniel bar-Tolmay (son of Tolmay or Ptolemy), was one of the Twelve Apostles. He went on a mission to India and is thought to have served in Ethiopia, Mesopotamia, Parthia, and Lycaonia. He brought Christianity to Armenia in the first century and is regarded, along with Saint Jude, as one of that country's patron saints. Bartholomew was martyred at the site of the Maiden Tower in Baku, Azerbaijan, where he was flayed alive and then crucified head-down. Michelangelo's *Last Judgment* in the Sistine Chapel of the Vatican shows Saint Bartholomew flayed and holding his own skin in his hand. The face on the skin in the painting is recognizable as that of Michelangelo.

After Bartholomew died, his body washed up on the island of Lipari off the coast of Italy, where pieces of his skin and bones are kept in the Cathedral of Saint Bartholomew the Apostle. Some of his relics were transported to the basilica of San Bartolomeo al'Isola in Rome in 983. Later, parts of his skull were transferred to Frankfurt and the Canterbury Cathedral in England.

The oldest extant hospital in England, Saint Bartholomew's Hospital, was founded in 1123 by Rahere, a court jester turned monk. In 1546, Henry VIII granted that hospital, along with Bethlem, Bridewell, and Saint Thomas', to the city of London as the four Royal Hospitals. William Harvey, discoverer of the circulation of blood, was appointed Hospital Physician at Saint Bartholomew's in 1609.

The memorial day of Saint Bartholomew in 1572 was the beginning of the massacre of tens of thousands of Huguenots (Protestants) throughout Paris and later, other parts of France. This event has come to be known as the Saint Bartholomew's Day massacre.

REFERENCES 9, 19, 42, 45

57

Basil the Great (Basil of Caesarea)

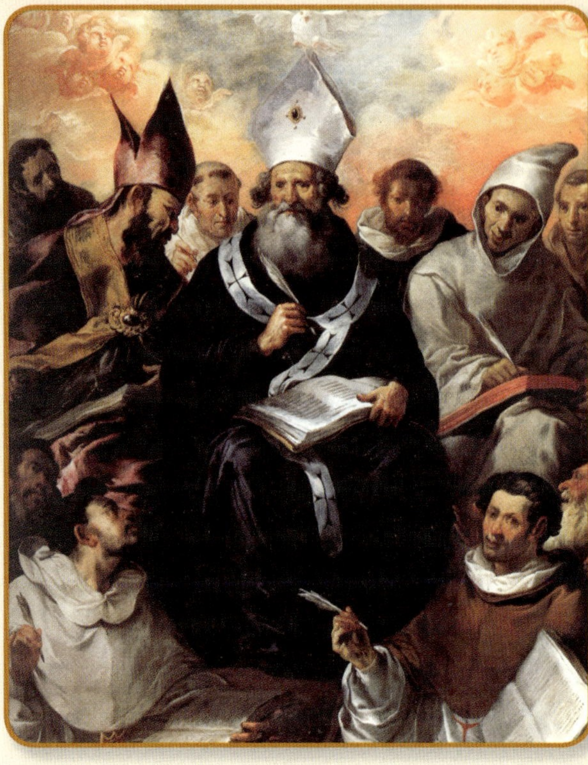

MEMORIAL DAY **January 1 (Anglican Church: January 2; Episcopal Church: June 14; Coptic Orthodox Church: January 14)**

PATRONAGE **Hospital administrators, educators, liturgists, Cappadocia**

LIFE & LEGEND

Basil, whose name is derived from Latin, meaning "kingly," was one of 10 children in a wealthy, pious Christian family in Caesarea, Cappadocia (now Kayseri, Turkey). He was born ca. 330 and had as siblings the theologian Gregory of Nyssa and the ascetic nun Saint Macrina the younger. Although many fourth-century Christians expressed reservations at or abhorrence of the idea of exposing young minds to the study of secular and pagan culture, Basil received an education thoroughly grounded in classical culture, including the study of medicine. He possessed the inclination and the means to pursue his studies in Caesarea, Constantinople, and Athens, where he became acquainted with the future emperor Julian (known later as Julian the Apostate) and formed an early friendship with the future theologian Gregory Nazianzus. Basil returned home in 356 with the intention of teaching rhetoric. However, under the influence of his sister Macrina, he entered the monastic life, in preparation for which he made a tour of the monasteries in Syria, Palestine, and Egypt. After his return, Basil and his brother Gregory organized the first large-scale monastery in Asia Minor. The Rule that Basil compiled for this monastery defines Eastern Orthodox monasticism to this day.

Ordained as a priest in 364, Basil succeeded Eusebius as bishop of Caesarea in 370. In his episcopal role, he effectively championed Nicene orthodoxy in the struggle against the Arian heresy (supported by the emperor Valens). The supporters of the Nicene Creed professed that the members of the Trinity were of one substance, whereas those ascribing to Arianism taught that Jesus was not of the same substance as God. Basil was the author of several important theologic treatises and commentaries on Scripture. His surviving correspondence (some 300 letters) provides a vivid picture of his life and times.

In the Byzantine East, the medical profession came to be regarded as the epitome of practical Christian charity—a perfect response to Christ's command to love one's neighbor. Partly toward this end, Basil established monasteries close to large population centers, where the monastics under his jurisdiction could extend their influence over large numbers of people. This influence included providing assistance to the poor, the aged, and the sick. Basil was certainly not the first bishop to establish a hospital in his jurisdiction, but the ptocheion (hospice for the poor) that he established was a model of its kind in accommodating the physical needs of the unfortunate. Described as a city within the city, the hospital portion of the ptocheion employed both physicians and nursing attendants. Basil himself was not averse to applying the medical knowledge he acquired in Athens to the needs of his spiritual children. By reason of these administrative talents, Basil is venerated as the patron saint of hospital administrators. The Roman Catholic Church named Basil a Doctor of the Church, and the Basilian fathers are of the Order of Saint Basil.

REFERENCES 19, 50

58

Baudelius

MEMORIAL DAY **May 20**

PATRONAGE **Pregnancy, childbirth, hernia, Nimes, Poitiers**

LIFE & LEGEND

Baudelius, who lived in the latter half of the third century and the early fourth century, is described by du Broc de Segange as a native of Orleans and by Butler as being of foreign origin. Both agree that Baudelius and his wife evangelized in southern Gaul and that he was martyred at Nimes for preaching Christianity on a day when the cult of Jupiter was being celebrated. After his head was severed, it bounced three times along the ground. At each place the severed head struck, springs emerged that still exist and have miraculous powers. On the site of the springs the oratory of the Three Fountains was built. Baudelius' wife had his body transported to Valsainte, where he was buried. A church, and later a monastery, were built there to honor him. The crypt of Saint Baudile at the corner of rue de Moulins and rue des Trois Fontaines in Nimes marks the spot where he was martyred. His cult flourished in several regions of France, as well as in Spain and Flanders.

REFERENCES 6, 9, 14, 16, 36

59

Bavo

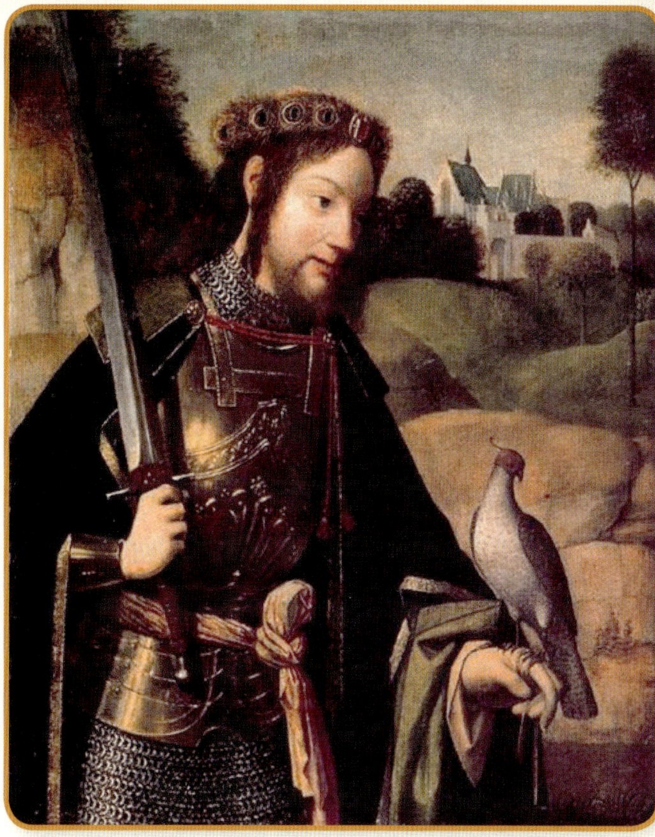

MEMORIAL DAY **October 1**

PATRONAGE **Whooping cough, Ghent, Haarlem**

LIFE & LEGEND

Bavo, who was born into a noble family in Brabant in 589, led a life selling slaves to the nobility until his wife died. At that point, he reformed and was converted to Christianity by Saint Amand and became a Benedictine monk. After his conversion, he distributed all his possessions among the poor and initially accompanied Saint Amand on missionary journeys through Flanders and France. He then withdrew to a hermitage in a beech tree in a forest near Ghent. He returned to Ghent where he died ca. 654. The memory of the holy hermit, who is supposed to be able to protect his votaries from whooping cough, is still greatly revered in Belgium and Holland.

REFERENCES 14, 47

60

Beatus (Beat, Bie)

MEMORIAL DAY **May 9**

PATRONAGE **Cancer**

LIFE & LEGEND

Beatus, whose name is derived from Latin, meaning "blessed," was born in Italy in the third century and devoted himself to converting infidel Gauls—first along the Garonne and subsequently in the regions of Vendomes, Nantes, and Laon. Another Saint Beatus evangelized in Switzerland and is known as the "Apostle of Switzerland." Later in life he lived as a hermit in a cave near Laon. The cavern had been inhabited by a dragon that Beatus slew by making the sign of the cross over it.

REFERENCES 16, 36, 42

61

Benedict the Moor

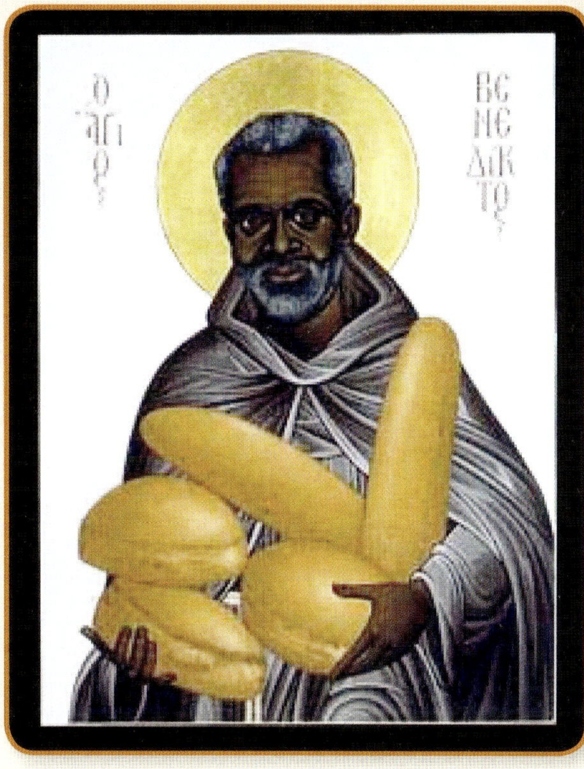

MEMORIAL DAY **April 4**

PATRONAGE **Labor, African Americans, Palermo**

LIFE & LEGEND

Benedict, which means "blessed," was born in 1526 to parents of African origin who lived as slaves at San Fratello, near Messina in Sicily. The landowner to whose estate they belonged promised to free the couple's firstborn child. As a firstborn, and because of his fortunate birth, Benedict the Moor became a patron saint of women in labor. Pious from his earliest years, Benedict was invited to join a band of men who lived a hermetic life in imitation of Francis of Assisi. When the band moved to Montepellegrino near Palermo, Benedict was chosen its superior. In 1562, Pope Pius IV declared that hermits must leave the idiosyncratic life and join an established order. Benedict, at age 38, joined the Franciscan convent of Santa Maria di Gesu near Palermo. Initially he served as its cook, but, in 1578, he was appointed superior—much against his inclination. Benedict was allowed to withdraw from the office after several years. He served for a time as novice-master and then returned to the kitchen, where his humble station did little to obscure public knowledge of his holiness and miracles. He died in 1589.

REFERENCES 6, 14, 16, 36, 46

62

Benedict of Nursia

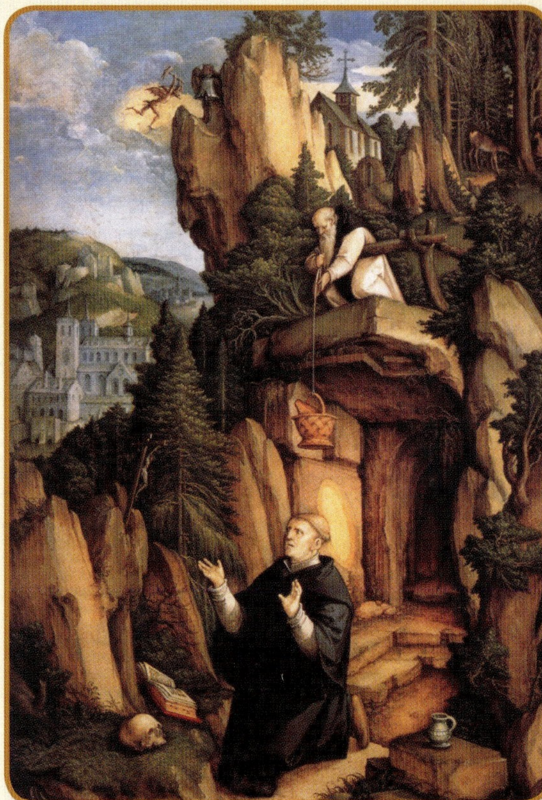

MEMORIAL DAY **July 11 (formerly March 21)**

PATRONAGE **Poison, erysipelas, fever, gallstones, kidney diseases, inflammatory diseases, calculi, monks, farmers, Europe**

LIFE & LEGEND

Benedict was the son of a Roman noble of Nursia (now Norcia in Umbria, Italy). His twin sister was Saint Scholastica. The first valid presentation of his life appeared in the second book of Saint Gregory's Dialogues. He was born ca. 480, and when he was about 19 years old he left his home and literary studies to settle in Enfide, near Subiaco. He became a hermit and lived in a cave for 3 years. Legend indicates that food was brought to him by a raven.

When the abbot of a neighboring monastery died, Benedict was recruited to replace him. Some of the resident monks were displeased and poisoned his drink. When Benedict blessed the cup, it shattered. When he prayed over the poisoned bread that the monks presented to him, a raven flew in and grabbed it from his hands.

Benedict built 12 monasteries in the area, and he remained the abbot of all of them. He recruited Saint Maurus and Saint Placid, two individuals involved in one of Benedict's miracles. He had a vision that Placid had fallen into the area's lake and dispatched Maurus, who rescued Placid from drowning.

Benedict moved to Monte Cassino, where he built a famous monastery, and it was there that he authored the famous Saint Benedict's Rule. The Rule, which was actually written for laymen and not clerics, contained precepts for monks, and Benedict is often regarded to be the founder of western Christian monasticism. The Rule that has guided more than 40,000 monasteries has been summarized as "pray and work." Under the Rule, a reasonable and equitable lifestyle was proscribed for the monks. The superior was elected, and the Rule served as a constitution for governance.

Benedict developed a fever and died at Monte Cassino ca. 547 and was buried in the same grave as his sister. He was canonized in 1220. In 1964, Pope Paul VI named him patron saint of Europe. In 2008, Pope Benedict XVI cited Saint Benedict's life work as integral to the development of European civilization and culture.

63

Bernard of Rodez

MEMORIAL DAY **October 9**

PATRONAGE **Pregnancy**

LIFE & LEGEND

Bernard was born in 1040 into a noble family of Rodez. He entered the monastery of Amance and became a disciple of the future Saint Gausbert, who left Amance to found the monastery at Mont-Sauve. On Gausbert's death, Bernard succeeded him as abbot, an office that he held for 30 years. He died in 1110 and is invoked by pregnant women, many of whom made the pilgrimage to the church at Monsalvy (Cantal), where his remains were entombed.

REFERENCES 16, 36

64

Bernardino of Siena

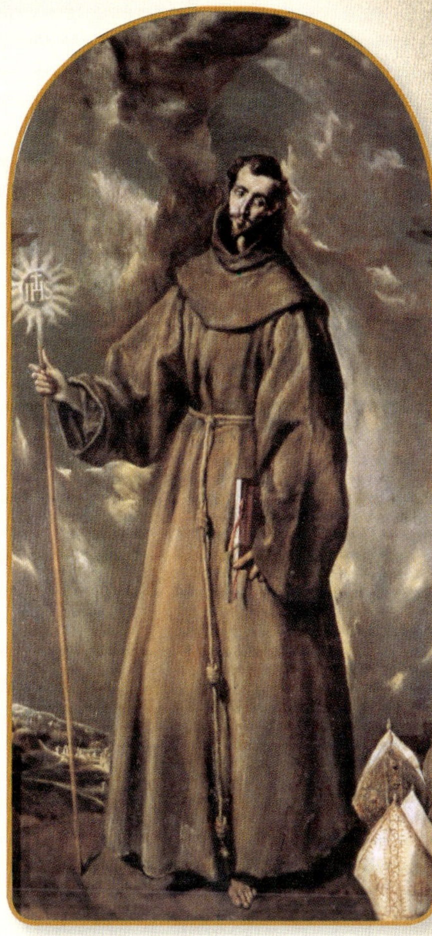

MEMORIAL DAY **May 20**

PATRONAGE **Lung problems, plague, gambling addicts, communication, public relations**

LIFE & LEGEND

Bernardino, whose name is derived from German, meaning "bear, brave," was born on September 8, 1380, into the noble family of Albizzeschi in the town of Massa, where his father was governor. Bernardino was orphaned at age eight and raised by his aunts. As a 17-year-old, he joined the Confraternity of Our Lady, attached to the Santa Maria della Scala hospital in Siena. During the outbreak of bubonic plague in Siena in 1400, Bernardino took care of the afflicted and for 4 months was in charge of the hospital. During that period his health was shattered (he may have contracted the plague), and he never completely recovered.

He joined the Friars Minor of the Franciscan order and was ordained in 1404. Shortly thereafter, Saint Vincent Ferrer, while preaching in Piedmont, predicted that someone in the audience would take over his evangelical mantle. About a decade later, Bernardino fulfilled the prediction and would eventually be referred to as the "Apostle of Italy." He preached to crowds of thousands throughout Italy. His sermons denouncing vice were accompanied by bonfires of vanities (such as cosmetics, mirrors, playing cards, and fine clothing). His attacks on usury led to the development of beneficial loan societies. He also persuaded warring factions in the cities to reconcile and strive for peace.

Bernardino was accused of heresy for false preaching but was exonerated and commended by the pope for his teaching. Bernardino was offered many bishopric positions, including Siena, but he declined these. In 1438, he was elected vicar-general of the Franciscan Order in Italy, a position he held for 4 years. In that role, he founded or reformed hundreds of convents and sent missionaries to the Orient. He died at L'Aquila, Abruzzi, in 1444. According to legend, his grave leaked blood until two factions of that city reached reconciliation.

Many miracles were attributed to Bernardino, who was canonized only 6 years after his death by Pope Nicholas V. Because of his selfless labors on behalf of the plague victims in Siena, Bernardino was invoked in times of plague. His career as an orator made him the patron saint of those with respiratory disorders. In 1472, his body was translocated to a church in Aquila, which had been built to receive it. That church was destroyed by an earthquake in 1703 and replaced by a structure that continues to enshrine Saint Bernardino's relics.

65

Bernulph (Bernold, Bernoul) of Utrecht

MEMORIAL DAY **July 19**

PATRONAGE **Infertility, pediatric tuberculosis**

LIFE & LEGEND

Bernulph was the parish priest in the village of Oosterbeck, near Arnheim, when he came to the attention of Emperor Conrad, who was struck by the simple priest's holiness. Conrad elevated Bernulph to the archiepiscopal throne of Utrecht in 1020. He died in 1054.

REFERENCES 16, 36

66

Bertha

MEMORIAL DAY **May 1**

PATRONAGE **Mental disorders**

LIFE & LEGEND

Bertha, whose name is derived from German, meaning "famous" or "bright," was born into a prominent family in Champagne, France. In accordance with an arrangement made by her parents, she married a young nobleman named Gombert. The young couple agreed to live together as brother and sister so that they might pursue holier lives. When Gombert came into his patrimony, the couple separated to dedicate themselves entirely to God. Gombert founded a monastery at Reims named in honor of Saint Peter. He later went to Ireland, where he founded a monastery that was destroyed by Nordic invaders, who beheaded him. Bertha, in the meantime, had built a convent in the Val d'Or near Annonay, where she served as abbess during the seventh century.

Gombert's nephews grew increasingly impatient over what they perceived as the waste of their family's wealth on the endowment of monasteries and other works of charity. A plot to murder Bertha was successfully executed by their sister (or perhaps cousin), Moncie. Following Bertha's death, her assassins were possessed by demons. Bertha appeared to the tormented Moncie several days after the murder to inform her that if she wished to be pardoned, she would have to devote all her means to retrieving the body of Gombert and burying it next to that of Bertha's in the convent in the Val d'Or. Moncie followed Bertha's instructions. Almost immediately, miracles occurred at the tomb of the holy couple, particularly among those with mental disorders.

REFERENCES 16, 36

67

Berthaldus (Bertaut) of Reims

MEMORIAL DAY **June 16**

PATRONAGE **Mental disorders**

LIFE & LEGEND

Berthaldus, who lived during the sixth century, was of royal Scottish lineage. With his companion, Amand, Berthaldus made a pilgrimage to Jerusalem. On their return, they passed through Champagne and met Saint Remigius, who ordained them both and engaged them to build a hermitage nearby. Berthaldus remained there for more than 50 years in a life of poverty, prayer, and chastity. Indulgences for pilgrimages to Berthaldus' shrine were granted during the fifteenth century.

REFERENCES 16, 36, 44

68

Berthilon

MEMORIAL DAY **April 26**

PATRONAGE **Fever**

LIFE & LEGEND

When Isaac the Good, bishop of Langres, reformed the abbey of Sainte Benigne in Dijon, he appointed Berthilon as its abbot ca. 855. The appointment corresponded with the intrusion of the Normans into Burgundy, and Berthilon eventually fell into the hands of the invaders, who destroyed his monastery and then beheaded him. When Berthilon's tomb was opened in the eleventh century, a pleasant fragrance emanated from the tomb, and his head was found reattached to his neck. His tomb afterward became a popular place of pilgrimage, and his assistance was frequently invoked by those with fevers.

REFERENCES 16, 36

69

Bertilia

MEMORIAL DAY **November 5**

PATRONAGE **Hernia, sore throat, cancer**

LIFE & LEGEND

Bertilia was the daughter of a noble family of Soissons, France. She was advised by Ouen, archbishop of Rouen, to enter the convent at Jouarre. When Queen Bathilde built the convent of Chelles, the abbess of Jouarre recommended that Bertilia be made its first abbess, a position that she held for 42 years. She died in 492.

REFERENCES 16, 36

70

Beuve (Bova)

MEMORIAL DAY **April 24**

PATRONAGE **Pregnancy, childbirth**

LIFE & LEGEND

Beuve and her brother, Saint Balderic, were the children of King Sigebert of Austrasia. She took the veil as a young woman in a convent established by Clotilde, queen of France. Later, Beuve became abbess of the monastery named in honor of Saint Peter that she and her brother founded at Reims ca. 639. Beuve remained abbess of Saint Pierre de Reims until her death, ca. 673, when she was succeeded by her niece, Saint Doda.

REFERENCES 16, 18, 36

71

Bibiana (Viviana)

MEMORIAL DAY **December 2**

PATRONAGE **Epilepsy, convulsive disorders, headache**

LIFE & LEGEND

Bibiana, whose name is derived from Latin, meaning "alive," was the daughter of Saint Flavianus (ex-prefect of the city of Rome) and Saint Defrosa. She was the sister of Saint Demetria. Following the death of these members of her family, ca. 363, an attempt was made to make Bibiana apostasize. When she refused, she was tied to a column and flogged to death. Her body was left in the open to be devoured by scavenging dogs. After 2 days, the corpse was buried by a priest named John. A church was built over the site of her tomb on the Esquiline in the fifth century.

REFERENCES 6, 18, 36, 46

72

Blase (Biagio, Blaise, Blasius, Blas)

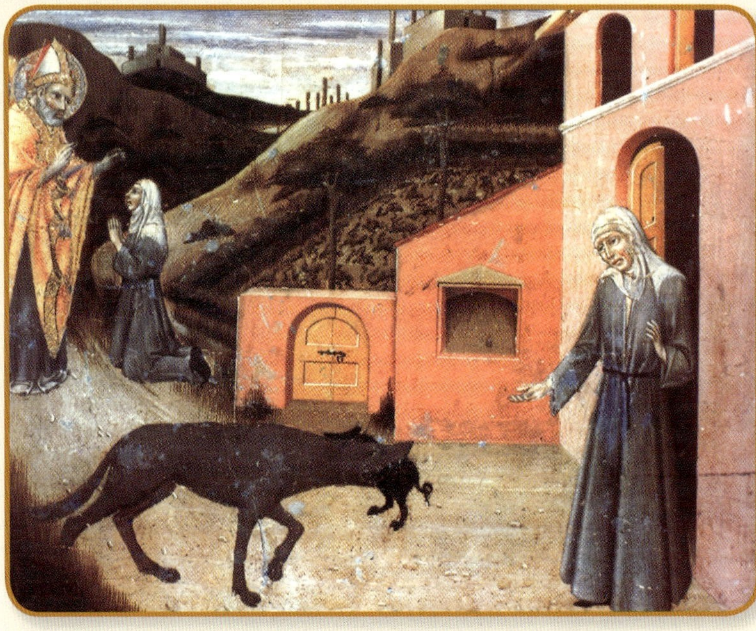

MEMORIAL DAY **February 3 (Oriental churches: February 11)**

PATRONAGE **Throat ailments, [otorhinolaryngology],* goiter, whooping cough, angina, tooth disorders, veterinarians, wild beasts, builders, carvers, stonecutters, wool combers and weavers, Anguillara, Montecatina Val di Cecina, Palombara Sabina, Pietrasanta, Sacrofano (Italy), Militello (Sicily), Dalmatia, Dubrovnik**

LIFE & LEGEND

Blase, whose name is derived from Latin, meaning "stuttering," was one of the most popular saints of the Middle Ages, and also one of the Fourteen Holy Helpers. He was born in Armenia, practiced as a physician, and became the

*Proposed patronage

bishop of Sebaste in Armenia. During the Diocletian persecution, Blase sought refuge in a cave in the woods, where birds brought him food. He ministered to animals and sick people who sought his help. After he was captured and in custody, a woman brought her son to him, who was in the terminal stage of strangulation because of a fish bone. Saint Blase cured the boy by prayer and the laying on of hands.

The first reference to this saint is in the medical writings of Aetius Amidenus, physician to Justinian I, in which Saint Blase's aid was invoked for treating objects stuck in the throat. Another legend indicates that Saint Blase miraculously had a wolf return a swine that it had stolen from a woman. That woman then brought a portion of the swine to Saint Blase with bread and candles, accounting for the saint's representation with two candles.

Blase suffered various forms of torture, including having his flesh torn with wool combs (leading to his patronage of members of the wool trade). He was thrown into a lake to drown, but stood on the surface while his persecutors drowned. He was eventually beheaded ca. 316.

There is an Armenian Order of Saint Blaise. Many German churches bear his name. In Cornwall, England, the village of St. Blazey takes its name from him. In 1222, the council of Oxford, England, forbade all work on his memorial day. In Dubrovnik, relics of his head, a bone from his throat, and bones from his hand are paraded on his memorial day.

REFERENCES 6, 9, 33, 45

73

Boetianus

MEMORIAL DAY **May 22**

PATRONAGE **Sick children**

LIFE & LEGEND

Boetianus was a monk of Irish origin who lived during the seventh century in seclusion near the village of Pierrepont, a short distance from Laon. He was murdered by barbarians of the neighborhood for his too-frequent criticism of their vices.

REFERENCES 16, 36

74

Bonitus (Bonet, Bont, Bond)

MEMORIAL DAY **January 15**

PATRONAGE **Gout, paralysis**

LIFE & LEGEND

Bonitus was born into a noble family of Auvergne and entered public service during the reign of Sigibert III, whom he eventually served as chancellor. In 677, he was appointed governor of Marseilles. Although Bonitus was a layman in public service, he succeeded his older brother, who later became Saint Avitus, as bishop of Clermont in 689. Bonitus sat on the episcopal throne for 10 years, but doubts regarding the canonicity of his election convinced him to resign the see and enter the monastery of Manglieu. On his return from a pilgrimage to Rome, he had a severe attack of gout. He died in 706 at Lyon.

REFERENCES 6, 14, 16, 36

75

Bonosa

MEMORIAL DAY **July 15**

PATRONAGE **Smallpox, skin pustules**

LIFE & LEGEND

Bonosa was beheaded for her faith in 207 at Porto Romano (near present-day Fiumicino) during the reign of Emperor Severus. She was martyred with her brother, Saint Eutropius, and her sister, Saint Zosim. Because she was so badly lacerated during the beatings that preceded her execution, she is the patron saint of those with scar-producing diseases of the skin, such as smallpox and other pustular manifestations. Details are lacking regarding her life, but remnants of the tomb of the sibling martyrs were discovered at Porto Romano early in the nineteenth century.

REFERENCES 18, 36

76

Bruno of Cologne

MEMORIAL DAY **October 6**

PATRONAGE **Plague**

LIFE & LEGEND

Bruno, whose name is derived from German, meaning "brown" or "armor," was born into the prominent Hartenfaust family of Cologne. He was sent to Reims at an early age to study at the cathedral school. In 1055, he returned to Cologne and was ordained to the priesthood. The following year he returned to Reims as a professor of theology. He assumed directorship of the school and remained in this position until 1074, when he was appointed chancellor of the diocese of Reims by Archbishop Manasses. Bruno was forced to flee Reims in 1080 because of difficulties with the corrupt archbishop, but he returned to the city after Manasses was deposed.

Although the people of Reims wanted Bruno to assume the vacant archiepiscopal throne, he had decided on a hermetic life. He went on a pilgrimage that resulted in his founding a monastery in the remote wilderness of the Chartreuse near Grenoble. The establishment of this hermitage with a handful of followers marks the beginning of the Carthusian order. Bruno was ordered to Rome in 1090 by Pope Urban II, one of his former pupils at Reims, who sought his counsel on church governance. The pope offered him the archbishopric of Reggio, but Bruno declined, choosing instead to resume the hermetic life in the monastery he founded in the forest of La Torre, near the present-day village of Serra San Bruno in Calabria. Although he led the life of a holy recluse, Bruno grew close to the Norman Count Robert Guiscard and his family. Bruno died at La Torre ca. 1101.

REFERENCES 6, 14, 36, 46

77

Burchard

MEMORIAL DAY **October 14**

PATRONAGE **Joint diseases, kidney diseases, calculi, rheumatism, urinary stones**

LIFE & LEGEND

A priest and native of Wessex, England, Burchard traveled to Germany, ca. 732, to join his countryman, Saint Boniface, in the evangelization of the Franks. Shortly thereafter, he was consecrated bishop of Würzburg by Saint Boniface. Burchard was among those sent to Rome by Pepin the Short in 749 to procure the pope's approval of Pepin's accession to the Frankish throne. In ca. 753, Burchard founded Saint Andrew's Monastery, which later bore his name, in Würzburg. In his later years, Burchard resigned his episcopal see and retired to a monastic life that he led until his death in 754.

REFERENCES 6, 14, 36

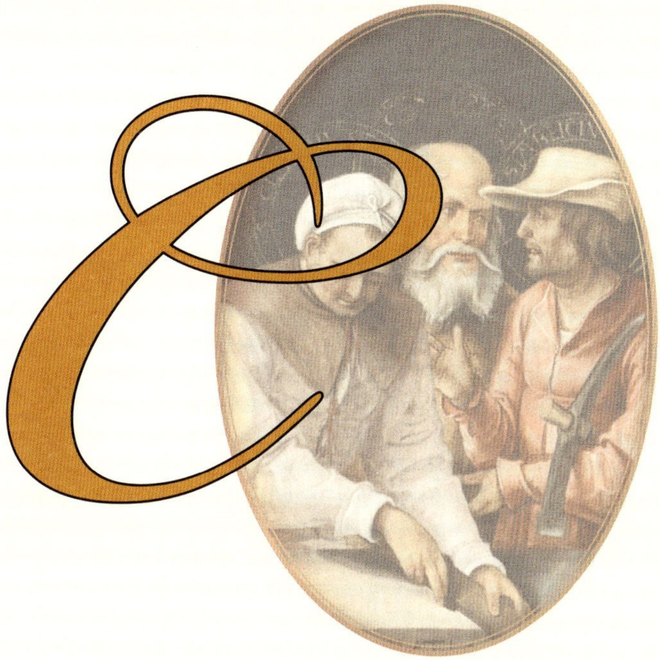

78

Cadoc of Llancarfan

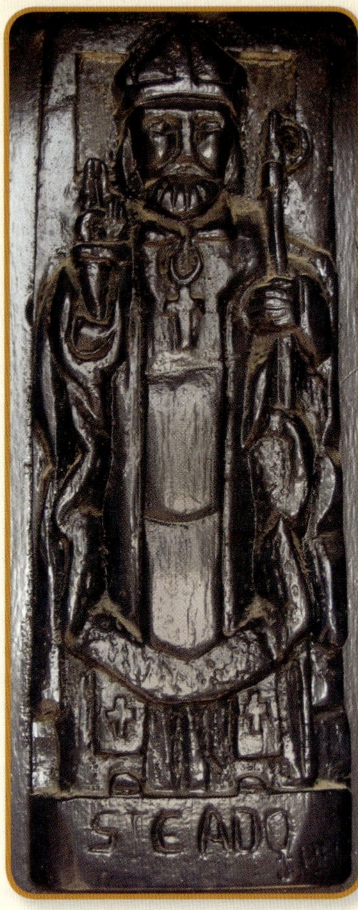

MEMORIAL DAY **September 24 (formerly January 24)**

PATRONAGE **Deafness, glandular disorders, scrofula, cramps**

LIFE & LEGEND

Cadoc, whose name is derived from Welch, meaning "battle," was one of the greatest of the Welsh saints. He was born toward the end of the fifth century in Wales, the son of Saint Gwynllyw, a regional king, and Saint Gladys, the daughter of another Welch king. The story of Saint Cadoc's life was first written by Lifris of Llancarfan about 1100 and is of questionable merit.

Cadoc's regal father stole a cow from the monk Saint Tathyw, who demanded its return. Because the king was impressed with the monk's courage, he entrusted his son to the monk's care and mentoring. Miracles were ascribed to Cadoc while he was still a boy. When Cadoc reached adulthood, he opted to serve Christ rather than follow his father's role as a tribal chief. Cadoc is said to have come into conflict with King Arthur and to have been one of the three keepers of the Holy Grail. He proselytized in Wales, where he built a hermitage at Llancarfan (south of Glamorgan) that became one of the most important monasteries in Wales; it was later destroyed. He also founded monasteries off the coast of Brittany, where his cult thrived. He made repeated visits to Rome and Jerusalem.

The circumstances and locale of his death are the subject of disagreement. It is held by some that he met a martyr's death ca. 580 near Weedon in Britain when he was speared by a Saxon while he was celebrating mass. Others say that he died in Italy. According to Butler: "Warned by an angel on the eve of Palm Sunday, he was transported in a white cloud to Benevento, Italy, where he was made bishop, and then met his death by martyrdom."

One of the tales associated with his life relates to a time of famine, during which Cadoc tied a string to the leg of a well-fed mouse, which then led him to a hidden granary that provided food for the starving monks. The basis for his patronage for deafness has as its origin the story of a bell that Saint Gildas had made for the pope. When Saint Gildas showed it to Cadoc, Cadoc was so impressed with the sound that he wished to possess it. But Saint Gildas took the bell to Rome where he gave it to the pope as intended. The bell would not ring for the pope, who released it to Cadoc, for whom it rang perfectly.

In the church on the island of Saint Cado in southern Brittany, there is an opening in the side of a stone wall into which people with impaired hearing squeeze their head and shoulders. The pilgrims then proceed to the Fountain of Saint Cado at the edge of the sea, where they drink from the fountain and introduce some drops of water into their ears, following which the hearing is improved.

REFERENCES 9, 48

79

Caesarius of Nazianzen

MEMORIAL DAY **February 25**

PATRONAGE **Physicians**

LIFE & LEGEND

Caesarius was born into a prominent Christian family of Cappadocia ca. 329. His father was Gregory the Elder, bishop of Nazianzen, and his brother was the theologian, Gregory Nazianzus. Despite this, Caesarius chose not to be baptized until shortly before his death. He was a man of notable character, charm, and intellect, had an inclination toward the sciences, and studied philosophy and medicine in Alexandria. His abilities drew the attention of the emperor, Constantius, who brought Caesarius to Byzantium as his principal physician. He retained that position during the reign of Julian the Apostate, even though Caesarius refused to renounce his faith. He continued in imperial service under Emperor Jovian, who appointed him quaestor of Bithynia.

In 368, Caesarius was buried in rubble after an earthquake in the city of Nicaea. Seeing the hand of God in his unlikely survival, Caesarius took the advice of his brother and of Basil the Great to forsake the honors of this world for the monastic state. Shortly after making this decision, Caesarius fell ill and died ca. 369. His wealth was distributed to the poor.

REFERENCES 16, 36, 50

80

Calogeros

MEMORIAL DAY **June 18**

PATRONAGE **Plague, hernia**

LIFE & LEGEND

Calogeros is a name derived from the Greek "ho kalos," meaning "beautiful man," and "ho geron," meaning "old man." The name was given to monks or hermits in Greece and southern Italy who were noted for their holiness. Thus we may not know the actual name of the Greek monk, supposedly from Constantinople, who lived a hermetic life in Sicily and was renowned for his power over demons. Biographic information on Calogeros suggests that there may have been more than one Sicilian saint of this name. Du Broc de Segange, for example, provides 486 as the year of Calogeros' death, whereas the "Santi Beati e Testimoni" website maintains that he was born ca. 466 and died ca. 561.

Calogeros is said to have subjected himself to an austere life and to the study of sacred literature from childhood. On a pilgrimage to Rome, he received permission from the pope to live in solitude in Sicily. With three disciples, Calogeros evangelized the Sicilians (and the inhabitants of the Aeolian islands), driving out the demons to whom they were subject and whom they worshipped. On Lipari, he cured many of their illnesses, using the waters of a mineral spring on the island. To this day a spring there bears his name. He later settled at Sciaccam where there was also a mineral spring and where he continued to evangelize and to expel demons from a nearby mountain dedicated to Kronos. Calogeros remains much venerated in Sicily.

REFERENCES 16, 36, 46

81
Camillus of Lellis

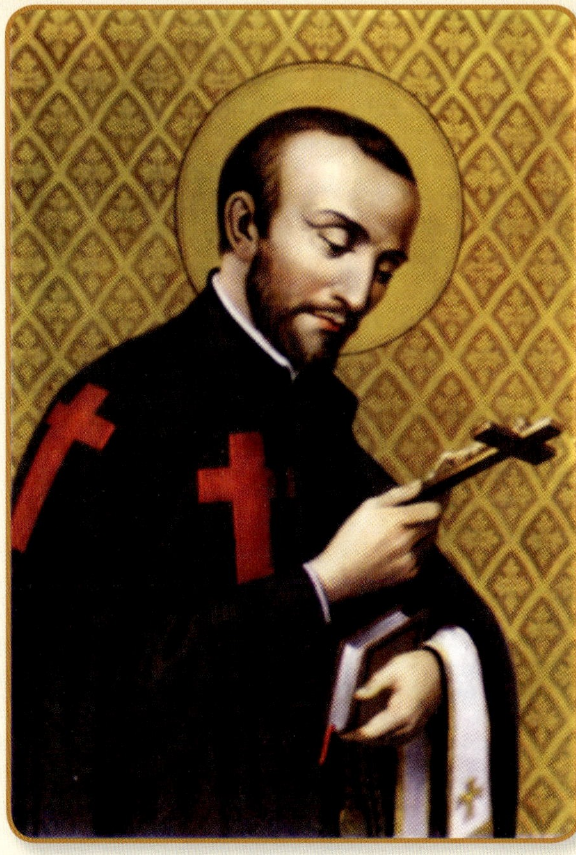

MEMORIAL DAY **July 14**

PATRONAGE **Sickness, hospitals, nurses, hospital workers, [palliation and end-of-life care],* against gambling**

LIFE & LEGEND

The name Camillus is derived from Latin, meaning "altar server." Camillus of Lellis was born the son of a military officer in 1550 at Bocchiavico, Abruzzi, a part of the kingdom of Naples, Italy. According to legend, his elderly (65-year-old) mother dreamed that an unborn son of hers would wear a red cross on his chest. It became the symbol of the Order of Ministers of the Sick (Order of the Brothers of a Happy Death), which was founded by Camillus in 1586. This was the first association between a red cross and any aspect of medical care.

Camillus initially served as a military officer fighting for the Venetians against the Turks, and later for Naples. Probably as a result of a military injury, for many years he suffered from a draining abscess above his ankle. Like his father, Camillus had an addiction to gambling that led to his dismissal from the army. He moved to Rome and worked at the San Giacomo Hospital for the incurable,

*Proposed patronage

where his leg wound had previously been treated, and he eventually became the hospital's administrator.

Lacking education, he began his studies at age 32 and was ordained in 1584. That year he founded the Congregation of the Servants of the Sick (Camillians), which expanded into several countries. The emblem of the red cross continues to be worn on the cassock and mantle by members of this order. During wars in Croatia and Hungary, the order established the first military ambulance service.

Camillus was also credited with ridding Rome of an episode of the plague and for a time was known as the Patron Saint of Rome. He died July 14, 1614, at Genoa and was buried near the high altar of the church of Saint Mary Magdalen in Rome. After he was canonized in 1742 by Pope Benedict XIV, his remains were moved directly under that altar.

REFERENCES 6, 9

82

Candida

MEMORIAL DAY **October 22**

PATRONAGE **Scrofula**

LIFE & LEGEND

The name Candida is derived from Latin, meaning "snowy white." Candida was a native of Tortosa, Catalonia, and was one of the companions of Saint Ursula, who lived during the fourth century. Although the story of Ursula and the 1000 virgins who were martyred with her at Cologne is a tenth-century legend, a Latin inscription dating from the late fourth or early fifth century in the church of Saint Ursula in Cologne confirms the martyrdom of "a group" of virgins in that city. Candida was purportedly one of that group.

REFERENCES 16, 36

83

Caprasius

MEMORIAL DAY **June 1**

PATRONAGE **Rheumatism, diseases of the nervous system**

LIFE & LEGEND

Caprasius was living a hermetic life in Provence when he became the spiritual father of Saint Honoratus during the fourth century. Caprasius accompanied Honoratus and his brother, Venantius, from Gaul to Greece, where they planned to establish a new community. When Venantius sickened and died in the Peloponnesus, Caprasius and Honoratus returned to Gaul and established a monastic community on the island of Lérins. Caprasius died ca. 430. Since the seventeenth century, a relic of Caprasius in the village of Chartèves (near Château-Thierry) has attracted pilgrims who invoke the saint for the healing.

REFERENCES 6, 14, 16, 36

84

Casilda (Casilla) of Toledo

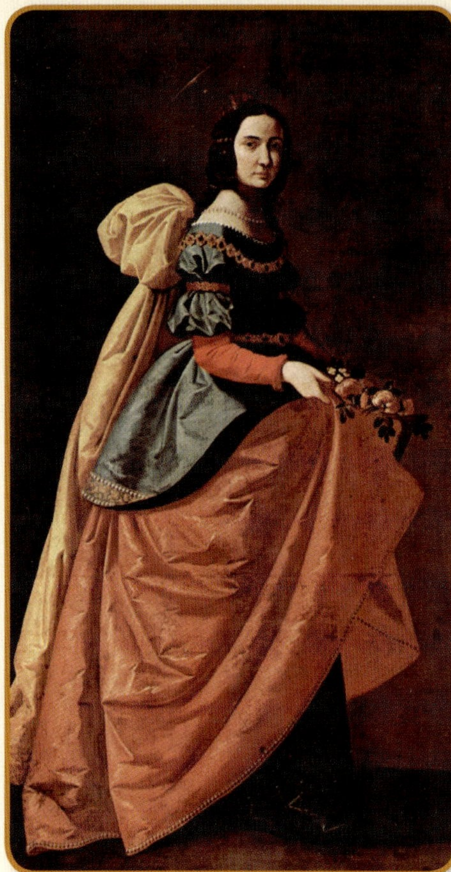

MEMORIAL DAY **April 9**

PATRONAGE **Hemorrhagic disorders, infertility**

LIFE & LEGEND

Casilda, who lived during the eleventh century, was the daughter of the Muslim governor, or emir, of Toledo, a city that had been captured by the Arabs in 711 and remained in Muslim hands until 1085. She was noted for her acts of charity, especially toward Christians held prisoner by her father. While carrying bread beneath her skirt to Christian prisoners, she was stopped by Muslim soldiers and asked to reveal what was beneath her skirt. She lifted her skirt and, rather than bread, a bouquet of roses was revealed. When she became ill with a hemorrhagic disorder that baffled her physicians, Casilda was advised by Christian acquaintances to bathe in a spring within the sanctuary of Saint Vincent near Burgos in Christian-held Castile. Casilda made this pilgrimage and was healed in the waters. She was baptized a Christian and proceeded to live a hermetic life in the vicinity of the spring in which she was healed. She was about 100 years old when she died.

REFERENCES 16, 36, 46

85

Casimir

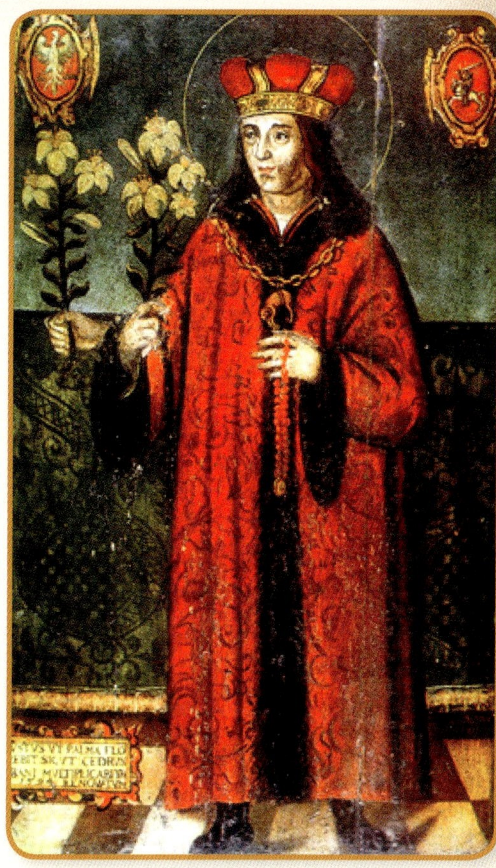

MEMORIAL DAY **March 4**

PATRONAGE **Plague, Poland, Lithuania**

LIFE & LEGEND

Casimir, whose name is derived from Polish, meaning "keeping the peace," was born in 1458, the second son and the third of 13 children of Elizabeth of Austria and King Casimir IV of Poland. Casimir was devout from childhood and followed an ascetic life, even while living in the Polish court. He performed remarkable acts of charity toward the poor, dispersing his own resources for their relief. In 1471, when disaffected members of the Hungarian nobility approached Casimir IV about placing his son on the Hungarian throne in place of King Mathias Corvinus, the king agreed and sent 15-year-old Casimir to the frontier with an army.

On learning that Mathias was himself approaching with a large army and that his own army had been depleted by desertions, Casimir heeded the advice of his officers and returned home. When Casimir refused to resume the campaign on the grounds of its essential injustice, his father was angered and confined the young prince to the castle of Dobzki. Casimir never again took up arms or governance, except once when acting as viceroy during his father's absence from Poland. He devoted himself thereafter to a life of study and prayer. He refused to marry, adding celibacy to the austerities he imposed on himself. He died in 1483 of lung disease at Vilna (Vilnius), aged 23. His holiness was widely known, and many miracles were reported at his tomb.

REFERENCES 6, 14, 16, 36

86

Castorius

MEMORIAL DAY **November 8**

PATRONAGE **Fever, stonemasons**

LIFE & LEGEND

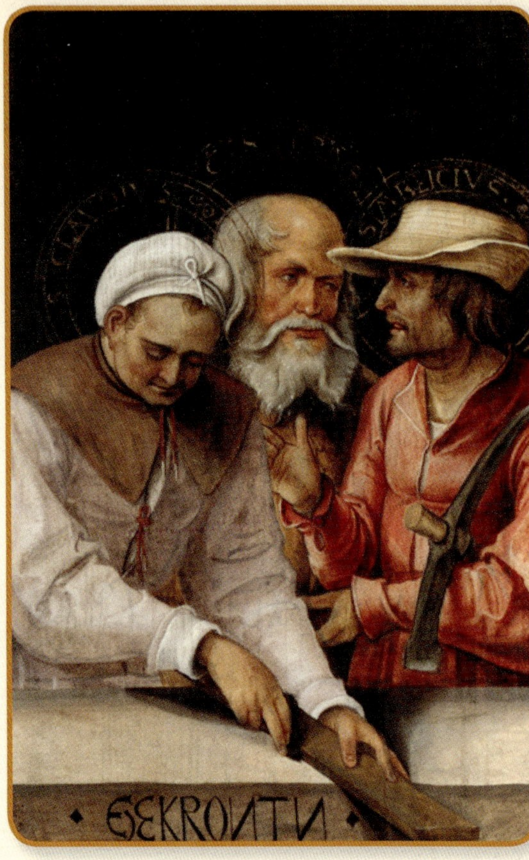

Castorius is the name given to one of the Four Holy Crowned Ones (Quatuor Coronati), of whom there are two distinct legends. One story describes them as stone carvers employed in the quarries at Sirmium in Pannonia. Their names are given as Claudius, Nicostratus, Simpronian, and Castorius. They came to Emperor Diocletian's attention not only because of their exceptional skill, but because, as Christians, they refused to carve a statue of the medical deity, Aesculapius. Diocletian was willing to overlook this first slight, but when the four later refused to sacrifice to the gods, they were arrested, sealed in leaden boxes, and cast into a river.

A second story describes the four as Christian soldiers who refused to sacrifice to Aesculapius when Diocletian was in Rome at the beginning of the fourth century. They were arrested, beaten to death, and thrown into a sewer. Butler states that the four martyrs were "buried on the Via Lavicana by Saint Sebastian and Pope Miltiades, who later directed, their names having been forgotten, that they should be commemorated under the names Claudius, Nicostratus, Simpronian, and Castorius." A basilica was erected on the Coelian Hill in their honor during the first half of the fifth century.

REFERENCES 6, 36

87

Catald of Taranto

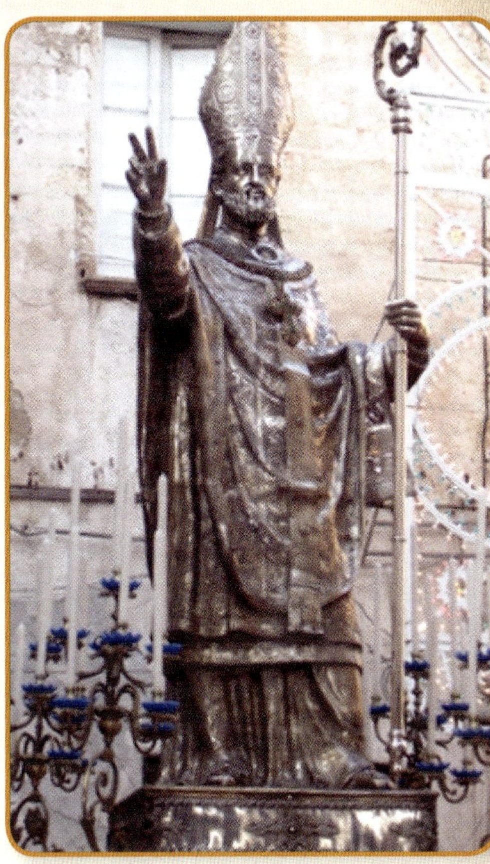

MEMORIAL DAY **May 10**

PATRONAGE **Blindness, epilepsy, hernia, paralysis, plague, storms, drought, Taranto (Italy)**

LIFE & LEGEND

Catald was born during the first half of the seventh century at Munster, Ireland. He studied at a monastery in Waterford under Saint Carthage. He later joined the school as a teacher and eventually became headmaster. Catald made a pilgrimage to Jerusalem, and on the way home he was shipwrecked by a storm near Taranto, Italy. His holiness impressed the populace of Taranto, and they made him their bishop. He consequently remained there for the rest of his life.

He was noted for his teaching and his care of his parishioners. He died in Taranto of natural cause ca. 685. His relics were found 250 years after he died during the renovation of the cathedral, where they remain. A remarkable number of diverse cures were associated with the exposure of his relics and the invocation of his name.

He was honored throughout Italy, Malta, and France but had no recognition in Ireland. This is because his Irish heritage was not appreciated until his relics were discovered and, with them, a cross of seventh-century Irish origin. This led to an investigation that identified Catald as a teacher and headmaster at the school of Lismore in Waterford.

REFERENCES 6, 9, 14, 16, 36, 45

88

Catherine of Alexandria

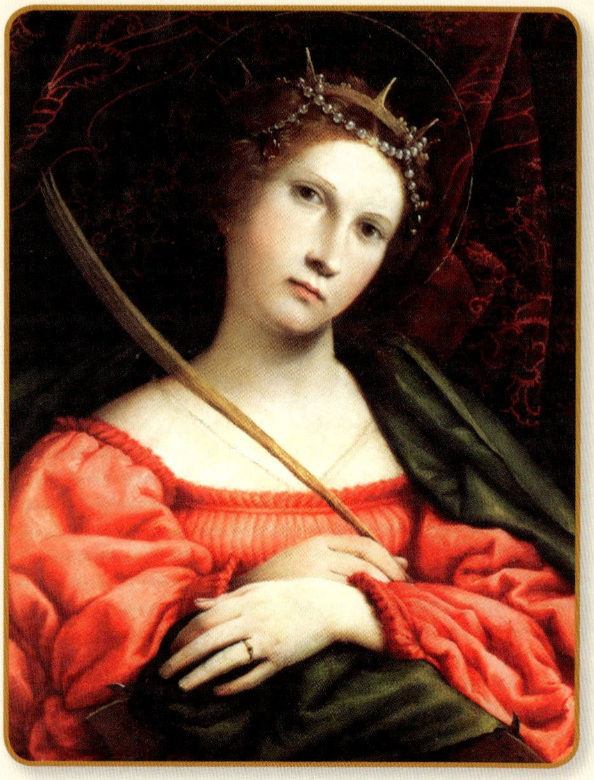

MEMORIAL DAY **November 25**

PATRONAGE **Sudden death, diseases of the tongue, those who work with a wheel, librarians, nurses, girls, female students**

LIFE & LEGEND

One of the Fourteen Holy Helpers, Catherine was born ca. 287, the daughter of Costus, governor of Alexandria. She became a Christian and censured Emperor Maximinus for persecuting Christians. Consequently, she was imprisoned. While in prison she converted the empress and the head of the emperor's troops. She was therefore condemned to die on the wheel, but when her body touched it, the wheel fell apart. The emperor then had her beheaded ca. 305. Angels carried her body to Mount Sinai, where, in the sixth century, a monastery and church were built. What is now called Saint Catherine's Monastery survives as a notable repository of early Christian art and manuscripts.

Saint Catherine and Saint Margaret were appointed advisors to Saint Joan of Arc, and Catherine is said to have appeared to Joan later. Her feast day was removed from the Roman Catholic calendar in 1969, but it was reinstated in 2002.

REFERENCES 9, 42

89

Catherine of Siena

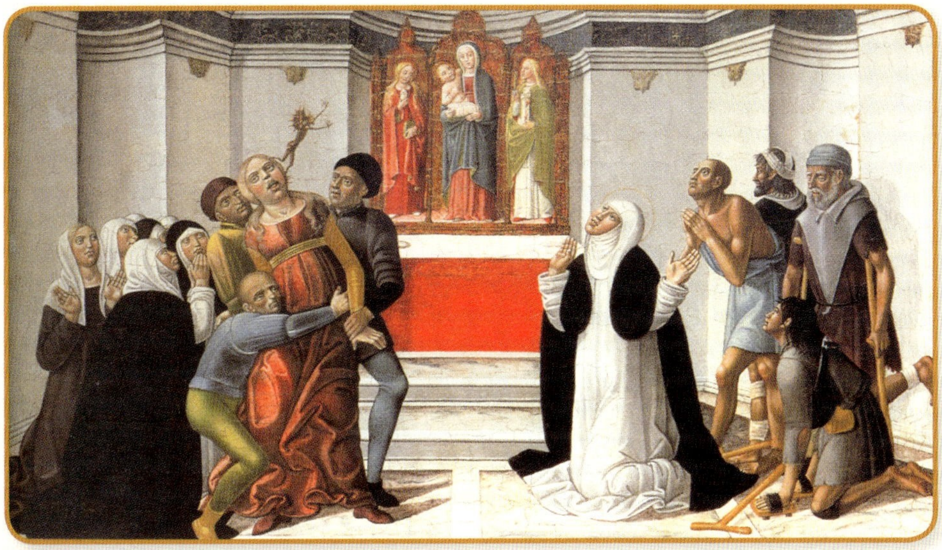

MEMORIAL DAY **April 29**

PATRONAGE **Sickness, plague, miscarriage, nurses, sexual temptation, fire, firefighters, fire prevention, Siena (Italy)**

LIFE & LEGEND

Catherine, whose name is derived from the Greek for "purity," was the twenty-fifth child born to Giacomo di Beneincasa and Lapa Piagenti of Siena. She was born in Siena on March 25, 1347, as a twin, although her sister died at birth. At age 6, she had a vision of Christ with the Apostles Peter, Paul, and John. On Shrove Tuesday, 1366, she had another vision in which she entered a mystical marriage with Christ, and the Infant Christ presented her with a wedding ring.

Catherine became a Dominican tertiary, initially devoting her time to caring for the sick in the city hospitals of Siena and to relieving sufferers during an outbreak of the plague. But she is best remembered as one of the most influential women in the history of the Roman Catholic Church. She served as a counselor to both Pope Gregory XI and Pope Urban VI. She tried to convince Pope Gregory XI to return the papacy to Rome from Avignon, where the popes resided for 74 years. During the Great Schism, which lasted from 1378 to 1418, she tried to heal the breach while she served as counsel to Urban VI in Rome. Her efforts persisted until she died from a mysterious illness at Rome in 1380 at age 33. On her deathbed, she brought about reconciliation between Pope Urban VI and the Roman Republic.

Although she could not write until later in life, and most of her writings were dictated, her works are considered among the classics in the Italian vernacular. Her major work is *The Dialogue of Divine Providence.*

She was canonized in July, 1461, by Pope Pius II and proclaimed a Doctor of the Church in October, 1970. In 1999, Pope John Paul II made her one of Europe's patron saints. Her body is buried in the Basilica of Santa Maria Sopra Minerva in Rome, and her head is entombed in the Basilica of San Domenico in Siena.

REFERENCES 6, 9

90

Catherine of Vadstena (Catherine of Sweden, Karin Ulfsdotter)

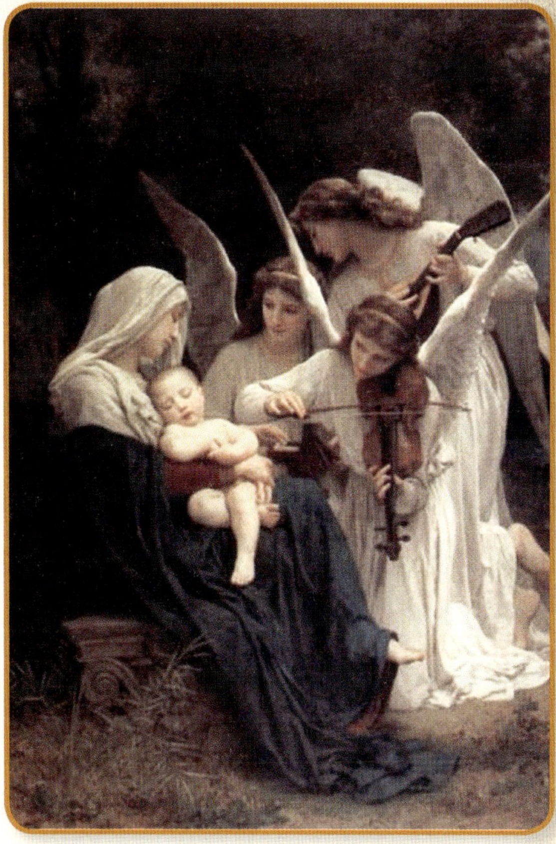

MEMORIAL DAY **March 24**

PATRONAGE **Miscarriage, premature birth, abortion**

LIFE & LEGEND

Catherine of Vadstena was fourth among the eight children of Saint Bridget. She was betrothed at an early age to a nobleman, Eggard von Kurnen, to whom she was devoted, but with whom she lived in chastity by mutual agreement. In 1350, she left Sweden to visit her mother, who, after being widowed, had founded a monastery at Vadstena in 1344. Catherine then moved to Rome, where she was noted for her monastic reforms, her charity to the poor, and her efforts to convince the pope to return from Avignon. Catherine remained in Rome, attending to various labors initiated by her mother. After the death of her husband in Sweden, the beautiful young Catherine was approached by several suitors, all of whom she refused—including a member of the powerful Orsini clan who then plotted (unsuccessfully) to kidnap her.

Catherine lived with her mother in a life of prayer and austerity. Together they made several pilgrimages to Assisi and a pilgrimage to the Holy Land. Bridget died in Rome after her return from Jerusalem in 1373. Catherine accompanied her mother's body back to Vadstena and then returned to Rome, where she pressed the papacy for Bridget's canonization. It was during this period in Rome that Catherine was approached by a woman who was pregnant an eighth time after having seven miscarriages. Catherine gave her a piece of Bridget's clothing and told the woman to keep it on her person at all times during her labor and delivery. The woman delivered a living child. After 5 more years in Rome, Catherine returned to Sweden, where she died in 1381 at Vadstena after a period of ill health.

REFERENCES 6, 15, 35

91

Ceranus

MEMORIAL DAY **September 27**

PATRONAGE **Toothache**

LIFE & LEGEND

Ceranus, the twenty-fifth bishop of Paris, held his see from at least 614, when he participated in a council of 69 French bishops convened in the city that year, until his death ca. 621-625. His remains are interred in the church of Sainte Genevieve de Paris.

REFERENCES 16, 36

92

César de Bus

MEMORIAL DAY **April 15**

PATRONAGE **Eye diseases**

LIFE & LEGEND

Born in Cavaillon (Provence) to Jean Baptiste de Bus, the consul de la ville, and his wife, Anne de la Marche, César was educated at the Jesuit college in Avignon. He was a pious child and early in life became a member of a lay order called the Compagnie des Pénitents Noirs. At age 18 he enlisted in the army formed by the Comte de Tende in Provence to combat the Huguenots. After the cessation of hostilities, César returned to Cavaillon and was preparing to participate in the siege of La Rochelle in a naval vessel commanded by his brother when he was suddenly taken ill. César convalesced in Paris, where he devoted the next 3 years to the pursuit of every pleasure the city offered. When he returned to Cavaillon, he initially persisted in these habits.

Under the influence of a pious widow and a humble sacristan, César gradually separated himself from his friends and the pleasures of this world to seek a manner of living more pleasing to God. He assumed a life of penitence and prayer and began theologic studies in Avignon. He was ordained to the priesthood in 1582 and was appointed canon of the cathedral in Avignon. He devoted much of his time to the spiritual and material needs of the poor. In the spirit of the Counter-Reformation and inspired by the example of Saint Charles Borromeo, César de Bus established two religious orders dedicated to the dissemination of Christian doctrine in a world unsettled by the Protestant Reformation. In 1592, he founded the Fathers of the Christian Doctrine, commonly known as the Doctrinaires, and a women's counterpart: the Daughters of the Christian Doctrine, an order that later became the Ursulines. At age 49, de Bus suffered an unspecified eye disease that eventually cost him his sight, but his sight returned 18 months before his death in Avignon in 1607. He was beatified by Pope Paul VI in April, 1975.

REFERENCES 16, 46

93

Cessator (Cossadre, Sadre)

MEMORIAL DAY **November 15**

PATRONAGE **Leprosy, scabies**

LIFE & LEGEND

Cessator was a bishop of Limoges who mobilized an army against Saracen forces in the Pyrenees in 730 and 731. The army of the warrior bishop was joined by that of Charles Martel, who put the finishing touch to the Saracen invaders. Cessator died in 732. The reasons for Cessator's patronage are unknown.

REFERENCES 16, 36

94

Charalampos

MEMORIAL DAY **February 10**

PATRONAGE **Plague, cholera**

LIFE & LEGEND

Charalampos was the bishop of Magnesia, Thessaly, late in the second century during the reign of Emperor Septimus Severus. He was arrested for his faith by Prefect Lucius, and he was stripped of his sacred vestments and flayed. When Lucius saw that Charalampos remained constant in his faith under torture, he began to strip off the bishop's skin with his own fingers, at which point Lucius' hands separated from his wrists and remained attached to the body of Charalampos. The bishop prayed that Lucius' hands might be restored to him, and they were—which did nothing to make the prefect reflect on the miracle nor to deflect his anger. Those who witnessed this miracle, including Charalampos' torturers (Porphyrius and Baptus), as well as three women, immediately converted to Christianity. Lucius ordered that they all be decapitated. Charalampos is invoked in times of plague and other epidemic diseases. In nineteenth-century Spain, he was invoked during outbreaks of cholera.

REFERENCES 16, 36

95

Charitina

MEMORIAL DAY **October 5**

PATRONAGE **Toothache**

LIFE & LEGEND

The virgin Charitina was martyred ca. 303 at Amisus in Asia Minor during the persecution of Diocletian. She died of exhaustion during her tortures, which included the extraction of her teeth with tongs. She is often depicted holding a pair of tongs.

REFERENCES 36, 46

96

Charles Borromeo

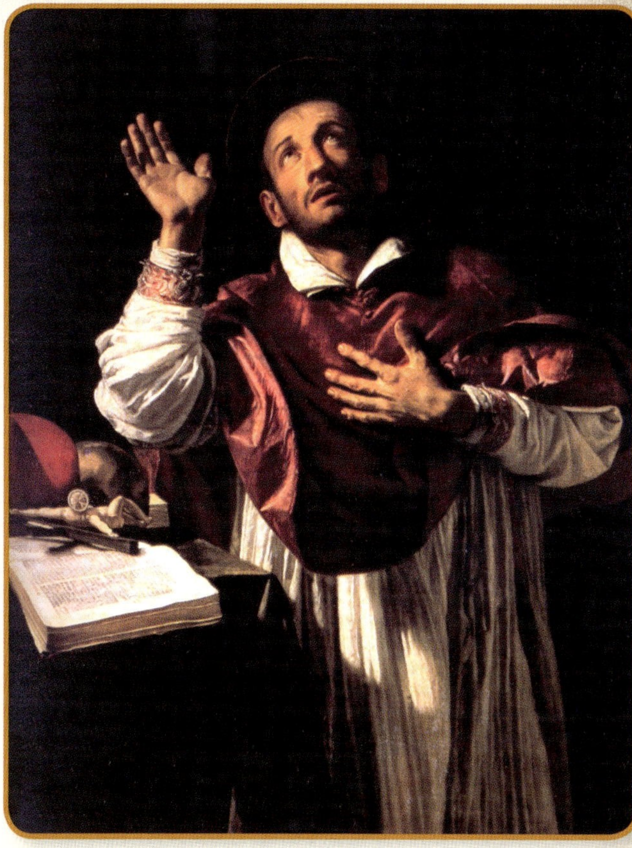

MEMORIAL DAY **November 4**

PATRONAGE **Stomach diseases, ulcers, intestinal disorders, colic, plague, Lombardy (Italy), Monterey (California), São Carlos (Brazil)**

LIFE & LEGEND

Charles Borromeo was born October 2, 1538, the son of the Count of Arona (bordering Lake Maggiore, Italy) and Margherita de'Medici. He studied civil and canon law at the University of Pavia and received a doctoral degree in 1559. At about that time, his mother's brother became Pope Pius IV, and Charles became one of the leading statesmen of the papal court. He was appointed administrator of the see of Milan, protector of Portugal, the Low Countries, and the Catholic cantons of Switzerland. He was also supervisor of the Franciscan and Carmelite orders, the Knights of Malta, and administrator of the Papal states.

He was a leader in the movement to combat the Protestant Reformation. He also played a major role in the resumption of the Council of Trent, which was directed at codifying Church doctrine and eradicating abuses. The council defined original sins and declared anathema against those who rejected the invocation of saints and veneration of their relics. It also dealt with Episcopal jurisdiction and the education and discipline of the clergy. In keeping with the decrees of the Council of Trent, he oversaw the clearance of ornate tombs from cathedrals and the division of naves into two sections to provide separation of the sexes. While at the papal court he founded a college in Pavia known as Almo Collegio Borromeo.

Charles entered the priesthood in 1563 and 3 months later was designated cardinal-priest and bishop of Milan. In that capacity he established schools, convents, and seminaries, in addition to reforming priestly functions. He founded the Confraternity of Christian Doctrine with its Sunday schools to teach the catechism to children. Historically, these are regarded as the first Sunday schools.

As Archbishop of Milan, he lived a humble life and supervised the care of the poor during the plague of 1576. As a consequence, he is frequently represented in art wearing a simple robe, barefoot, carrying the cross of an archbishop, a rope around his neck, and raising a hand in blessing. He died in Milan in 1584 and was canonized by Pope Paul V in 1610. His crypt is in the Duomo di Milano, and a 60-foot-high statue stands high on a hill overlooking Arona.

REFERENCES 9, 26

97

Charles the Good

MEMORIAL DAY **March 2**

PATRONAGE **Fever**

LIFE & LEGEND

Count of Flanders and Amiens, Charles the Good received his cognomen from his subjects. After the murder of his father, Canute, the king of Denmark, Charles' mother (Adele of Flanders) took her son, at age 5, to the court of her father, Robert, the Count of Flanders. When old enough to take up arms, Charles joined his uncle on a crusade to the Holy Land, where he distinguished himself in combat. He then returned home to fight against the English.

Robert was succeeded as Count of Flanders by his son, Baldwin, who, being childless, designated his cousin heir. On Baldwin's death, Charles assumed the title Count of Flanders, although not without objections and armed resistance from others claiming priority in the family lineage.

Respected by his subjects for the justness of his reign and his concern for the poor, Charles was nonetheless murdered one morning in 1127 while attending mass at the church of Saint Donat in Bruges. He was the victim of a conspiracy among those who resented his interference with their profitable grain-hoarding during famines and other unjust practices. Du Broc de Segange relates that febrile invalids who drank water from Charles' skull were cured of their malady. After the French Revolution, his remains were transferred to the cathedral in Bruges.

REFERENCES 6, 16, 36

98

Christine of Saint Trond (Christina the Astonishing)

MEMORIAL DAY **July 24**

PATRONAGE **Incurable diseases, contagious diseases**

LIFE & LEGEND

Born to a peasant family at Brusthem near Liège, Christine suffered a seizure at age 22 that seemed to have resulted in her death, and she was placed in a coffin. As the Agnus Dei was being sung during her requiem mass, Christine sat up in her coffin and soared to the rafters of the church, where she remained until coaxed down by the priest at the end of the service. She related that she had indeed been dead, had visited hell, purgatory, and heaven, and had been allowed to return to earth to pray for the souls of those she had seen in purgatory. She also stated that she had flown to the rafters to escape the smell of human beings, an unpleasant scent that she made great effort to avoid thenceforth.

Christine adopted a mode of life that led many of her contemporaries to conclude she was mad. Others regarded her unconventional and often offensive behavior as the mark of a holy woman. All efforts to restrain or confine Christine failed as she wandered about in holy madness. Toward the end of her life, she entered the convent of Saint Catherine in Saint Trond, where she died in 1224, aged 74. She is known as a teaching apostolate.

REFERENCES 6, 14, 36

99

Christopher

MEMORIAL DAY **July 25 (Orthodox Church: May 9)**

PATRONAGE **Epilepsy, toothache, deafness, paralysis, plague, travelers, mariners, motorists, lightning, archers, bookbinders, gardeners, storms, Saint Kitts**

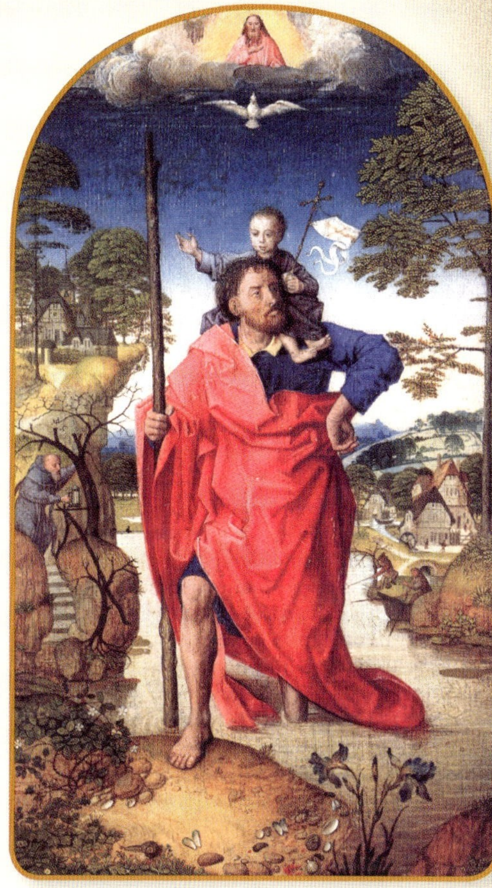

LIFE & LEGEND

Saint Christopher's biography is based on no historical evidence and varies with the source. According to the Roman Catholic Church, he was born in Canaan and named Reprobus or Offero. An unusually large man, he ferried people on his back across a river. Legend states that one day he carried a small child who was disproportionately heavy. The child revealed that he was Jesus Christ, and that this apparent weight was because of the sins of the world. Christ baptized Reprobus in the river and conferred on him the name Christopher, meaning "Christ bearer" ("phererein" means "to carry" in Greek).

At Christ's command, Christopher planted his staff in the ground, and a fruit tree miraculously emerged. This became the focal point of many conversions, thereby irritating Emperor Decius, who had Christopher tortured and beheaded ca. 251.

The Eastern Orthodox view indicates that during the reign of Decius, Christopher was captured in combat in Egypt. He was baptized and began to preach. He was imprisoned, survived torture and several attempts at execution, and was eventually martyred. He was said to have been a cannibal and is depicted with the head of a dog rather than a man. But this representation might only reflect the sentiment that all persons who lived outside the Greco-Roman-Persian world were bizarrely different.

Little factual material is known, and, although Christopher was one of the Fourteen Holy Helpers, his feast day was downgraded to a local commemoration in 1969 because of lack of authentication, but he was not decanonized.

REFERENCES 6, 9, 42, 45

100
Chrysolius

MEMORIAL DAY **February 7**

PATRONAGE **Fever**

LIFE & LEGEND

Born to Christian parents (perhaps of royal lineage) in Armenia, Chrysolius had been well educated and was so esteemed in his province that he was appointed bishop or archbishop of one of its cities. Chrysolius later journeyed to Rome, perhaps during the persecution of Diocletian, where he was favorably received by Pope Marcellus. He was later among a party of missionaries sent to evangelize in Gaul. Settling in Comines, Chrysolius preached in the region of the Lys and Scheldt rivers.

While preaching one day in the present-day village of Verlinghem, Chrysolius was arrested by a party of soldiers, who flogged him and then split his skull with the blow of an ax. Left on the ground in a pool of his own blood, Chrysolius revived, picked up the part of his cranium severed by the ax, and made his way back to Comines. Overcome by thirst on the difficult journey home, Chrysolius miraculously made a spring of pure water rise from the earth. The waters of this spring were long after regarded as a remedy for fever. Chrysolius died after his return from Verlinghem ca. 302.

REFERENCES 16, 36

101

Clare of Assisi

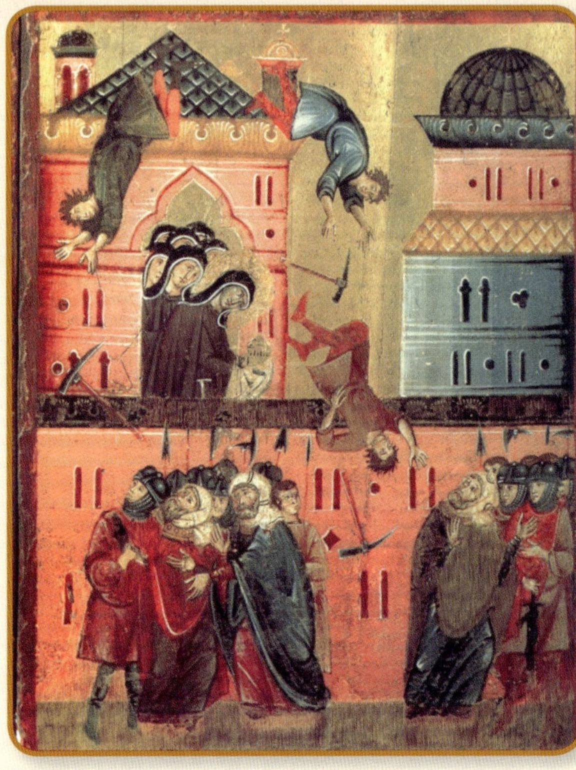

MEMORIAL DAY **August 11**

PATRONAGE **Eye diseases, [telemedicine],* goldsmiths, needle workers, good weather**

LIFE & LEGEND

Clare, whose name is derived from Latin, meaning "clear" or "bright," was born Chiara (a variant of Clare) Offreduccio on July 16, 1194, in Assisi, Umbria, the eldest daughter of the Count of Sasso-Rosso and Ortolano, a member of the noble family of Fiumi. As a child, she was devoted to prayer and sought a spiritual life.

When she was 18, she attended a Lenten course that was preached by Francis of Assisi in the Church of San Giorgio, and sought him out to aid her in her quest to follow a life dedicated to Christ. That year, when her parents committed her to marry a wealthy man, Clare sought refuge from Saint Francis, who had her hair cut off, clothed her in a simple tunic and veil, and admitted her to the service of Jesus Christ. She initially entered a nearby Benedictine nunnery with her sister, Agnes, but moved to the church of San Damiano after a brief period. San Damiano was part of a network of women's religious houses, and it became the focal point of Clare's activities.

*Proposed patronage

During her life, Clare worked as a member of the Order of San Damiano and eventually became its abbess for nearly 40 years. The order became known as the Order of Saint Clare, usually referred to as Poor Clares, 10 years after her death. She regarded Francis of Assisi as her spiritual leader, aided him, and took care of him during his terminal illness until he died in 1226.

Clare and the members of her order rarely left the confines of the church, and they devoted themselves to poverty, humility, and manual labor. In 1234, when the army of Frederick II entered San Damiano, Clare raised the Blessed Sacrament in front of the advancing troops, who then took flight. Later, when a force led by General Vitale di Aversa attacked Assisi, Clare and her associates issued prayers to save the town. A storm developed that destroyed the advancing army's tents and panicked the troops.

Toward the end of her life, when she was too ill to attend mass, she was miraculously able to hear and see the mass in her cell. This was the basis of her formal designation as the patron saint of television by Pope Pius XII in 1958.

Clare died on August 11, 1253, and was canonized by Pope Alexander IV 3 years later as Saint Clare of Assisi. Her remains were interred in the Basilica of Saint Clare, which was constructed in 1260. A new shrine was built in 1872, which continues to permit viewing of her relics. Pope Urban IV officially changed the name of the Order of Poor Ladies to the Order of Saint Clare.

REFERENCES 9, 42, 45

102

Clarus of Albi (Clair de Lectoure)

MEMORIAL DAY **June 1**

PATRONAGE **Eye diseases**

LIFE & LEGEND

Little is known of Clarus other than he is regarded as the first bishop of Albi (ancient Albiga) on the Tarn River northeast of Toulouse. Clarus was later sent to evangelize in Aquitaine. While preaching at Lectoure, the sound of his voice is said to have pulverized the statues of the gods. Seized by the indignant locals, Clarus was beheaded in 469 before an altar of Diana.

His relics were preserved at Lectoure for seven centuries before being transferred to the church of Saint Eulalie in Bordeaux. His patronage for eye diseases might be because the name Clarus is derived from Latin, meaning "clear."

REFERENCES 16, 36

103

Clarus of Vexin

MEMORIAL DAY **November 4**

PATRONAGE **Eye diseases, blindness**

LIFE & LEGEND

Born in Rochester, England, Clarus left England for France after entering the priesthood. On the road from Cherbourg, where he had disembarked, Clarus miraculously healed the servant of two hermits who had been attacked on the road with an ax and left for dead. Clarus spent 2 years in relative obscurity in the monastery at Mandun, when he was located by the hermits whose servant Clarus had healed. Much was made of this miracle, so Clarus sought greater solitude and withdrew to a hermitage still in the neighborhood of the monastery. Even there, the holiness of his life and his additional miracles drew unwanted attention, including a new problem presented by a noblewoman who was intent on seducing the holy man. This time Clarus and his disciple Cyrinus withdrew even farther into the wilderness in the ancient district of Vexin in Normandy. In 894, his spurned seductress found Clarus and sent two men into the forest to murder him. After killing Clarus, they severed his head. According to legend, Clarus then picked up his head and carried it back to the hermitage, where he deposited it at the feet of his disciple, Cyrinus.

The origin of his patronage stems from Clarus' healing of a man who had been blind from birth. Three years after Clarus' death, the blind man made a pilgrimage to the saint's tomb, where he fell asleep. In a dream, an angel told him to gather earth from Clarus' grave and rub it onto his eyes. When the man awoke, he did this and was immediately able to see.

REFERENCES 16, 36

104

Claude of Besançon

MEMORIAL DAY **June 6**

PATRONAGE **Convulsions in children, fever, disabled people**

LIFE & LEGEND

Claude, whose name is derived from Latin, meaning "disabled," was born in 607 into a prominent family of Franche-Comté. He initially embraced the profession of arms, a calling he abandoned at age 20. He was ordained into the priesthood at Besançon, served as canon of its cathedral, and retired 12 years later to the monastery of Saint Oyand at Condat in the Jura Mountains (the present-day monastery of Saint Claude). Claude was made abbot, introduced the Benedictine Rule, and restored the monastery's buildings.

In 685, he was made bishop of Besançon, an office he held for 7 years before returning to Condat, where he died in 699. The cult of Saint Claude dates from the twelfth century, when his tomb was opened and his remains were found incorrupt. Numerous miraculous healings occurred at his tomb.

REFERENCES 6, 14, 16

105

Clodoald (Cloud)

MEMORIAL DAY **September 7**

PATRONAGE **Scrofula, carbuncles, furuncles**

LIFE & LEGEND

Clodoald was born in 522 in Gaul, the youngest of the three sons of Clodomir, who was the second son of Clovis, king of the Franks. Clodoald's name is derived from Old English, meaning "out of the mist." After the death of their father, the three sons of Clodomir were raised in Paris by their grandmother, Clotilda, the widow of Clovis. Their uncles, Childebert and Clotaire of Soissons, decided to murder the three boys (Clodoald was 8 years old at the time) and divide their portion of the kingdom between them. The two older boys were stabbed to death, but Clodoald escaped and was removed to the South of France beyond the reach of his uncles. When he came of age, Clodoald made no attempt to claim his inheritance, but chose instead to place himself under the discipline of Saint Severinus, who lived as a hermit near Paris. Clodoald later established a hermitage near Nogent-sur-Seine. He died of natural causes in 560.

REFERENCES 6, 36, 45

106
Clotilda

MEMORIAL DAY **June 3**

PATRONAGE **Sick children, fever, paralysis**

LIFE & LEGEND

A native of Burgundy and a Christian from birth, Clotilda was married to Clovis, the pagan king of the Franks. In a battle against the Alemanni on the plains of Tolbiac that his army was plainly losing, Clovis vowed to "the God that Clotilda worships" that he would convert to Christianity if his army should triumph. The battle was won, and Clovis was baptized in 496 at Reims. Clotilda was a widow for 34 years, during which period she witnessed a murderous struggle for the Frankish throne that resulted in the execution of two of her grandchildren (see *Clodoald*), civil war between two of her sons, and the unhappy marriage of her daughter to the Visigoth, Amalaric. Eventually Clotilda withdrew from Paris to Tours, where she devoted herself to prayer, supporting religious institutions, and assisting the poor. She died from fever in 545.

REFERENCES 6, 16, 36

107

Colette (Nicolette)

MEMORIAL DAY **March 6**

PATRONAGE **Eye diseases, infertility, childbirth, headache, fever**

LIFE & LEGEND

Colette, whose name is derived from Greek, meaning "victory of the people," was the daughter of Robert Boellet, a carpenter at the abbey of Corbie in Picardy. Her mother was nearly 60 years old when she gave birth to her in 1381. After the deaths of her parents, Colette assumed an ascetic life in a cell beside the church of Corbie provided her by the abbot.

She became a Franciscan tertiary and is noted to have had visions, including one in which Francis of Assisi charged her to restore to its original purity the women's branch of the Franciscan order established by Saint Clare. Seeking authority to do so effectively, Colette sought out Pope Benedict XIII, the pope recognized by the French during the schism, who was so impressed by the young woman that he bestowed on her the habit of the Franciscan order and made her superior over all the Minoress convents. As a sign of divine approbation, Colette was made blind for 3 days before beginning her reforming mission.

She traveled through Flanders, France, Savoy, and Spain in her mission to reform the order—meeting much opposition along the way. She successfully reformed many existing convents and established 17 new ones. Colette died at the convent she established in Ghent in 1447.

REFERENCES 6, 14, 16, 36

108

Colman of Stockerau

MEMORIAL DAY **October 13**

PATRONAGE **Plague, Austria**

LIFE & LEGEND

In 1012, while journeying down the Danube on his way to Jerusalem, the Irish or Scots pilgrim Colman was arrested and hanged as a spy at the village of Stockerau. His patience under unjust sufferings was taken as a proof of his sanctity. This was reaffirmed by the incorruption of his exhumed body, which was associated with many miracles.

REFERENCES 6, 14, 36

109

Columba of Sens

MEMORIAL DAY **December 31**

PATRONAGE **Eye diseases, Sens (France)**

LIFE & LEGEND

Columba, whose name is derived from Latin, meaning "dove," was a native of Spain who lived during the third century. She was martyred at Sens in Gaul at age 16. When Emperor Aurelian came to Sens, he ordered Columba and her companions to be put to death. She was initially defended from dishonor by one of the bears belonging to the amphitheater. She was beheaded at the fountain of Azon on the road to Meaux and was buried by a man who had recovered his sight by invoking her name.

REFERENCES 6, 36

110
Columban

MEMORIAL DAY **November 21 or November 23**

PATRONAGE **Mental disorders, imbecility**

LIFE & LEGEND

Born in the western part of Leinster, Ireland, Columban began an ascetic life on the island of Cluain Inis, and subsequently spent many years in the monastery at Bangor. About 585, Columban was one of a dozen monks sent as missionaries to Gaul, where much of the population was still pagan, and where the existing Christian dioceses were in disorder.

In ca. 590, Columban built his first monastery at Annegray in the Vosges Mountains. He later established a monastery at Luxeuil and a third at Fontaine. Columban raised the ire of many of the Frankish bishops for imposing the strict practices of Celtic monasticism in their dioceses, for dating Easter according to the Irish and Eastern practice, and for the independent status he assumed within their jurisdictions. Columban's position became untenable when he criticized King Theodoric II of Burgundy for the latter's refusal to take a queen and for keeping concubines. Theodoric expelled Columban and all Irish monks from his realm in 610. When the ship carrying Columban and his party of exiled monks back to Ireland ran aground just off the coast, Columban took the opportunity to disembark and make his way to Metz, where he was welcomed by King Theodebert. The king supported Columban in evangelizing the pagans in the region of Zurich and around Lake Constance. When Theodebert was defeated in battle by the Burgundian king, Theodoric, ca. 612, Columban fled from his old enemy by crossing the Alps into Italy, where he established a monastery at Bobbio. Columban died ca. 615.

REFERENCES 6, 14, 36, 46

111

Conrad of Piacenza

MEMORIAL DAY **February 19**

PATRONAGE **Hernia**

LIFE & LEGEND

A nobleman of Piacenza, Conrad, whose name has a Germanic derivation meaning "experienced advisor," was hunting one day when he and his beaters set fire to some brush to drive out the game. The fire turned into a conflagration, spreading to neighboring fields and threatening the surrounding villages. When a poor man found in the area was accused of having set the fire, a guilt-ridden Conrad confessed his role in the fire's origin. The authorities ordered Conrad to make restitution to those whose crops and property had been destroyed—a fine that consumed most of his wealth and his wife's dowry. Reflecting on having been stripped of their worldly possessions so suddenly, Conrad's wife decided to become a Poor Clare, and Conrad attached himself to the third Order of Saint Francis. His new life brought the pious Conrad attention that was unwelcome to one who had decided to turn his back on the world. Conrad migrated to Noto in Sicily, where he lived a hermetic life in the region for the next 30 years. He died in 1351. Many miracles were attributed to him, especially by those with hernias.

REFERENCES 6, 14, 16, 36

112

Consortia

MEMORIAL DAY **June 22**

PATRONAGE **Hemorrhage**

LIFE & LEGEND

Consortia belonged to a family of saints. She was the daughter of Saint Eucher, the young bishop of Lyon, who, before entering holy orders, had married Saint Galle. From this marriage issued two sons, Saint Veron and Saint Serlone, and two daughters, Saint Tullie and Saint Consortia.

After the death of her father, Consortia sought the approval of Clotaire, king of the Franks, to establish a hospital and church. Having been informed of the holiness of the virgin's life, Clotaire begged Consortia to heal his daughter, who was then gravely ill. The princess was healed of her malady through the prayers of the saint, who thus obtained the grateful king's protection. After Clotaire's death, however, Consortia attracted the attention of Hecca, governor of the province of Marseilles, who obtained royal permission to marry her. Shortly before the ceremony took place, Hecca was met by Consortia leading a procession of the poor, who were singing psalms. He was so taken by the moment that he tripped stepping off his ship and was impaled on his own spear. Consortia died in 468.

REFERENCES 16, 18, 36

113
Cornelius

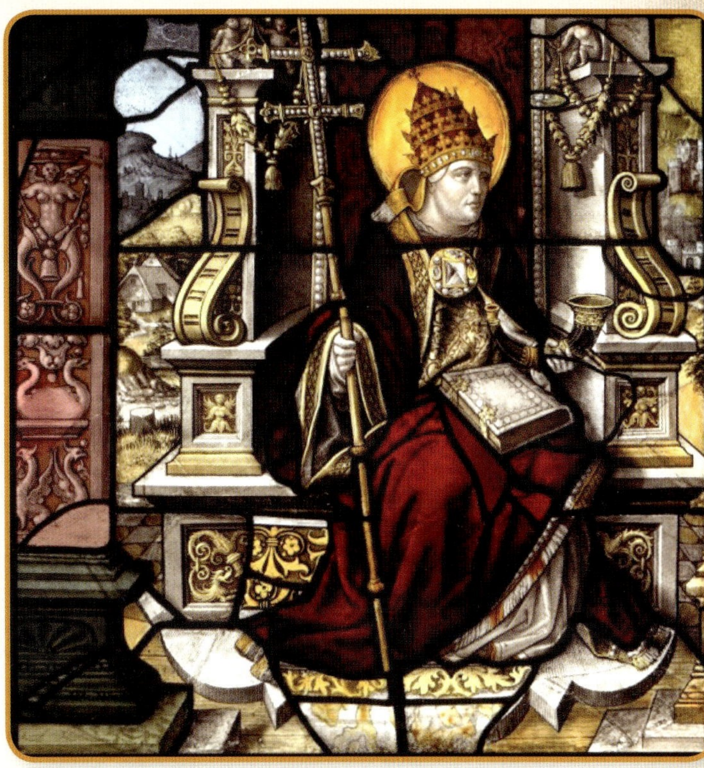

MEMORIAL DAY **September 16**

PATRONAGE **Earache, epilepsy, convulsive disorders, fever**

LIFE & LEGEND

Cornelius, whose name is derived from Latin, meaning "horn," was the twenty-first pope. He was elected in 251, at a time when persecution of Christians was rampant and papal ascension represented a virtual death sentence. Cornelius was elected by 16 bishops convening in Rome. During his papacy, the size of the Church of Rome consisted of 46 priests and about 50,000 Christians.

After Cornelius' election, the Roman priest, Novatian, made himself antipope, thereby creating a schism in the Church. The difference between the two camps related to apostasy. Cornelius proclaimed that the Church had the power to forgive apostates after they had performed specific penances. The Novatians indicated that lapsed Christians could not be pardoned. The bishops upheld Cornelius. Two years into Cornelius' papacy, the persecutions were reinstituted by Emperor Gallus, and Cornelius died a martyr's death. His remains were buried at the cemetery of Saint Callistus in Rome.

REFERENCES 42, 45

114

Cosmas and Damian

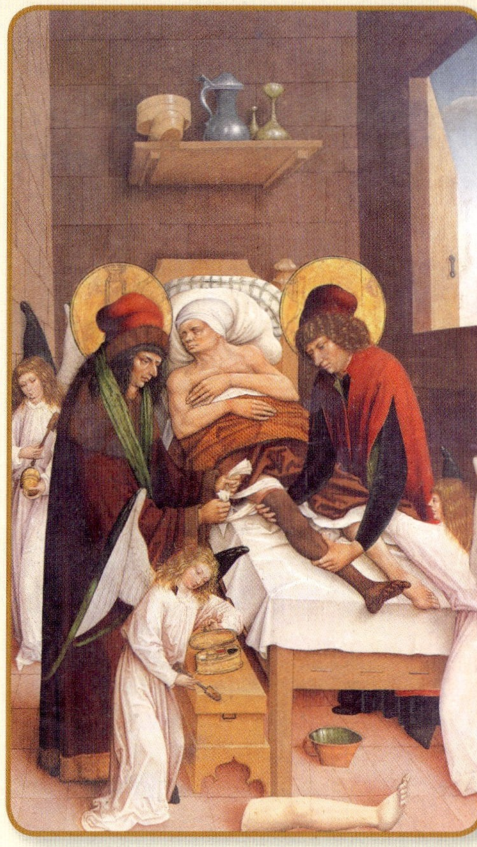

MEMORIAL DAY **September 26 (Oriental and Eastern Orthodox Churches: July 1, October 1, November 1)**

PATRONAGE **Surgeons, physicians, [transplantation],* pharmacists, dentists, midwives, blindness, epidemic diseases, barbers, hairdressers, Gaeta (Italy)**

LIFE & LEGEND

Cosmas and Damian, whose names have Greek derivations, meaning "universe" and "to tame," respectively, were twin brothers who were born in Arabia and practiced as physicians in the seaport of Ægea (modern Ayash) in the Gulf of Iskanderun and later in the Roman province of Syria. They accepted no payments for their services and therefore were named "anargyroi" or "the silverless (non-mercenaries)." As such, they were successful proselytizers for Christ.

The most famous of the miracles ascribed to the twin physicians was the successful replacement of the cancerous leg of a man with the leg of a recently deceased Ethiopian they exhumed from the grave. As a consequence, they are regarded as the patron saints of organ transplantation.

*Proposed patronage

During the Diocletian persecution, Prefect Lysias ordered them to recant their Christianity. They refused despite torture. Attempts were made to kill them by stoning, drowning, and arrows. All miraculously failed, and the vehicles of torture were turned on the perpetrators. On September 27, 287, Cosmas and Damian, together with their three brothers, Anthimus, Leontius, and Euprepius, were beheaded.

The remains of the martyrs were buried in Cyrus in Sicily. Emperor Justinian I restored the city in their honor in gratitude for his having been cured of a serious illness by the invocation of their names. In Rome, Pope Felix IV erected a church in their honor. The mosaics of that church survive and are among the most valuable arts of the city. The skulls of the twins, the gift of Maria, daughter of Emperor Charles V, are venerated in the convent of the Clares in Madrid. Their relics are also said to be enshrined in the church of Saint Michael in Munich. In Brazil, where the twin saints are regarded as the protectors of children, the names of Saint Cosmas and Saint Damian are borne by the oldest of the country's churches, located in Igarassu, Pernambuco.

In the thirteenth century, the College of Saint-Côme was organized as a Paris guild, divided into clerical barber surgeons of "the long robe" and lay barber surgeons "of the short robe." The barbers were admitted to the practice of minor surgery in 1372. Ambroise Paré, the greatest surgeon of the sixteenth century, was eventually admitted into the College.

REFERENCES 6, 9, 33

115

Crescentia

MEMORIAL DAY **June 15**

PATRONAGE **Toothache**

LIFE & LEGEND

Crescentia, whose name comes from Latin, meaning "growing," was the nurse of Saint Vitus. She fled from Sicily to Lucania and then to Rome with both the adolescent wonderworker and her husband, Modestus, who was the boy's tutor. This was brought about by Vitus' refusal to respond to his father's insistence that he renounce Christianity, a faith he had probably acquired from his tutor.

According to legend, Vitus' miraculous powers became known to Emperor Diocletian, who asked Vitus to cure the illness of his child. Vitus did so, but he refused to sacrifice to the gods, thus incurring the emperor's wrath. Vitus, Modestus, and Crescentia were arrested, tortured, and slated for execution. An angel is said to have led the threesome back to Lucania, where they died peacefully ca. 300.

REFERENCES 6, 16, 36

116

Cunégonde

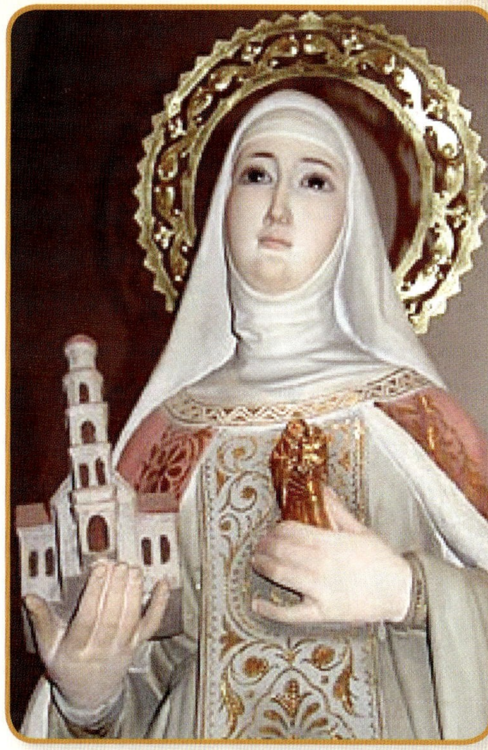

MEMORIAL DAY **March 3**

PATRONAGE **Childbirth, critically ill infants**

LIFE & LEGEND

Cunégonde was the daughter of Siegfried, count of Luxembourg, and his wife, Hedwig. She was married to Saint Henry II, duke of Bavaria, who in 1002 was crowned king and in 1013 was crowned Holy Roman emperor. Cunégonde was crowned empress at Paderborn 2 months later. In 1014, the imperial couple was received and crowned by Pope Benedict VIII in Rome. Cunégonde led a life of exemplary piety and charity, and she was responsible for the foundation of the monastery and cathedral at Bamberg. After her husband's death in 1024, Cunégonde renounced the world and entered the convent she had established at Kaufungen. There she remained until her death in 1040. Some sources maintain that Cunégonde and Henry, though married, had taken a vow of celibacy. A frequently chronicled episode in the life of the imperial couple focuses on Henry's momentary suspicion of his wife's infidelity. To prove her innocence from the calumnies circulating in court, Cunégonde walked barefoot unharmed over red-hot iron. She was buried next to her husband at Bamberg Cathedral.

REFERENCES 6, 16, 46

117
Cunera

MEMORIAL DAY **June 12**

PATRONAGE **Throat diseases, respiratory disorders**

LIFE & LEGEND

Cunera was one of the companions of Saint Ursula, who, in the eighth century, escaped the slaughter of the 11,000 virgins at Cologne through the agency of Rabdad, a nobleman from the region of Utrecht. Returning home, Rabdad placed Cunera in the care of his wife, who, suspecting that her husband had become enamored of the young girl, had her strangled, accounting for her patronage.

REFERENCES 16, 36

118

Cuthbert of Lindisfarne

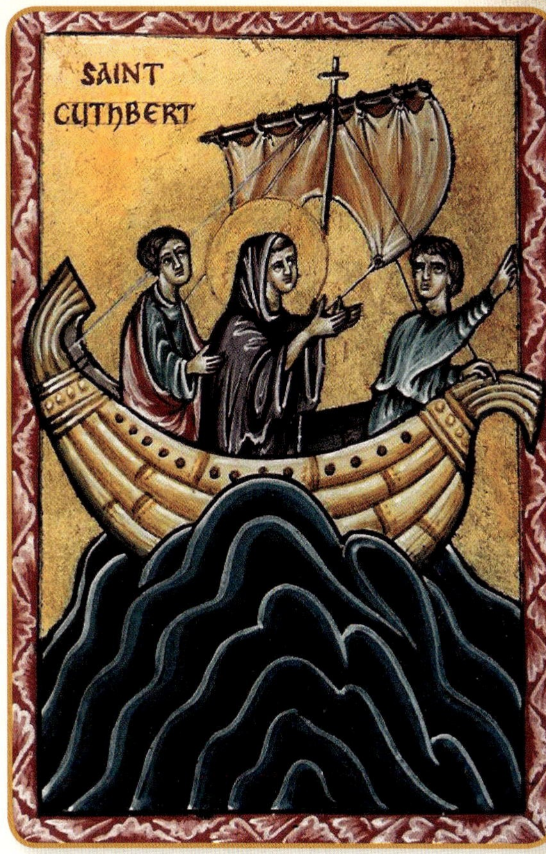

MEMORIAL DAY **March 20**

PATRONAGE **Plague, sailors, shepherds, England, Northumbria, Durham**

LIFE & LEGEND

Cuthbert, whose name means "famous and clever," was born about 634 and was orphaned at an early age. He became a Benedictine monk at the monastery of Melrose. Because of a dispute regarding liturgical practices, he left for Lindisfarne, where he became abbot and eventually the bishop. While on the Farne islands, he instituted the first bird protection laws, which were directed at preserving eider ducks, which are often called cuddy ducks (Cuthbert's ducks). He worked with plague victims and was noted for his ability as a prophet. He died of natural causes in 687, and his body was removed to Durham Cathedral. His name is associated with many miracles, and Cuthbert was revered as one of the most popular saints of England before the twelfth century.

REFERENCES 9, 33, 42

119

Cyriacus

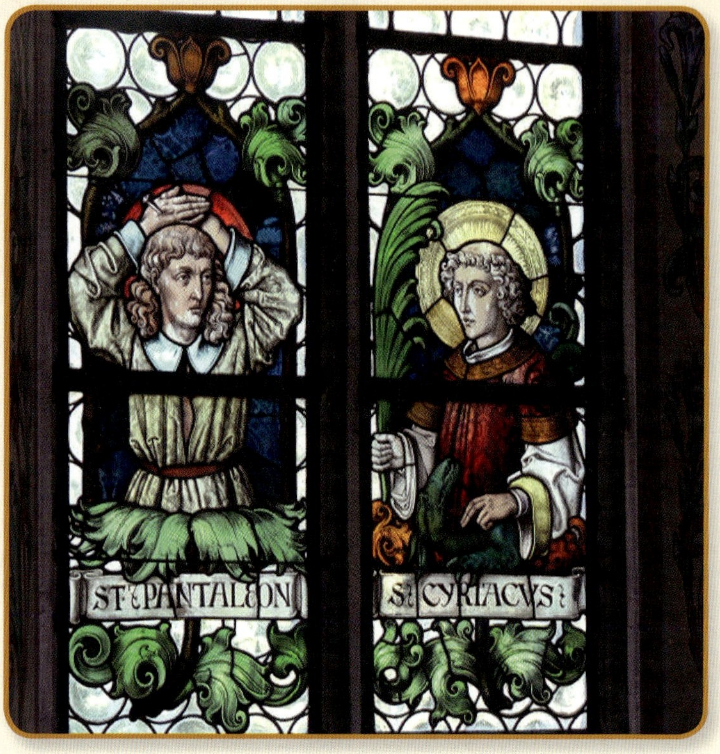

MEMORIAL DAY **August 8**

PATRONAGE **Eye diseases, diabolic possession, temptation**

LIFE & LEGEND

Cyriacus, whose name is derived from Greek, meaning "belonging to God," is one of the Fourteen Holy Helpers. He was born of Roman nobility during the third century. He converted as an adult, at which time he gave away his wealth to the poor. Cyriacus included in his ministry the slaves who built and tended the baths of Emperor Diocletian. He converted Diocletian's daughter, Artemisia, and her mother, Saint Serena. He also converted the entire household of King Sharpur I of Persia. He was tortured and beheaded on the Salarian Way in Rome ca. 303. His relics were translated to the church of Santa Maria in Rome and to Saint Cyriacus Abbey in Alsace, France.

REFERENCES 6, 9

D

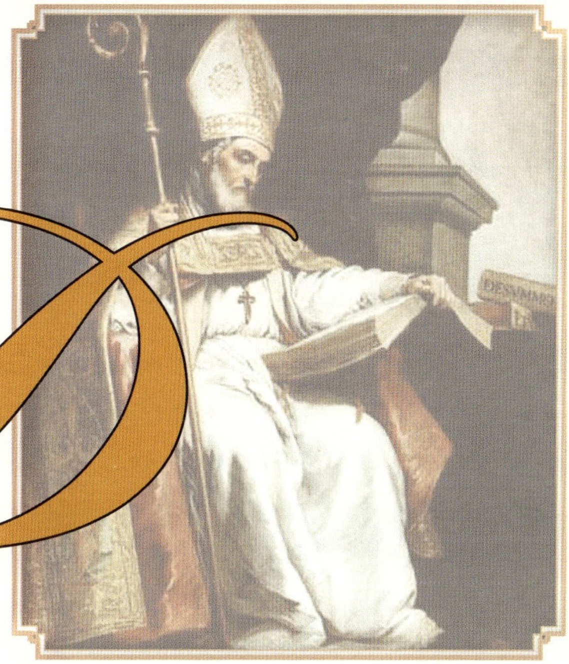

120

Dalmatius Moner

MEMORIAL DAY **September 24**

PATRONAGE **Toothache, infant dentition**

LIFE & LEGEND

Dalmatius was born in 1291 into a noble family at Santa Coloma in Catalonia. He was educated at nearby Girona, and later at the University of Montpellier. At age 25 he returned to his homeland and entered the Dominican monastery in Girona. Although active as a teacher and director of novices, Dalmatius was noted for his life of silence and prayer. He later asked to be transferred to Marseilles, where he lived a hermetic life of even greater austerity and became known for his humility, his commerce with angels, and his ability to perform miracles. Dalmatius returned to the Dominican house at Girona for the last 4 years of his life. His relics are preserved there in a silver reliquary and are said to have cured tooth diseases. Immediately after his death in 1341, he was invoked particularly against toothache. One of his teeth was preserved in the sacristy of the monastery, encased in a silver reliquary. It was the custom of mothers to bring their infants in contact with Dalmatius' relics to facilitate dentition.

REFERENCES 14, 16, 36, 46

121

Damasus

MEMORIAL DAY **December 11**

PATRONAGE **Fever**

LIFE & LEGEND

Damasus, the son of a Roman cleric, served as a deacon in the church where his father was priest. At age 60, Damasus was elected Bishop of Rome, an election that was bitterly contested and resulted in the election of Antipope Ursinus by a disaffected minority. The latter was eventually exiled by Emperor Valentinian. The papacy of Damasus was noted for his attempt to correct the increasingly luxurious lifestyles of the Roman clergy, his opposition to Arianism, his encouragement of Saint Jerome in the translation of the Bible into Latin, and his effort to restore the catacombs and burial places of Christian martyrs as pilgrimage sites. Damasus may also be regarded as the first pope who sought to make Christianity a distinctly Roman religion, with Rome and its bishop at Christendom's center. He died ca. 384.

REFERENCES 6, 14, 36

122
Daniel of Padua

MEMORIAL DAY **January 3**

PATRONAGE **Childbirth**

LIFE & LEGEND

Daniel, whose name is derived from Hebrew, meaning "God is my judge," was a converted Jew who was ordained a deacon by the bishop of Padua. He was martyred in the fourth century during the reign of Diocletian, but his existence was unknown until the discovery of his burial place in 1075.

According to legend, Daniel appeared to a blind man and told him to pray for the restoration of his sight in the oratory of Saint Prosdicimo in Padua, where Daniel's tomb was hidden. When the miracle was reported, a search for the tomb was begun, resulting in the discovery of a sarcophagus inscribed with his name. In Spain and Italy, Daniel is regarded as the protector of women separated from their husbands by war and of women in childbirth.

REFERENCES 16, 36, 46

123

Danio

MEMORIAL DAY **May 12**

PATRONAGE **Childhood hernia**

LIFE & LEGEND

Danio was a priest in Bologna who was esteemed by the people. After his death in 1184, the mothers of infants and children with hernias would take their offspring to Danio's tomb to be healed.

REFERENCES 16, 36

124

Defendens (Defendente)

MEMORIAL DAY **January 2**

PATRONAGE **Epilepsy, cholera**

LIFE & LEGEND

Defendens was a soldier in the Theban Legion, a unit recruited in Egypt and dispatched to Gaul under the command of Saint Maurice. Before breaking camp at Agaunum (present-day Saint-Maurice-en-Valais, Switzerland), the legionnaires were ordered to make customary sacrifices to the gods. The Christian soldiers in the legion represented most of its complement and refused the order. To break what he perceived as mutinous behavior, Emperor Maximian ordered one soldier in ten to be flogged and decapitated—a continuous decimation that resulted in the execution of all or most of the legion ca. 268.

In 380, Theodore, the bishop of nearby Martigny, discovered the cemetery that was thought to contain the remains of the Theban Legion and erected a church on the site. Du Broc de Segange maintains that the execution of the Theban Legion occurred near Marseilles, and that Theodore was bishop of that city, near which he built a no-longer-extant church to commemorate the martyred soldiers. Du Broc de Segange and others maintain that the saint venerated as Defendens in the Valais, and as Defendente in northern Italy, are different saints than the martyr of the Theban Legion. In 1884, Defendens was invoked by the bishop of Marseilles during an outbreak of cholera in that city.

REFERENCES 16, 36, 46

125

Denis (Dionysus)

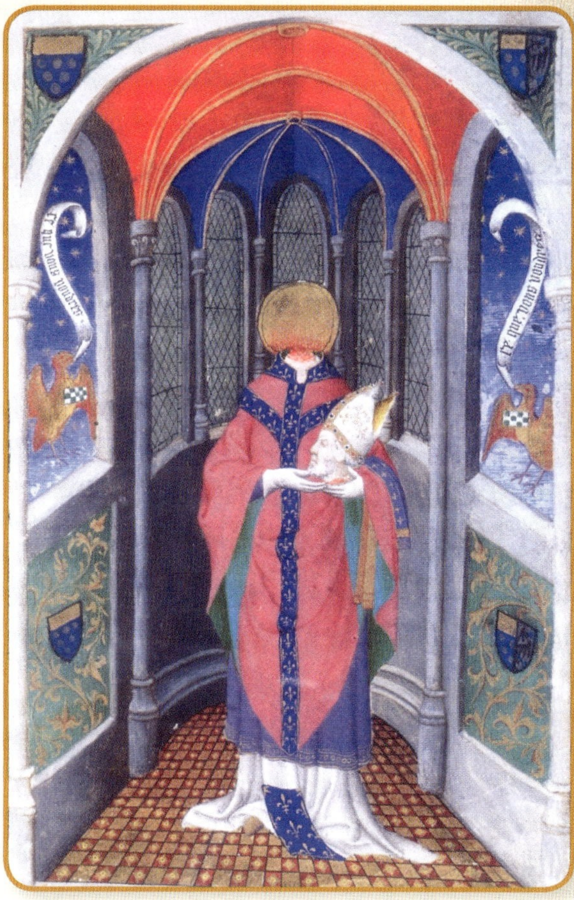

MEMORIAL DAY **October 9**

PATRONAGE **Rabies, hydrophobia, headache, diabolic possession, France, Paris**

LIFE & LEGEND

Denis, whose name is derived from that of Dionysus (the Greek god of wine), was born in Italy, and little is known about his early life. He was sent by Pope Fabian (236-250) with other missionary bishops to Gaul to restore the faith at a time when the Church suffered significantly under the persecution of Emperors Decius and Valerian.

He and his fellow bishops settled on an island in the River Seine in the city that was to become Paris. A church was built and many were converted, leading to the wrath of the Roman governor, Fescenninus Sisinnius. Saint Denis, along with Saint Rusticus and Saint Eleutherius, were seized, tortured, and put to death ca. 258 at Montmartre, giving that site its name, which means "mountain of martyrs." Saint Denis, who is considered the first bishop of Paris, was beheaded. One legend indicates that his body carried the severed head for some distance. Saint Denis is one of the Fourteen Holy Helpers. The Basilique Saint Denis, located in a suburb of Paris, is the burial place of all but three of the French monarchs.

REFERENCES 6, 9, 11

126

Deodatus (Dié, Didier)

MEMORIAL DAY **June 19**

PATRONAGE **Plague**

LIFE & LEGEND

Deodatus was a native of Gaul who became bishop of Nevers ca. 655. He resigned the episcopate several years later to become a hermit—first in the Vosges Mountains and later in the forest of Hagueneau near Strasbourg. The latter community was the origin of the monastery at Ebersheim. Deodatus later returned to the Vosges, where he attracted followers whom he organized in a monastery called Jointures because of its location at the juncture of the Rothbach and Meurthe rivers. Deodatus served as abbot there until his death ca. 679. Saint-Dié-des-Vosges is where the naming of America took place when a narrative and accompanying large map first presented the name, which honored Americus Vespucci.

REFERENCES 6, 14, 16, 36

127

Desideratus (Dirié, Dizié)

MEMORIAL DAY April 30

PATRONAGE Toothache

LIFE & LEGEND

Desideratus was a monk who lived in the fifth or sixth century at Gourdon in Provence. Renowned for his saintliness, Desideratus was particularly successful in healing those with diseases of the teeth.

REFERENCES 16, 36

128

Desiderius (Didier, Dizier, Désiré) of Langres

MEMORIAL DAY **May 23**

PATRONAGE **Childbirth, Langres**

LIFE & LEGEND

A native of Liguria, Desiderius is venerated in France. He was the third bishop of Langres, succeeding Saint Juste in that office. Both du Broc de Segange and Kerler place him in the third century, although Desiderius is mentioned by Saint Athanasius as present at the Council of Sardica in 346. When an army of Germanic barbarians besieged Langres (ca. 356), Desiderius offered his own life to the barbarian commander if he would spare his flock. Desiderius was subsequently beheaded and remains one of the patron saints of Langres.

REFERENCES 16, 36, 46

129

Desiderius of Vienne

MEMORIAL DAY **May 23 or May 26**

PATRONAGE **Fever**

LIFE & LEGEND

Desiderius was born at Autun, educated in Vienne, and ordained to the diaconate and priesthood by Verus, bishop of Vienne. At Verus' death, Desiderius succeeded him in the episcopate. Desiderius was much esteemed by Gregory the Great, who exonerated him after a formal complaint made to Gregory by Queen Brunhildis, queen of Austrasia and widow of Sigisbert. Brunhildis was angry at Desiderius' public criticism of the immorality of her court. By means of a council called and manipulated by Brunhildis, Desiderius was banished from Vienne. He returned several years later, only to attract the attention and ire of King Theodoric of Burgundy. Desiderius was subsequently murdered in 607, according to some accounts, by three men on Theodoric's orders. According to others, one impulsive soldier acted alone while he was escorting Desiderius to his second banishment from court. The place of Desiderius' death is marked by the present-day village of Saint Didier sur Chalaronne.

REFERENCES 6, 14, 16, 36, 46

130

Dinoaldus (Dinault)

MEMORIAL DAY **August 11**

PATRONAGE **Epilepsy**

LIFE & LEGEND

As a child who lived during the fifth century in an area of France known as Beauvoisis, Dinoaldus was confronted in a field by mounted Huns who inquired what god he worshipped. When Dinoaldus responded that he worshipped Jesus Christ, the Huns beheaded the boy. In the fifteenth century, his relics were transferred from the village church of Milly to the abbey of Saint Lucien, where the child martyr was invoked for the cure of epilepsy.

REFERENCES 16, 36

131

Dizaint

MEMORIAL DAY **June 26**

PATRONAGE **Paralysis**

LIFE & LEGEND

Dizaint succeeded Saint Leger as bishop of Saintes (Charente-Maritime) in the seventh century. On the walk from the city of Ardres, known as Pas de Calais, in the middle of a meadow there is a spring named after Saint Dizaint, where they bathe children who have weak limbs that are unable to support them or allow ambulation. These waters have provided miraculous cures.

REFERENCE 16

132 Dominic of Silos

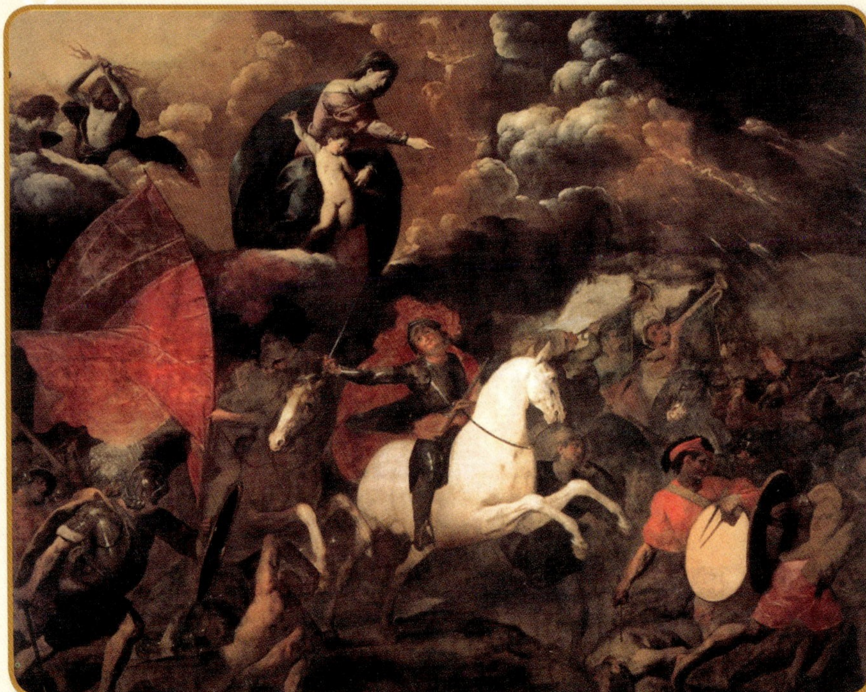

MEMORIAL DAY **December 20**

PATRONAGE **Labor, rabies**

LIFE & LEGEND

Dominic, whose name is derived from Latin, meaning "Lord," was born at Cañas in Navarre, Spain. He was a humble shepherd before entering the Benedictine monastery at San Millán de la Cogolla. He eventually became abbot, but was driven from his post by the king of Navarre over matters of property and money. After leaving Navarre, Dominic was received by the Catalonian king, who made him abbot at the San Sebastián monastery in Silos, an establishment that was in moral and physical disarray. Dominic restored both the monastery's buildings and its reputation as a spiritual center. He was known for his holiness, for his many efforts to ransom Christians from the Moors, and for the many miracles attributed to his name. He died of natural causes in 1073. Butler notes, "Until the revolution of 1931, it was the custom for the abbot of Silos to bring the staff of Saint Dominic to the royal palace whenever a queen of Spain was in labor and to leave it by her bedside until the birth had taken place."

REFERENCES 6, 36, 46

133

Dominic of Sora

MEMORIAL DAY **January 22**

PATRONAGE **Snakebite, rabies, toothache, fever**

LIFE & LEGEND

A native of Foligno in Umbria, Dominic was born in 951 and was educated at the Benedictine monastery of San Silvestro near his native city. He later entered the monastery of Santa Maria di Pietrademone (Sabina), where he was ordained into the priesthood. Thus began a long career in which Dominic vacillated between a coenobitic (community) and hermetic lifestyle. He founded monasteries at Scandriglia, L'Aquila, Sangro, Sora, Trisulti, and other places. In each monastery he founded, Dominic appointed another monk as abbot so that he could resume the hermetic life. Dominic is buried at the monastery at Sora, where he died in 1031.

REFERENCES 6, 16, 36, 46

134
Domitian of Maestricht

MEMORIAL DAY **May 7**

PATRONAGE **Fever**

LIFE & LEGEND

A native of France, Domitian was elected bishop of Tongres (or Tongeren, Belgium), an episcopal see that was later moved to Maestricht. He was known for the many conversions he performed in the Meuse Valley during the sixth century, for the churches and hospices he built, for his relief of the poor in times of famine, and for slaying the dragon that desolated the countryside and poisoned the wells of the town of Huy.

REFERENCES 6, 14, 16, 36

135

Donanus

MEMORIAL DAY **April 17**

PATRONAGE **Fever, scrofula**

LIFE & LEGEND

Donanus was abbot of a monastery in Scotland during the eleventh century. According to du Broc de Segange, "We know practically nothing about him, other than the fact that Duncan, King of Scotland, had great esteem for him, and that his staff had the power to cure fevers and scrofula. This staff was destroyed by the heretics."

REFERENCES 16, 36

136
Donatus

MEMORIAL DAY **June 30**

PATRONAGE **Fever, hail, electric storms, fire**

LIFE & LEGEND

There are many saints with the name Donatus, which is derived from Latin, meaning "given by God." The earliest noted Donatus is the second-century martyr whose tomb was discovered in the catacomb of Saint Agnes at Rome in the mid-seventeenth century. The exhumed relics of the saint were carried to Germany and elsewhere.

REFERENCES 16, 36

137

Drogo (Droyon)

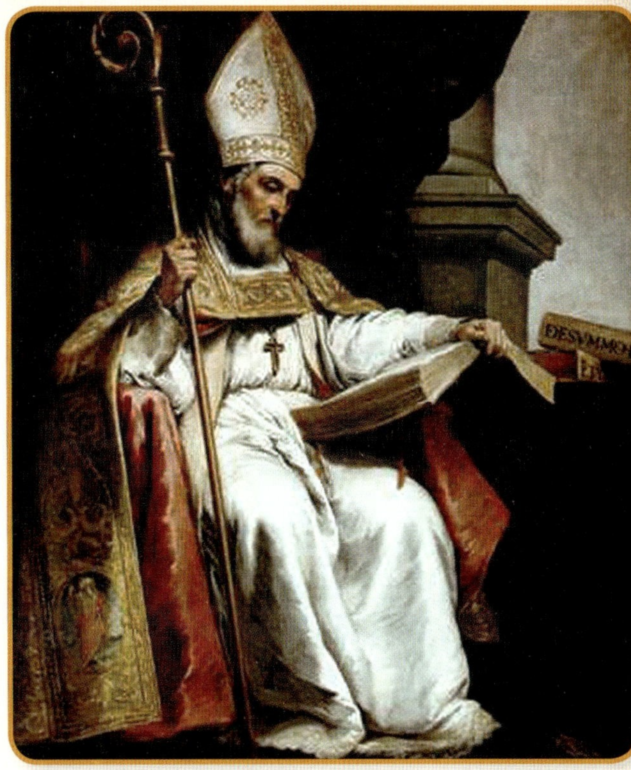

MEMORIAL DAY **April 16**

PATRONAGE **Physically repulsive people, deafness, dumbness, hernia, gallstones, mental illness, labor, pregnancy, calculi, fractures, sprains, shepherds, coffee**

LIFE & LEGEND

Drogo was born into a Flemish noble family in 1105 in Sebourg, France. His mother died when he was born, which later gave him a profound sense of guilt. When his father died and left Drogo an orphan while still in his teens, he rid himself of all his property and became a pilgrim. He traveled to Rome about nine times and, while at home, tended sheep. He was said to be able to bilocate—witnesses attested to seeing him in the fields and going to mass on Sundays at the same time.

On one of his pilgrimages, Drogo became ill and was left with a repugnant physical appearance, which frightened the townspeople. He was isolated from human view in a cell attached to a church. He subsisted on barley, water, and the Eucharist for 40 years. He died in Sebourg in 1185.

REFERENCES 6, 16, 36

138

Dulcidius (Doucis, Doux) of Agen

MEMORIAL DAY **October 16**

PATRONAGE **Palpitations, stomach problems, fever**

LIFE & LEGEND

Dulcidius succeeded Saint Phoebadius as bishop of Aginnum (present-day Agen, Lot-et-Garonne), a bishopric since the fourth century. He died ca. 475.

REFERENCES 36, 46

139

Dymphna

MEMORIAL DAY **May 15**

PATRONAGE **Epilepsy, neurologic disorders, insanity, mental disorders, psychiatrists, rape victims, sleepwalkers**

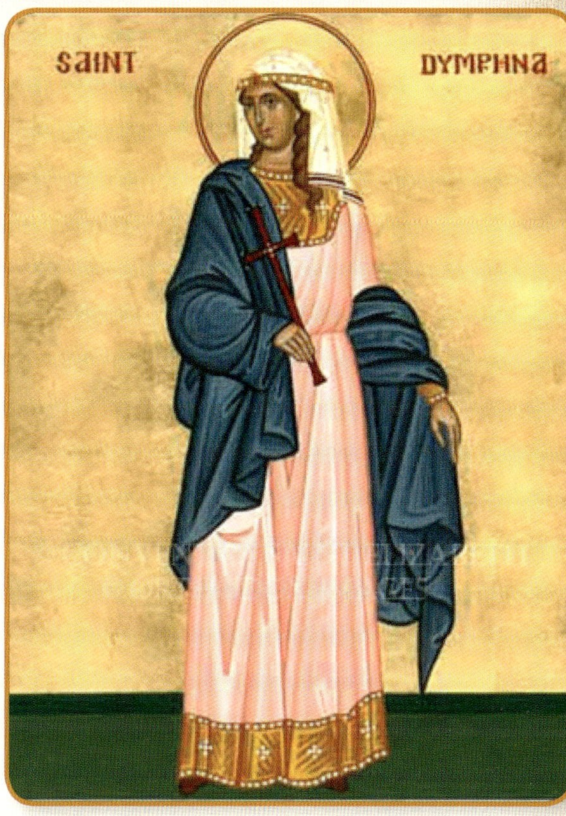

LIFE & LEGEND

Dymphna, whose name means "young deer" in Gaelic, was born in the seventh century into the family of a pagan Irish chief named Damon. When her mother died, her father made advances on her. She fled with her confessor, the elderly Saint Gerebernus, to Belgium, where they took refuge in a church in the region of Gheel near Antwerp. Her father caught up with her, and when she refused to return to Ireland, he decapitated both her and her confessor. She was buried in the area of Gheel, and her remains are now maintained in a reliquary of the church. The burial place purportedly has been the site of miraculous cures of mental illnesses, and a sanatorium that was built in the region persists to the present. The sanatorium is unique in that treatment incorporates shelter in the homes of local inhabitants.

REFERENCES 6, 9, 42

E

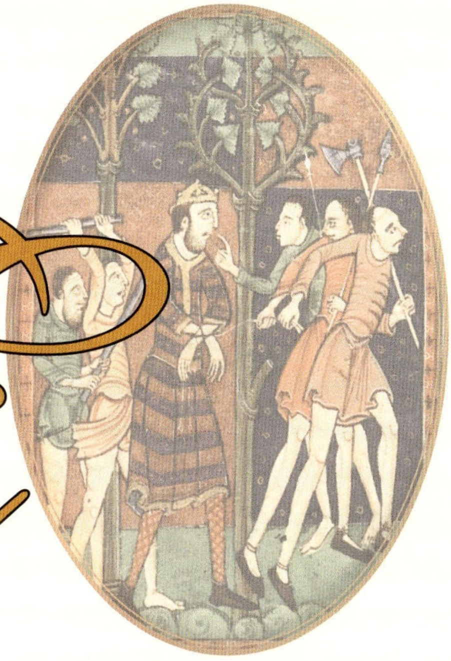

140

Ebrulf (Evroult)

MEMORIAL DAY **December 29**

PATRONAGE **Epilepsy, fever, mental illness**

LIFE & LEGEND

A native of Bayeux in Normandy, France, Ebrulf was born in 626 and raised in the court of King Childebert I. Although he was attached to the court, Ebrulf and his wife agreed to separate so that she could become a nun and he a monk. For a time Ebrulf lived at a monastery in Bayeux. He later left this community to pursue a more reclusive life in the forest of Ouche in Normandy. But even in this dense forest, Ebrulf could not find complete solitude. He was soon joined by disciples, including repentant bandits who had previously hidden in the forest. Ebrulf thus established a monastery in the forest, of which he became abbot. He died in 706, and his relics were translated to Depping, England, during the eleventh and twelfth centuries.

REFERENCES 6, 14, 36

141

Edmund the Martyr

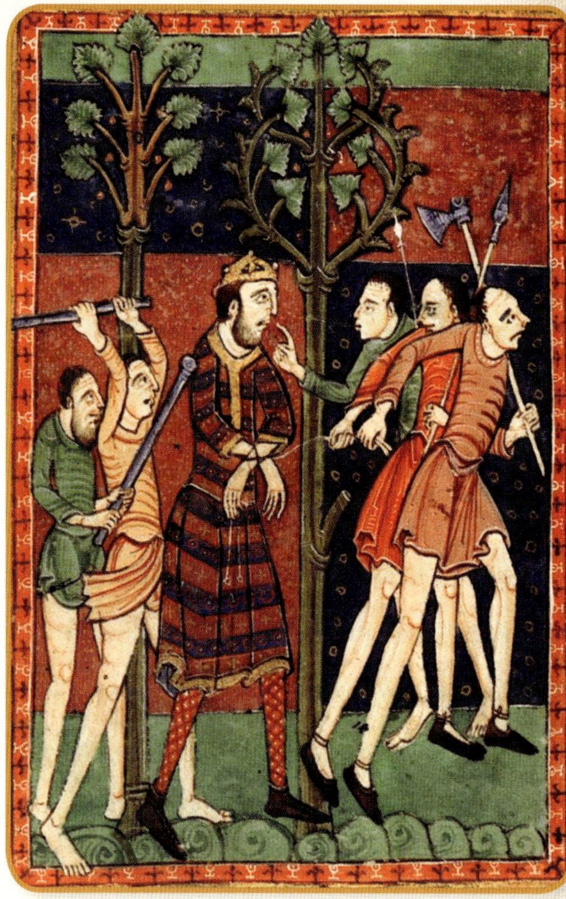

MEMORIAL DAY **November 20**

PATRONAGE **Plague, wounds, torture victims, kings, England (replaced by Saint George)**

LIFE & LEGEND

Edmund, a name that has an English derivation and means "prosperous protection," was born ca. 841. His place of birth and origin are open to question. Some indicate that he was of Old Saxon origin and was born in Nuremberg, whereas others believe that his father, whom he succeeded, was King Æthelweard of East Anglia. Edmund became king of East Anglia on December 25, 855. He was highly regarded for his just treatment of his subjects, and he was dedicated to Christianity, as evidenced by his retirement to his royal tower for 1 year to learn the entire Psalter so that he could recite it by heart. In 869, an army of pagan Danes marched through East Anglia and killed Edmund. It is said that he refused to renounce Christ and died a martyr's death—beaten, shot with arrows, and ultimately beheaded at Hoxne, Suffolk, England.

According to legend, his head was thrown into the wood, and when his troops called out seeking him, the head answered. The head was found protected by a wolf. After the head and body were buried, subsequent exhumation revealed the body and head joined and the absence of any arrow wounds. The body was ultimately interred at Bury Saint Edmunds. The shrine was destroyed in 1539 during the English Reformation. Many English churches are dedicated to Saint Edmund's memory, the most notable being Christopher Wren's Saint Edmund the King and Martyr in London. A recent failed attempt was made by BBC Radio Suffolk to restore Saint Edmund to his original status as patron saint of England, replacing Saint George.

REFERENCES 6, 9, 42, 45

142

Edward the Confessor

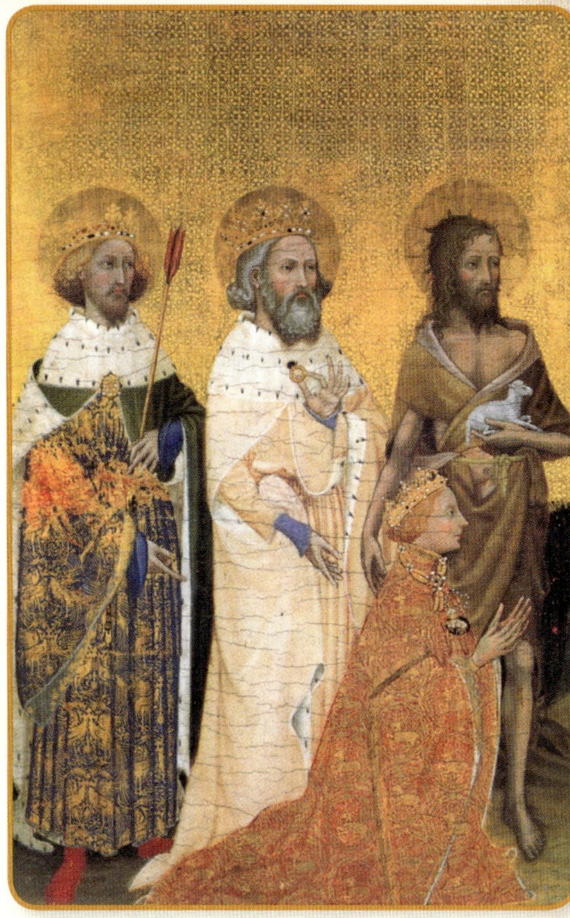

MEMORIAL DAY **October 13 (January 5 in England)**

PATRONAGE **Scrofula, leprosy, the Royal Family of England**

LIFE & LEGEND

Edward, which literally means "protector of wealth," was born in 1004 at Islip, England, the son of Ethelred II, the Unready. Some historians have suggested that he was an albino with white hair. To avoid the Danish invasion of England, he was taken by his mother to Normandy in 1016, where he spent more than 25 years and developed his piety. After one abortive attempt, he returned to England in 1041 and ascended to the throne the following year. He married but had no children, leading to the suggestion that he had taken a vow of chastity. His reign was marked by peace and prosperity, but during that time the territorial earls aggrandized more power, and England increased its association with Normandy, making Edward the penultimate Anglo-Saxon king of England.

Edward founded Westminster Abbey between 1045 and 1050. It began as the Abbey of Saint Peter on Thorney Island and was known as the West Minster to distinguish it from the other cathedral, Saint Paul's. During his reign, Edward was the first king to "lay his hand on" as treatment for scrofula, which became referred to as “the king’s evil.” Legend indicates that he was responsible for many cures for that disease as well as leprosy.

Edward died of natural causes in 1066. A century later, Osbert de Clare, prior of Westminster, wrote about the life of Edward, whom he considered to be a holy man as a consequence of the healing that he performed with his touch. Osbert went to Rome and argued for Edward’s canonization, which took place in 1161 under Pope Alexander III. Because Edward died of natural causes, perhaps a stroke or brain hemorrhage, he was named Edward the Confessor to distinguish him from his canonized predecessor, Edward the Martyr. In 2005, Edward’s remains were found under the pavement in front of the high altar of Westminster Abbey.

REFERENCES 6, 9, 42

143

Eligius (Eloi)

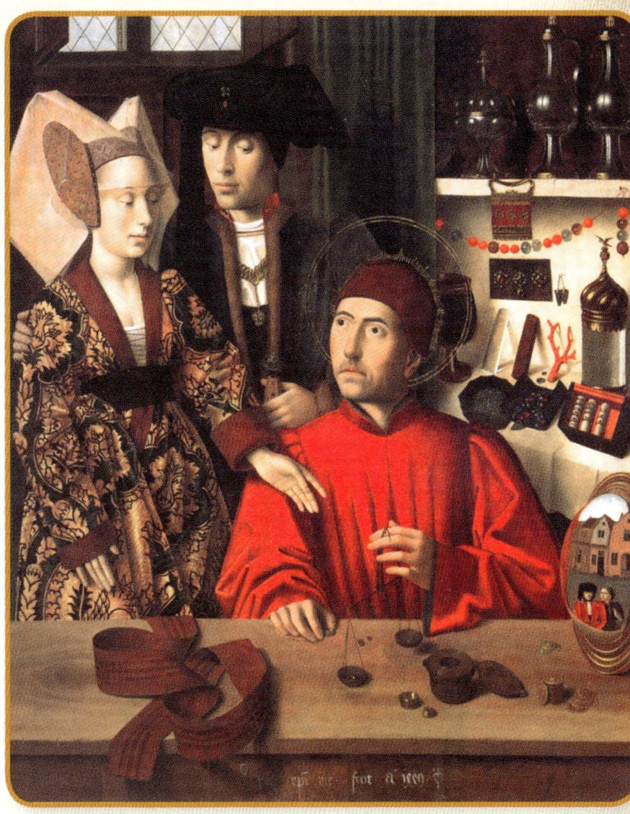

MEMORIAL DAY **December 1**

PATRONAGE **Scrofula, epidemics, jewelers, goldsmiths, horse-drawn cabs**

LIFE & LEGEND

Eligius, whose name is derived from Latin, meaning "selected," was born ca. 688 at Chaptelat near Limoges and was apprenticed by his father to a goldsmith in Limoges. On completion of his apprenticeship, Eligius journeyed to Paris, where he was employed by the treasurer of King Clotaire II. Not only through his skill as a goldsmith, but also for his nobility of character, Eligius came to the attention of Clotaire, who made him master of the royal mint. His name can be seen on gold coins stamped during the period. Eligius was also a skillful artificer of reliquaries and other objects made of precious metals. Although he adopted the elegant style of the court in his dress and manner, Eligius remained unaffected by the money and power surrounding him. He was generous to the poor and sought the company of learned and holy men, some of whom later became bishops and saints. Eligius remained in royal favor when Dagobert succeeded his father Clotaire to the throne.

Dagobert retained Eligius as a counselor and ambassador, and gave Eligius property at Solignac near Limoges for the foundation of a monastery. Eligius also built a major convent in Paris during Dagobert's reign. Eligius was also made bishop of Noyons in 640. He was particularly active in the evangelization and conversion of the pagans inhabiting the region of Tournai and present-day Flanders. Miraculous healings were attributed to Eligius even during his lifetime, and many more after his death in 660. There is a legend that he removed the leg of a horse to facilitate shoeing it and then put the leg back in place.

REFERENCES 6, 9, 36, 41, 42, 45

144

Elizabeth of Hungary

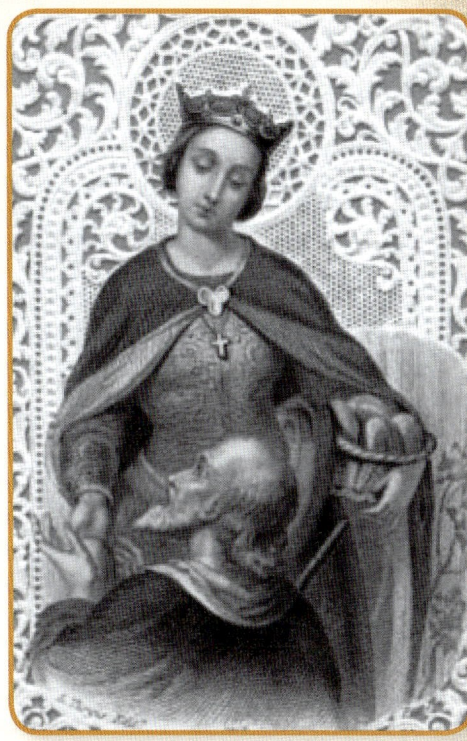

MEMORIAL DAY **November 19**

PATRONAGE **Toothache, hospitals, hospice**

LIFE & LEGEND

Elizabeth, whose name is derived from Hebrew, meaning "worshiper of God," was born in 1207, the daughter of King Andrew II of Hungary. At age four she was brought to the court of the Landgrave of Thuringia (at Wartburg near Eisenach) as the betrothed of his son, Ludwig. In 1221, Ludwig succeeded his father and married Elizabeth, then age 14. During a marriage portrayed as idyllic, Elizabeth bore Ludwig three children and became renowned for her great charity to the poor, which included the construction of a hospital. This earned Elizabeth much criticism from other members of the court, although her husband sanctioned her largesse. Ludwig joined the army of Emperor Frederick II on the sixth crusade, but died of a contagious disease at Otranto in Puglia before leaving Europe. His grieving wife was subsequently forced out of Wartburg by her brother-in-law, who usurped the title of Landgrave.

After making provision for her children, Elizabeth joined the tertiaries of the Franciscan Order in 1228. She lived at Marburg, where she built a small hospice for the care of the sick and the poor, and she came under the spiritual direction of her often-criticized confessor, Conrad of Marburg. After 2 years, Elizabeth's health began to fail, and she died at Marburg, aged 24. She was canonized by Pope Gregory IX within 4 years of her death.

REFERENCES 6, 14, 36, 42, 45, 46

145

Emerentiana

MEMORIAL DAY **January 23**

PATRONAGE **Pregnancy, colic, stomach disorders**

LIFE & LEGEND

Emerentiana was the foster sister of Saint Agnes. In one account of her martyrdom, Emerentiana was stoned to death ca. 304 by fanatic pagans while praying at the burial place of her foster sister 2 days after her martyrdom. In another version, she was stoned at Agnes' funeral 8 days after the latter's demise and was buried in the same location by Agnes' parents. In both versions, Emerentiana is described as a catechumen, (as yet unbaptized), warranting Saint Ambrose's remark that she was baptized in her own blood. Her name now appears only on local calendars.

REFERENCES 6, 16, 36, 46

146

Emilien (Milan)

MEMORIAL DAY **June 25**

PATRONAGE **Headache, calculi, urinary stones, hernia**

LIFE & LEGEND

As bishop of Nantes, Emilien successfully organized armed resistance to Muslim armies that had penetrated into the Bourgogne, until he was captured and beheaded by the enemy in 725.

REFERENCES 16, 36

147

Engelmund

MEMORIAL DAY **June 21**

PATRONAGE **Toothache**

LIFE & LEGEND

Engelmund was born in England at the end of the seventh century. He became a Benedictine monk and one of the companions of Saint Willibrord in converting the pagans of what is now North Holland and Friesland. He based his missionary activity in present-day Velsen (north of Haarlem), where he died ca. 720 and was buried. During his life, Engelmund created a spring in Velsen, the waters of which were regarded as effective in healing toothache.

REFERENCES 6, 14, 16, 36

148

Engratia (Encratis)

MEMORIAL DAY **April 16**

PATRONAGE **Headache**

LIFE & LEGEND

Engratia was the daughter of a Christian prince of what is now Portugal. She was accompanied by 18 horsemen to Saragossa, where she was to be married to a notable figure of Gallia Narbonensis (Provence). Engratia arrived in Saragossa during the persecution of Christians by Diocletian. She was arrested by Governor Dacian, who subjected her to various tortures, including having a nail driven into her skull, accounting for her patronage. Engratia eventually died from her many wounds ca. 304. Her 18 companions were beheaded outside the city.

REFERENCES 14, 16, 36

149

Enimia

MEMORIAL DAY **October 5**

PATRONAGE **Leprosy, skin diseases, tinea**

LIFE & LEGEND

Enimia was the beautiful daughter of Clotaire II, king of France. After taking a vow to remain a virgin, Enimia prayed that her beauty might be disfigured when her father announced her betrothal. Her prayer was answered in the form of leprosy that ended all question of marriage. Enimia remained afflicted with this disease for several years, until being instructed by an angel to wash herself in the fountain of Burle at Gevaudan (Lozere). Enimia did so and was healed of her affliction. She subsequently founded a convent near Gevaudan in the seventh century and became its first abbess.

REFERENCES 4, 36

150

Erasmus (Elmo)

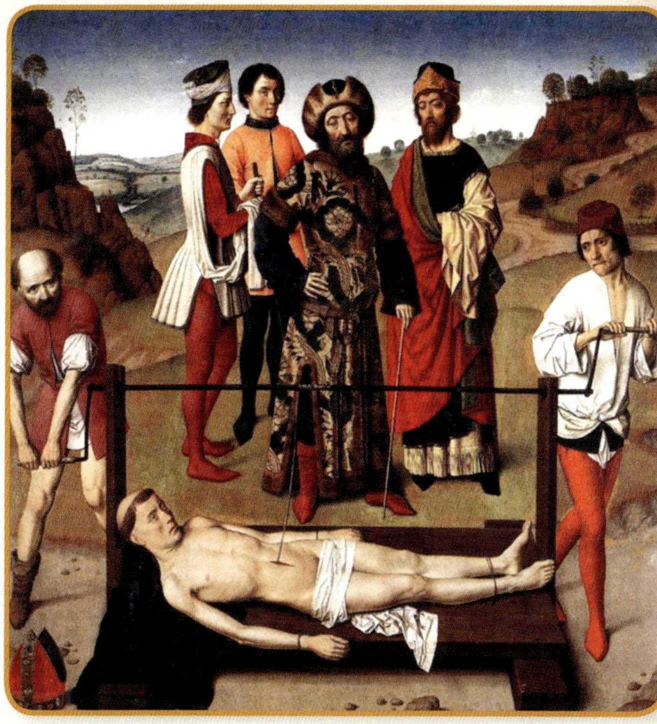

MEMORIAL DAY June 2

PATRONAGE Colic in children, intestinal ailments, labor, appendicitis, sea sickness, sailors, explosives workers, cattle pests, Formiae, Gaeta, Italy

LIFE & LEGEND

The name Erasmus is derived from Greek, meaning "lovely." The name Elmo is a corruption of "ermo," a contraction of Erasmus. Erasmus, whose date of birth is unknown, was the bishop at Formiae, overseeing all of Campania in Italy.

He was one of many targets during the Diocletian persecutions. According to legend, he was beaten with heavy metal hammers and then thrown into a pit of vipers. At that point thunder and lightning came and electrocuted all but Erasmus. Subsequently, the Western Roman Emperor, Maximian, had Erasmus covered by pitch and hot oil, but to no avail. Erasmus was then placed in a barrel full of spikes and rolled down a hill. He emerged unaffected. After his teeth were pulled out and he was roasted on a grill, he remained unscathed and fled to Mount Lebanon, where the ravens brought him food. He was recaptured ca. 303 in the Roman province of Illycrium, at which time his abdomen was cut open and his intestines were wound around a windlass and extracted.

This ultimate torture that resulted in his martyrdom and death (the windlass) was the basis of his patronage of sailors and also intestinal ailments. The legend that he continued preaching while lightning struck the ground around him was the probable reason for his becoming the object of prayers by sailors confronted with storms at sea. The electrical discharges at the mastheads of ships were considered a sign of his protection and took his name, "Saint Elmo's Fire."

His relics were initially maintained in the cathedral of Formia. After that location was destroyed by the Saracens in 842, the relics were removed to Gaeta, where he continues to be honored individually and as one of the Fourteen Holy Helpers.

REFERENCES 6, 9, 42, 45

151
Ethelburga (Aubierge)

MEMORIAL DAY **July 7**

PATRONAGE **Pregnancy, rheumatism**

LIFE & LEGEND

An illegitimate daughter of Anna, king of East Anglia, Ethelburga and her half-sister, Sethrida, entered the religious house in the forest of Brie (Gaul) founded by Saint Fara, or Burgundofara. Sethrida succeeded Burgundofara as abbess at Faremoutiers, and Ethelburga succeeded her sister in that office. Ethelburga died in 664. When her body was exhumed, it was incorrupt.

REFERENCES 6, 14, 16, 18, 36

152

Etheldreda (Audrey)

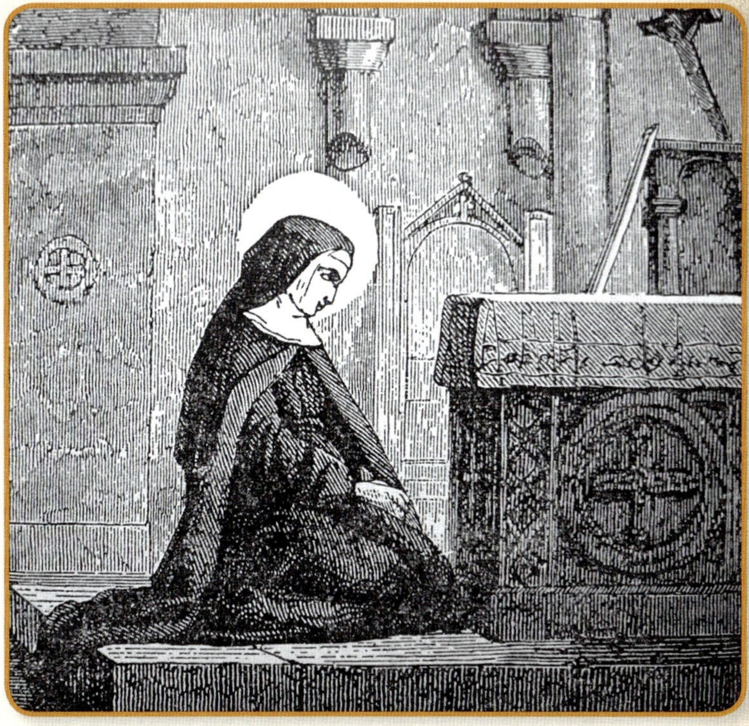

MEMORIAL DAY **June 23**

PATRONAGE **Eye disease**

LIFE & LEGEND

Born at Exning in Suffolk, Etheldreda, or Audrey, which is derived from English, meaning "noble strength," was one of the daughters of Anna, king of East Anglia. She lived in celibacy with her husband Tonbert (Tonbercht), who died 3 years into their marriage. Etheldreda then retired to the island of Ely, where she lived for 5 years in reclusion and prayer. Once again, however, she was pressed to marry—this time to Egfrid, the younger son of the king of Northumbria. Egfrid, who was younger than Etheldreda, at first agreed to maintain a celibate relationship with his wife. Later, however, he demanded his conjugal rights. With the support of Saint Wilfrid, archbishop of York, Etheldreda withdrew to the convent of Coldingham, where she took the veil. A year later she returned to Ely, where she established a convent, of which she was abbess until her death 7 years later in 679. During the later years of her life, she developed a large tumor in her neck.

He body was reinterred in 694 and was found incorrupt. In 1194, it was reinterred in the cathedral at Ely, and was again found incorrupt. Before the Reformation, the cult of Saint Audrey was widespread throughout England. In the Middle Ages, a festival called Saint Audrey's Fair was held on her feast day. The merchandises, particularly neckerchiefs, were shoddy, contributing to the origin of the word "tawdry."

REFERENCES 6, 16, 36

153

Eugenia (Ouine)

MEMORIAL DAY **June 7**

PATRONAGE **Ear diseases, insanity, deafness**

LIFE & LEGEND

Eugenia, whose name is derived from Greek, meaning "of noble descent," lived during the sixth or seventh century and was the virgin martyr of Mans. She may have been of Cornish origin—possibly one of the daughters of King Judhael of Domnonée. Eugenia is famous for the miracles that have taken place at her tomb in the crypt of the chapel at the priory of Saint Victor. Many individuals were cured who were deaf or had diseases of the ear. It is for this reason that she is called "Ouine"—from the French ouie (ear) or ouir (to hear).

REFERENCES 16, 36

154

Eulalia of Barcelona (Alausia, Olaire, Ouille)

MEMORIAL DAY **February 12**

PATRONAGE **Pregnancy, childbirth, dysentery**

LIFE & LEGEND

Eulalia, whose name is derived from Greek, meaning "elegant," was a native of Barcelona. She was tortured and executed in her native city during the persecution of Christians by the Emperor Diocletian. She was martyred the same year as Saint Eulalia of Merida, ca. 304, with whom she is sometimes confused.

REFERENCES 14, 16, 18, 36

155

Eustace (Eustachius)

MEMORIAL DAY **September 7**

PATRONAGE **Sick children, fever, eye diseases, fire, family discord**

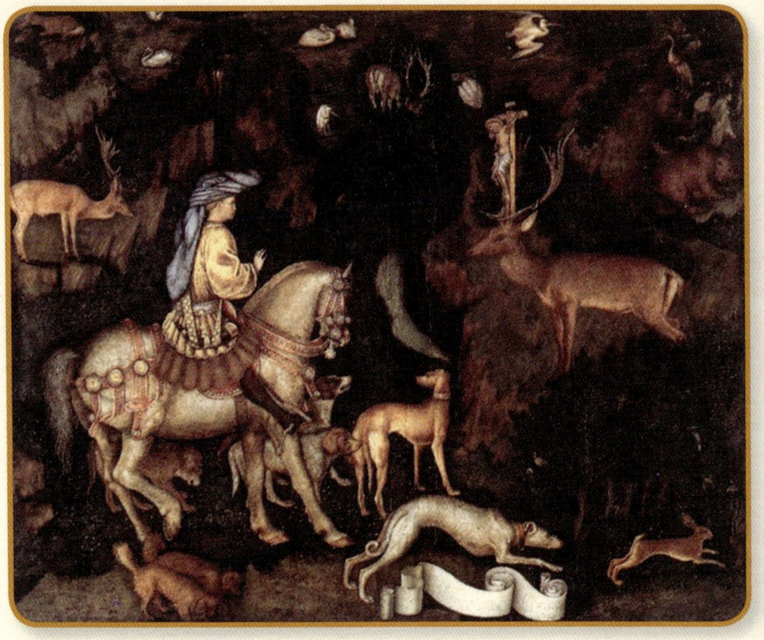

LIFE & LEGEND

Eustace, whose name derives from the Greek, meaning "rich," was born near Beauvais. He was ordained by the bishop of Beauvais and served there until joining the Benedictine Order at the monastery of Saint-Germer-de-Fly. He was later elected abbot of this monastery. Eustace was dispatched by Pope Innocent III to the South of France to combat the Albigensian heresy, and he served as apostolic legate to England. Eustace died in 1211. Not far from Canterbury, there is a spring blessed by the saint that is noted for the healing properties of its waters.

Saint Eustachius is the name of an island in the Caribbean Sea where the first shot confirming the independence of the United States was fired.

REFERENCES 14, 16, 36, 42, 45

156
Eutropius

MEMORIAL DAY **April 30**

PATRONAGE **Headache, dropsy, lameness, tumors, and sickly infants**

LIFE & LEGEND

Eutropius was probably a companion of Saint Denis on his mission to evangelize the inhabitants of Gaul during the third century. He became the first bishop of Saintes (Charente-Maritime), although he was expelled by its citizens and lived in a cell outside the city. When the Roman governor discovered that Eutropius had converted his daughter Eustella, he asked the butchers of Saintes to slay Eutropius. Eutropius' corpse was discovered by Eustella with the head split open by the blow of an ax.

Du Broc de Segange maintains that Eutropius was a first-century missionary to Gaul. According to this legend, Eutropius was the son of a Persian monarch who, while visiting the court of Herod, heard the preaching of Jesus of Nazareth. He became one of Jesus' disciples, and after learning of the crucifixion, ordered all the Jews in his father's realm to be put to death. Eutropius later visited Rome, where he was ordained to the episcopate by Pope Clement, who dispatched him to Gaul. All sources are agreed on the matter and manner of his martyrdom.

REFERENCES 6, 14, 16, 36

157
Exsuperius

MEMORIAL DAY **September 28**

PATRONAGE **Fever**

LIFE & LEGEND

Born at Arreau in the Hautes-Pyrenees, Exsuperius was made bishop of Toulouse ca. 405. He was widely known and respected. Exsuperius requested and received from Pope Innocent I what is regarded by Biblical scholars as an important list of what were the canonical books of Scripture at a period when the canon was being settled. Exsuperius was also known for his charity. Saint Jerome dedicated his commentary on Zacharias to Exsuperius in gratitude for his assistance to the monks of Palestine and Egypt. Exsuperius died in 412.

REFERENCES 6, 14, 16, 36

158

Ezekiel Moreno y Diaz

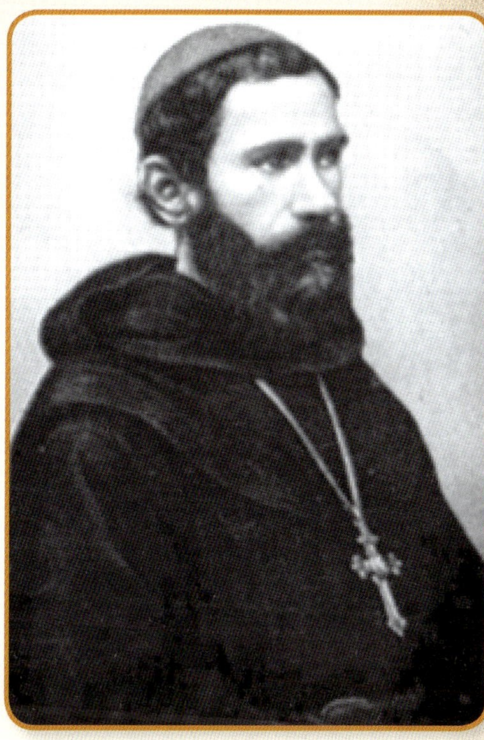

MEMORIAL DAY **August 19**

PATRONAGE **Cancer**

LIFE & LEGEND

Ezekiel, whose name is derived from Hebrew, meaning "God's strength," was born on April 9, 1848, into a pious but poor family at Alfaro, Trazona, Spain. He made his vows as an Augustinian Recollect when he was 16 years old, and he was ordained in Manila, Philippines, in 1871. He gained a reputation for his missionary work during the ensuing 15 years. He was called back to Spain to serve as rector of the College of Novitiare of Monteagudo.

In 1888, Ezekiel went to Colombia to continue his missionary activities. In 1894, he became the first vicar apostolic of Casnare and bishop of Pasto. He served in that role until he was diagnosed with cancer of the palate, which caused him to return to Spain, where he died on August 19, 1906. He was beatified by Pope Paul VI in 1975 and canonized by Pope John Paul II in 1992. Several miracles involving cancer cures were associated with his beatification and canonization, accounting for his patronage.

REFERENCES 9, 11

F

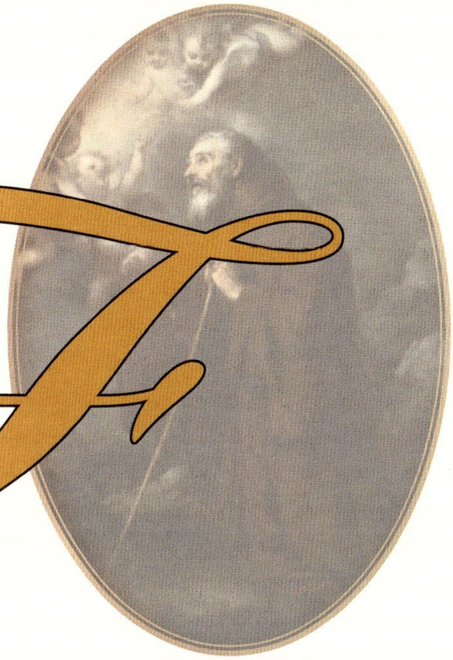

159

Faith (Fides, Foi)

MEMORIAL DAY **October 6**

PATRONAGE **Pregnancy, infertility**

LIFE & LEGEND

Faith was probably born, and was certainly martyred, at Agen (ancient Aginum) on the Garonne River in southwest France. As a young girl, ca. 303, Faith was arrested by the procurator, Dacian, who ordered her to sacrifice to the traditional Roman gods. She refused, was tortured on a red-hot grill, and was beheaded. Some sources maintain that Faith died during her tortures on the grill.

REFERENCES 6, 18, 36, 46

160

Fara (Burgundofara)

MEMORIAL DAY **December 7**

PATRONAGE **Eye diseases, blindness**

LIFE & LEGEND

Born at Poincy, near Meaux, Fara was the daughter of Agneric, a prominent officer in the court of Theodebert II, king of Austrasia. Three of Agneric's children were to attain sainthood: Cagnoald of Laon, Faro of Meaux, and Fara. At an early age, Fara vowed to remain a virgin and devote herself to God. When her father sought to arrange her marriage, Fara became seriously ill—an illness that was relieved only when Agneric agreed to respect his daughter's vow. Agneric was not faithful to his promise, however, and again tried to arrange his daughter's marriage.

On this occasion, Fara fled the paternal household and sought refuge in the sanctuary of a church. Bishop Eustasius intervened, brought Agneric to reason, and himself gave Fara the veil. Agneric subsequently presented to his daughter an estate, on which she erected Evoriacum, a monastic community that would attain great renown. Fara was abbess of this foundation for nearly 40 years. She died in 657.

Legend relates that Fara shed so many tears during the disagreements with her father that she eventually went blind. Her vision was miraculously restored by Bishop Eustasius.

REFERENCES 6, 18, 36, 46

161

Félix of Bourges

MEMORIAL DAY **January 1**

PATRONAGE **Eye diseases, fever**

LIFE & LEGEND

Although much esteemed by his contemporaries, little is known of the life of Félix, whose name comes from Latin, meaning "happy." Saint Germain of Paris officiated at his consecration as bishop of Bourges. Félix attended the Council of Paris in 573. He died ca. 580 and is still venerated at Bourges. Those who drank water mixed with dust from the slab covering his tomb reported miraculous cures.

REFERENCES 6, 16, 36

162

Félix of Nantes

MEMORIAL DAY **July 7**

PATRONAGE **Plague, fractures**

LIFE & LEGEND

A nobleman of Aquitaine, Félix was a married man when he was named bishop of Nantes in 549. His wife became a nun when Félix assumed his episcopal role. He was esteemed for his great charity, for evangelizing the rural population of his diocese, and for completing the cathedral begun by his predecessor at Nantes. He died ca. 582.

REFERENCES 6, 14, 36

163

Felix of Nola

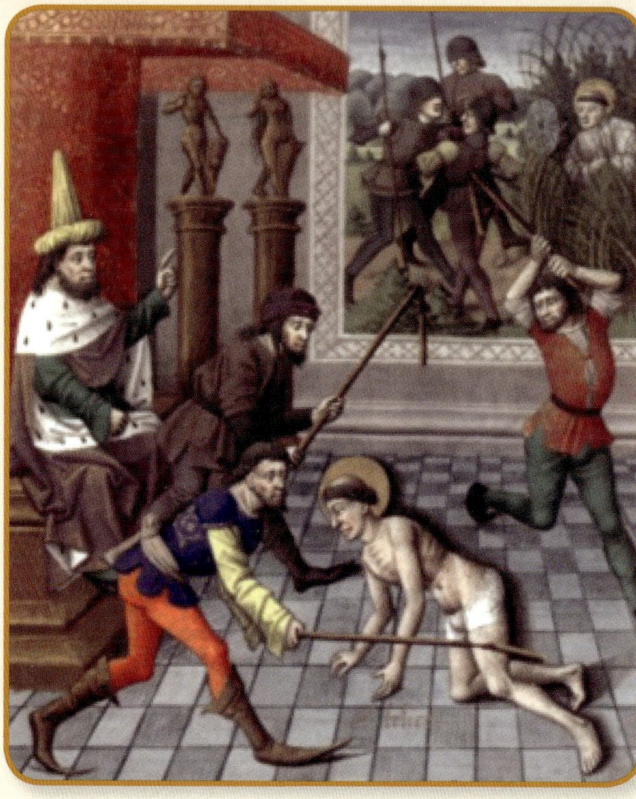

MEMORIAL DAY **January 14**

PATRONAGE **Eye diseases**

LIFE & LEGEND

Felix lived during the third century, the son of a Syrian soldier who had retired to Nola near Naples, Italy. His biographies, which were written by Saint Gregory of Tours and the Venerable Bede, were based on the fifth-century writings of Saint Paulinus of Nola, who served as a porter to one of the churches in Nola dedicated to Saint Felix.

After his father died, Felix distributed his goods among the poor, and he was ordained by Bishop Maximus of Nola. In 250, at the onset of the Decian persecution, the bishop fled, and Felix was tortured and chained in prison. One night, an angel released Felix from his chains, opened the prison door, and dispatched Felix to the aid of Bishop Maximus. After Felix hid himself and Maximus, a spider wove a web over the entrance of their hideout and thus convinced pursuers that the area was abandoned. Felix died a natural death ca. 255, but he is regarded as a martyr because of his trials. Five churches were built in his honor near Nola.

REFERENCES 9, 42, 45

164

Felix of Split (Salona, Spalatum, Spello)

MEMORIAL DAY **May 18**

PATRONAGE **Sick children**

LIFE & LEGEND

Felix of Split was bishop of Salona in Dalmatia (present-day Split, Croatia) when he was martyred ca. 304 during the persecution of Christians by Emperor Diocletian. Several sources place Felix in the Umbrian city of Spello rather than the Dalmatian city of Salona or Spalatum. This confusion is attributable to the assonance of the Latin place names Spalatum and Spoletium, the latter being the Umbrian city where these sources believe Felix's remains were transferred after his initial burial outside the walls of nearby Spello (ancient Hispellum).

REFERENCES 16, 36, 46

165

Ferreolus

MEMORIAL DAY **September 18**

PATRONAGE **Rheumatism**

LIFE & LEGEND

Ferreolus was a tribune with the Roman army stationed at Vienne in Gaul. He was a Christian and was arrested by Governor Crispinus for his refusal to cooperate in the persecution of Christians during the reign of Diocletian, and for his prior association with Saint Julian of Brioude. Ferreolus miraculously escaped from prison but was reapprehended, tortured, and beheaded ca. 304.

REFERENCES 6, 14, 36, 46

166

Fiacre (Fiachra)

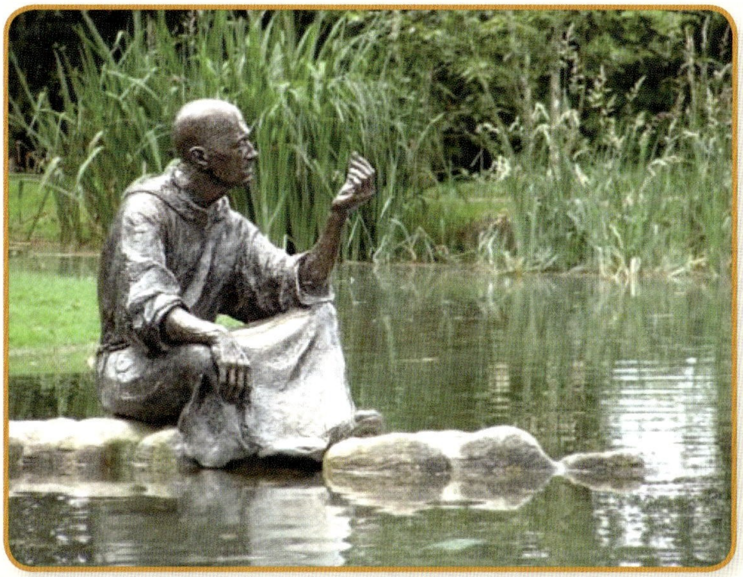

MEMORIAL DAYS **August 18, August 30, September 1**

PATRONAGE **Fistula-in-ano, hemorrhoids, [proctology],* venereal diseases including syphilis, sterility, calculi, cancer, colic, dysentery, gangrene, headache, hemorrhage, rectal diseases, ulcers, gardeners, florists, box and tile makers, taxicab drivers**

LIFE & LEGEND

Fiacre, which is derived from a word meaning "raven" or "jet-black," was born in Ireland in the seventh century and raised in a monastery, where he became proficient in the use of herbs for healing medical ailments. After he was ordained, he initially retired to an isolated hermitage on the banks of the Nore River in the area of Kilfiachra (Kilfera, County Kilkenny), which preserves the memory of his name. His therapeutic successes brought him an ever-increasing following that interfered with his isolation and time, which he preferred to save for a focused

*Proposed patronage

dedication to God. Consequently, he fled to France and arrived at Meaux in 628 where he, now named Fiacre, was warmly received by Saint Faro, the bishop at the time.

Fiacre was granted land at Brogillum (Breuil) by the bishop; this land was central to a legend that is associated with his life and eventual canonization. Purportedly, Fiacre was granted as much land as he was able to surround with a furrow in one day. He proceeded to turn up the earth, fell trees, and remove bushes and dense weeds using only the point of his staff, rather than a spade, with miraculous speed. The legend continues that a local woman, who witnessed the event, was convinced that this was witchcraft and that Fiacre was possessed of the devil. On learning of the accusation and that it had been reported to the bishop, Fiacre ceased his work and sat on a stone to meditate, whereupon the stone became soft as a pillow and, when Fiacre eventually stood up, an impression of his buttocks remained. When the entrenchments and the stone were viewed by the bishop, he accepted Fiacre as a man to whom the Lord gave great merit.

Fiacre built a church and monastery in that region and died there on August 18, 670. His remains were interred in the church at Breuil, which is still a site of pilgrimage for the cure of bodily ailments. In 1479, his relics were removed to the cathedral church at Meaux. In 1617, a part of the relics was given to the duke of Tuscany, and 20 years later Cardinal Richelieu received part of the vertebrae.

The stone of the legend remains and has been used to effect cures of a variety of anal disorders. This has led to his patronage for the cure of fistula-in-ano, which has been given the name "le fic de Saint Fiacre," and hemorrhoids. This is also responsible for Fiacre being referred to as the patron saint of proctology.

Anne of Austria, the wife of Louis XIII and mother of the Louis XIV, the Sun King, attributed the recovery of her husband from a serious illness to meditation invoking the powers of Saint Fiacre, and before Louis XIV's famous operation for fistula-in-ano, Saint Fiacre's powers were invoked. Anne made a pilgrimage to the shrine in 1641. She also acknowledged the saint's role in the birth of her son.

Fiacre's reaction to the accusations of the woman who suggested that he was possessed of the devil was to prohibit all women from entering his church. Those who transgressed suffered visible consequences. Even Anne of Austria was forced to offer her prayers outside the door of the church. His aversion to women accounts for his patronage of venereal disease and sterility.

The miraculous clearing of land by Fiacre led to his patronage on the part of gardeners and florists. Fiacre also had the patronage of hackney and taxicab drivers, and French cabs were called "fiacres," stemming from the fact that the first establishment to provide coaches for hire in Paris in the middle of the seventeenth century was in the rue Saint-Martin near the Hôtel Saint-Fiacre.

REFERENCES 9, 33, 42

167

Fidelis of Spello

MEMORIAL DAY **April 25**

PATRONAGE **Children's diseases**

LIFE & LEGEND

Nothing is known of the life or "actes" of Fidelis, whose name is derived from Latin, meaning "faithful." He is venerated in the Umbrian town of Spello.

REFERENCES 16, 36

168

Firminus

MEMORIAL DAY **September 25**

PATRONAGE **Fever, convulsions, rheumatism, scurvy, dropsy, tremors, erysipelas, neurologic disorders**

LIFE & LEGEND

Born into a prominent pagan family of Pamplona in Navarre, Firminus, whose name is derived from Latin, meaning "strong," was both baptized a Christian and consecrated as bishop of Toulouse by Saint Honoratus. Firminus wandered far into northern Gaul as a missionary bishop, basing his activity at Ambianum (Amiens), where he was ultimately arrested for his faith and martyred ca. 303. A church was built at Amiens over Firminus' tomb by his successor, also named Firminus—one of three saints of that name from Amiens. Firminus' feast day is observed in Pamplona on July 7. The encierro, or the traditional running of the bulls, takes place in Pamplona during the week-long festival that celebrates Navarre's patron, San Fermin.

REFERENCES 6, 14, 16, 36, 46

169
Flamina

MEMORIAL DAY **May 2**

PATRONAGE **Eye diseases**

LIFE & LEGEND

Little is known of the virgin martyr of Nicomedia, except that she lived in the fifth century and that her relics were transferred to France during the Middle Ages. It is stated that her patronage has been sought since time immemorial.

REFERENCES 16, 36

170

Flavitus (Flavy)

MEMORIAL DAY **December 18**

PATRONAGE **Fever**

LIFE & LEGEND

Venerated in France as Saint Flavy, Flavitus is supposed to have been either a slave or a prisoner in Italy when he was sold to a certain Montanius, who employed him at his estate Marcelliacum (present-day Marcilly-le-Hayer), south of Nogent-sur-Seine. Flavitus was made steward of the estate and married Aponia. At one point, he was a victim of false accusations of sexual advances toward Montanius' wife, but he was cleared.

On being manumitted, Flavitus was tonsured and then ordained a priest. He remained in the neighborhood of Marcelliacum, where he led a hermetic life, and Aponia received the veil from Saint Lupus. Flavitus died of natural causes in Gaul ca. 630. Although he was venerated in several areas of France, the cult of Saint Flavy remains centered at Marcilly-le-Hayer, where the waters of one of two fountains associated with the saint are known for their miracle-working power.

REFERENCES 16, 36, 46

171
Florentius

MEMORIAL DAY **June 1**

PATRONAGE **Plague**

LIFE & LEGEND

Florentius, whose name is derived from Latin, meaning "blossoming," was beheaded at Perugia for his faith during the reign of Emperor Decius, ca. 250. He and his companions in martyrdom (Cyriacus, Faustinus, Julianus, and Marcellinus) are venerated on June 1 or June 5. The relics of Florentius were reported to have been carried in procession through the streets of Perugia, preserving its inhabitants from horrible outbreaks of plague in 1358, 1400, and 1629.

REFERENCES 16, 36

172
Forannan

MEMORIAL DAY **April 30**

PATRONAGE **Rabies, tooth diseases**

LIFE & LEGEND

Forannan was bishop of a now unknown diocese named Domhnach-Mor before leaving Ireland in response to a dream in which an angel showed him a place of great beauty that he was to seek. Forannan sailed up the Meuse River with 12 companions, settling at the abbey of Waulsort (Wasour)—the place of his vision. He was made abbot of Waulsort in 962. On his return from a journey to Rome, Forannan visited the monastery at Gorze in Lorraine, where he studied the Benedictine Rule by which he was to reform Waulsort on his return. Numerous miracles were reported to have occurred at the tomb of Forannan in Waulsort.

Du Broc de Segange maintains that Forannan was bishop of Armagh before his departure from Ireland. He also relates that when Forannan and his companions found no ship that might take them from Ireland, they mounted two pieces of wood found on the shore in the form of a cross that carried them across the sea.

REFERENCES 6, 14, 16, 36, 46

173

Fortunatus of Fano

MEMORIAL DAY **June 8**

PATRONAGE **Plague**

LIFE & LEGEND

Fortunatus was bishop of Fano (the ancient Fanum Fortunae) in the Marche sometime during the sixth century, and he is one of the city's four patron saints. His name was invoked by Fano's inhabitants in times of plague.

REFERENCES 36, 46

174

Fourteen Holy Helpers

MEMORIAL DAY **August 8 (dropped in 1969)**

LIFE & LEGEND

The Fourteen Holy Helpers were defined as a group sometime between 1346 and 1349 in the Rhineland of Germany, when the plague was devastating Europe. Each of the 14 saints had been invoked effectively by victims of the plague and other diverse afflictions.

The 14 saints, their memorial days, and the situations for which each is invoked are:

Achatius	**May 8**	*Headache*
Barbara	**December 4**	*Fever, sudden death, plague, lightning, fire*
Blase	**February 3**	*Diseases of the throat, tooth disorders, goiter, whooping cough, angina*
Catherine of Alexandria	**November 25**	*Diseases of the tongue, sudden death*
Christopher	**July 25**	*Plague, sudden death, epilepsy, toothache, deafness, paralysis, lightning, storms*
Cyriacus	**August 8**	*Diseases of the eye, diabolic possession, temptation at the time of death*
Denis (Dionysus)	**October 9**	*Headache, diabolic possession, rabies, hydrophobia*
Erasmus (Elmo)	**June 2**	*Stomach and intestinal ailments, colic, labor, appendicitis*
Eustace (Eustachius)	**September 7**	*Sick children, fever, eye diseases, family discord, fire*
George	**April 23**	*Herpetic diseases, skin diseases, leprosy, plague, syphilis*
Giles	**September 1**	*Plague, epilepsy, disability, breast feeding, breast cancer, leprosy, panic, madness, nightmares*
Margaret of Antioch	**July 20**	*Childbirth, backache, sterility, kidney diseases*
Pantaleon	**July 27**	*Consumption*
Vitus	**June 15**	*Epilepsy, lethargy, poisonous bites, storms*

In 1774, the Basilika Vierzehnheiligen was built to honor the Fourteen Holy Helpers in Bad Staffelstein, near Bamberg. In 1969, Pope Paul VI dropped Barbara, Catherine of Alexandria, Christopher, and Margaret of Antioch from the list of saints for universal veneration. In 2004, Pope John Paul II reinstated Catherine of Alexandria as an optional memorial.

175
Fraimbaud

MEMORIAL DAY **August 16**

PATRONAGE **Headache**

LIFE & LEGEND

Fraimbaud was born into a noble family in the province of Arvernes. Through his father's connection with King Childebert, the young Fraimbaud was placed at court, where he was educated. Despite this promising beginning, Fraimbaud chose to withdraw from the court and the world to pursue a hermetic life. Initially he lived in a cave near present-day Ivry-sur-Seine. He later entered the abbey of Micy near Orleans, where he was ordained to the priesthood.

Fraimbaud's holiness attracted numerous pilgrims, who sought his spiritual counsel and on occasion the miraculous healing of their maladies. This attention convinced Fraimbaud to once again withdraw into the wilderness and establish a hermitage near Mayenne.

Fraimbaud is said to have played a prominent role at the fourth Council of Orleans, to have been active in the evangelization of pagans, and to have been conspicuous in the performance of many healing miracles. He died ca. 532.

REFERENCES 31, 36

176

Framechildis (Frameuse)

MEMORIAL DAY **May 17**

PATRONAGE **Headache**

LIFE & LEGEND

Framechildis was descended from a powerful German family and was married to Badefroi (Woldefroi), a noble lord in the court of King Dagobert II. She was the mother of Saint Austreberta. She died ca. 685 and was buried in the church of Marconne, which she had built. Her name is invoked in the diocese of Amiens, of which Marconne is a part.

REFERENCES 16, 18, 36

177

Franca of Piacenza

MEMORIAL DAY **April 25**

PATRONAGE **Eye diseases**

LIFE & LEGEND

Franca, whose name is derived from Latin, meaning "free man," was born in 1170 into the noble Vitalta family of Piacenza. She was placed by her father in the Benedictine convent of San Siro at age 7. She made her profession at age 14, and in 1198 she was elected abbess. The strictness of her reforms met with opposition from within the convent and also from members of the Piacentine nobility. For this reason, and because of her desire for a more spiritual life, Franca left San Siro and joined a newly formed Cistercian community at Montelana in 1214. The community later moved to Pittolo, where Franca died in 1218. Her tomb was the object of much veneration and the site of numerous miracles. Once, a band of armed men was intent on plundering the monastery when its chief was suddenly struck blind. He recovered his sight only when he invoked the intercession of the deceased Saint Franca.

REFERENCES 16, 18, 36, 46

178

Francis of Paola

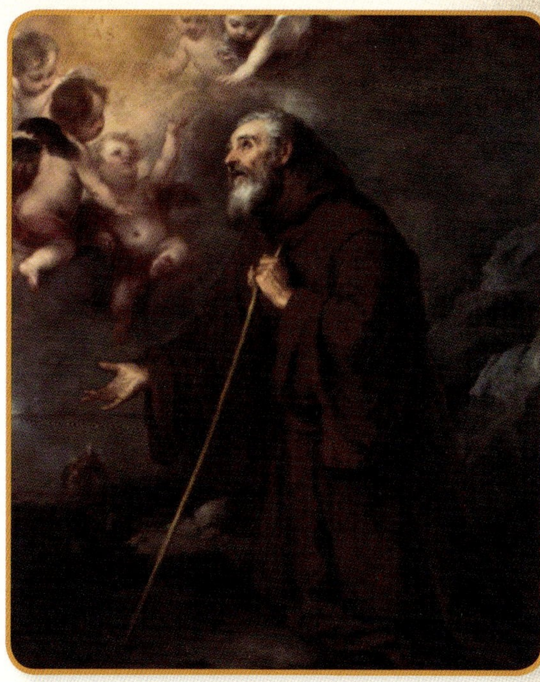

MEMORIAL DAY **April 2**

PATRONAGE **Plague, sterility, mariners, Calabria (Italy)**

LIFE & LEGEND

Francis, who was named after Saint Francis of Assisi, was born in Calabria in 1416. He made a pilgrimage to Rome and Assisi as a teenager, after which he became a hermit in a cave near Paola. He attracted many followers, and in 1452 he founded the Hermits of Saint Francis of Assisi, which was approved by the Holy See in 1474. In 1492, they were renamed the Franciscan Order of Minim Friars. Penance, charity, and humility were the rule. In addition, the order observed perpetual Lent and also abstained from eggs and milk.

Francis gained a reputation as a prophet and a miracle worker. In 1464, he wanted to cross the Straits of Messina to visit Sicily. When a boatman refused him passage, Francis placed his cloak on the water and fashioned a sail using his staff, which allowed him to cross the strait. This legend inspired a piece of music by Franz Liszt, "Walking on the Waves."

In 1481, a dying King Louis XI of France appealed to Pope Sixtus IV to send Francis to heal him. Francis did not heal the king but prepared him to accept death. Louis' son, Charles VIII, continued to use Francis for counsel and built a monastery for Francis' followers in Plessis and another for French monks in Rome. Francis spent 25 years in France and died there in 1507. His relics were distributed to many churches and were credited with many miracles. Saint Francis was canonized in 1519 by Pope Julius II.

REFERENCES 6, 42, 45

179
Francis de Sales

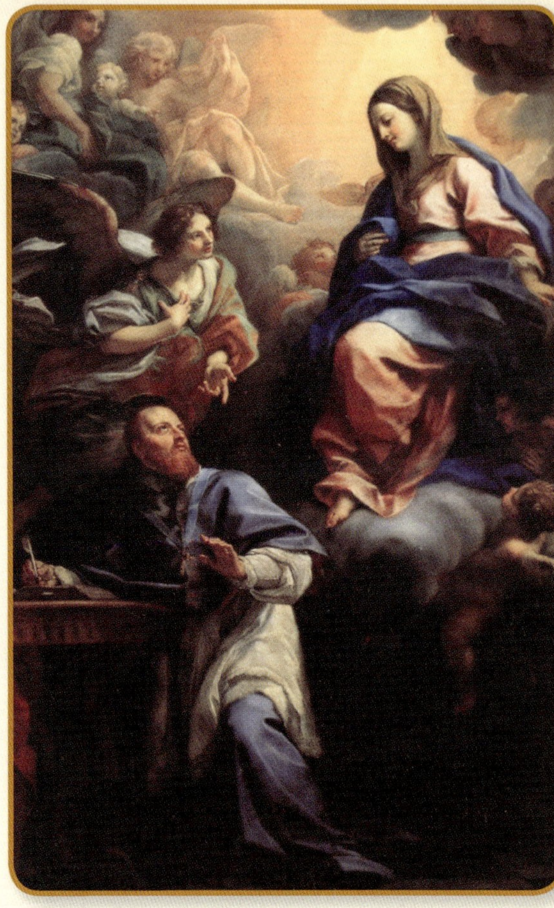

MEMORIAL DAY **January 24 (formerly January 29)**

PATRONAGE **Deafness, writers and journalists, the dioceses of many cities**

LIFE & LEGEND

Francis, whose name is derived from Italian, meaning "Frenchman," was born into a Savoyard noble family at the Chateau de Thorens in what is now France. His early education was conducted at La Roche and Annecy under the guidance of Jesuits. At age 12, he proceeded to Clermont College in Paris, where his education continued. A year later he developed deep despair after a discussion about predestination. This persisted for almost a decade, until he had an epiphany at the Church of Saint-Étienne-des-Grès (Saint Stephen) when he realized that he was destined to dedicate his life to God.

He transferred to the University of Paris, where he received doctorates in both law and theology. A series of experiences led Francis to become a priest. While riding a horse, his sword fell, crossing another sword on the ground to make the sign of the cross. After his ordination, Francis became provost of the cathedral chapter of Geneva, Switzerland. He was very successful in his evangelism in the heavily Calvinist city. In 1602, Francis became bishop of Geneva and enhanced his reputation as a speaker, writer, and friend of the poor.

He helped found the women's Order of the Visitation of Holy Mary with Saint Frances de Chantal. Francis was a prolific writer; the most famous of his books is *Introduction to the Devout Life.* He also developed a sign language to teach a deaf man, thus accounting for his patronage by the deaf.

Francis died in Lyon on December 28, 1622, while accompanying the Court of Savoy to France. He was buried at the Basilica of the Visitation in Annecy, but the relic of his heart was kept in Lyon. It was removed to Venice during the French Revolution, where it remains. Saint Francis de Sales was beatified by Pope Alexander VII in 1661 and canonized by the same pope in 1665.

The Oblates of Saint Francis de Sales was founded in 1830 to honor him. He was also honored in 1858 by the naming of the Order of the Salesians of Don Bosco. Blessed Pius IX declared Saint Francis a Doctor of the Universal Church. In 1923, Pope Pius XI proclaimed Saint Francis de Sales patron of writers and journalists. His feast day now coincides with the day he was buried.

REFERENCES 6, 9, 42, 45

180

Francis Xavier

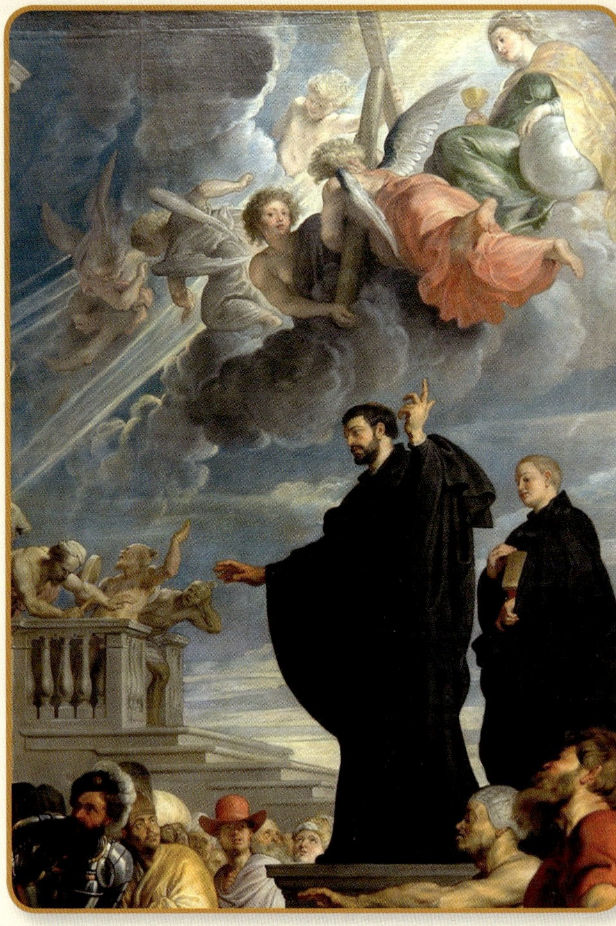

MEMORIAL DAY **December 3**

PATRONAGE **Plague, leprosy, hospital administrators, Australia, New Zealand, China, Japan, Goa, India**

LIFE & LEGEND

Francis was born in 1506 near Pamplona in the Kingdom of Navarre, at the family castle of Xavier, the name of which was derived from Basque, meaning "new house." He went to Paris to study, and there he met Pierre Favre and Saint Ignatius Loyola, who had been planning the formation of the Society of Jesus. The three were joined by Lainez, Salmerón, Rodríguez, and Bobadillia. On August 15, 1534, this group made the vow of Montmartre that eventually led to the formation of the Society of Jesus.

In 1537, Francis Xavier and Ignatius Loyola received their Holy Orders in Venice and left for Rome. The Society was formally approved in 1540. Francis was appointed to evangelize in the East Indies by King John III of Portugal. He arrived at Goa in 1542 and preached and ministered to the sick and poor for 3 years throughout western India. He continued his efforts in Malacca, the Molucca Islands, and the Philippines. He worked throughout Japan for two and a half years, and, in 1552, he sailed to the island of Sancian in anticipation of extending his work to mainland China. He took ill while on the island and died that year.

In the course of only 10 years, Francis developed the reputation of being a miracle worker, healer, and prophet. He baptized more than 40,000 people and is considered by the Roman Catholic Church to have converted more people to Christianity than anyone other than Saint Paul. This earned Francis the designation of the Apostle of the Far East.

Francis' body is interred in a silver casket in the Basilica of Bom Jesus in Goa. His right forearm was detached and is displayed at the main Jesuit church in Rome, Il Gesú. He was beatified by Pope Paul V in 1619 and canonized by Pope Gregory XV in 1622 at the same time as Ignatius Loyola. Francis' name identifies many schools and institutes of higher learning in the United States and throughout the world. Xavier University of Louisiana, founded as a high school by Saint Katherine Drexel of Philadelphia and the Sisters of the Blessed Sacrament in 1915 and expanded to become a college in 1925, is the only historically black Catholic university in the Western Hemisphere.

REFERENCES 9, 11, 40

181

Fredegand

MEMORIAL DAY **July 17**

PATRONAGE **Plague**

LIFE & LEGEND

Fredegand was an Irish-born monk who accompanied Saint Foillan in his missionary journeys to England and later to modern-day Belgium during the seventh century. He became abbot of the Kerkeloder abbey (Kerkedor te Deurne) near Antwerp.

REFERENCES 36, 46

182
Friard

MEMORIAL DAY **August 1**

PATRONAGE **Fever, kidney diseases**

LIFE & LEGEND

Friard was born at Besné (Loire-Atlantique). He lived the hermetic life on an island in the Loire (Vindunitta) near Nantes with his companion in spiritual labor, Saint Secundel, under the protection of Saint Félix, bishop of that city. On an occasion when Friard was attacked because of his piety, his attackers were held off by a swarm of wasps. Friard prayed for his enemies, and the wasps disappeared. Friard died ca. 557.

REFERENCES 16, 36, 45, 46

183
Frisius

MEMORIAL DAY **June 24**

PATRONAGE **Epilepsy**

LIFE & LEGEND

Frisius was a son of the Fries king, Radbod. His mother was the sister of Charles-Martel. After Frisius was killed in combat by infidel Goths during the eighth century, his body was recovered by his Christian friends and placed in a sarcophagus that was submerged in a nearby spring. His body was discovered by peasants of the neighborhood, who placed it in a chapel that was consecrated to the saint. Cures of epilepsy were reported to have occurred at that site.

REFERENCES 16, 36

184
Fursey

MEMORIAL DAY **January 16**

PATRONAGE **Eye diseases, fever, paralysis, calculi, heart diseases, dropsy, colic, hernia, scabies, other skin diseases**

LIFE & LEGEND

Fursey was born ca. 567 at Munster on the western coast of Ireland near Lough Corrib. His father was an Irish prince, Fintan, and his mother was Gelges, the only daughter of another powerful lord. The infant Fursey was baptized and named by Saint Brendan, who also accepted him into the monastic life. Fursey established a monastery at Rathmat that attracted many new members, and he also served as an itinerant preacher evangelist. After 12 years of preaching in Ireland, Fursey settled in East Anglia with his brothers, Saint Foillan and Saint Ultan. They were welcomed by King Sigebert, who gave them land to erect a monastery. Fursey was given to visions, summarized by the Venerable Bede, that focused on the fate of the soul after death and on the struggle between demons and angels over the souls of those just departed.

Between 640 and 644, Fursey made the decision to cross the channel into Gaul, where he was received by King Clovis II and was given land to build a monastery at Lagny-sur-Marne. While in France, he worked with Saint Blitharius as a successful evangelist, and raised the son of a court nobleman from the dead. Fursey died near Mezerolles in 648 while journeying through the area of Somme. When his relics were translated in 654, the body was incorrupt. Many miracles were reported to have occurred at his tomb.

REFERENCES 6, 14, 16, 36, 45, 46

G

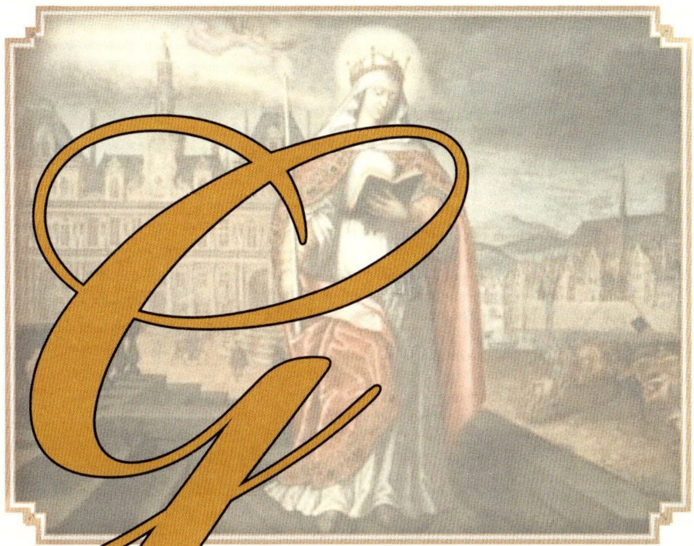

185

Gall of Clermont

MEMORIAL DAY **July 1**

PATRONAGE **Fever, plague**

LIFE & LEGEND

Not to be confused with the renowned Irish saint of this name, Gall, whose name is derived from Latin, meaning "rooster," was born ca. 486 into one of the first families of Clermont in Auvergne. His father intended to marry his son to the daughter of an imperial senator, but Gall fled the paternal household to enter the monastery at Cournon d'Auvergne. He was later ordained a deacon by Quintianus, the bishop of Clermont, and later still became a cantor in the chapel of King Theodoric because of his fine voice. When Quintianus died in 527, Gall succeeded him as bishop. Gall was the uncle of Saint Gregory of Tours, and was much involved in his nephew's upbringing and education. Gall was notable as a miracle worker and one whose meekness and humility attracted converts. He died of natural causes ca. 554.

REFERENCES 6, 16, 36, 45

186

Gaucherius (Galtier, Walter)

MEMORIAL DAY **April 9**

PATRONAGE **Fever**

LIFE & LEGEND

Born at Meulan-sur-Seine, Gaucherius made the decision at age 18 to become a recluse. With a like-minded friend named Germond, Gaucherius withdrew into the forest near present-day Aureil in the Limousin region (Haute-Vienne). The reputation of these holy men eventually attracted disciples and led to the building of a monastery. Gaucherius also founded a religious house for women nearby. He died at age 80, ca. 1140, after falling from his horse while returning to Aureil from Limoges. Du Broc de Segange notes, "The invocation of Gaucherius against fever is justified by the cures effected by his intercession—a number too large to be counted."

REFERENCES 6, 14, 16, 36

187

Gebhard of Konstanz

MEMORIAL DAY **August 27**

PATRONAGE **Childbirth, Konstance (Switzerland)**

LIFE & LEGEND

The son of Count Ulrich of Bregenz, Gebhard, whose name is derived from German, meaning "brave gift," was born in Austria in 949 and was educated at the cathedral school in Konstanz. He was elected bishop of that city in 979 and in 983 founded the Benedictine monastery at Petershausen, where he is buried at the abbey. He died in 995.

REFERENCES 36, 46

188

Gebuinus of Lyon (Gébuin, Jubinus)

MEMORIAL DAY **April 17**

PATRONAGE **Calculi, gout, joint diseases**

LIFE & LEGEND

Gebuinus was the son of Hugues III, count of Dijon. He was archdeacon to Raynaud de Bas, bishop of Langres, when he was chosen in 1076 to replace the deposed Humbert as bishop of Lyon. As a close ally of Pope Gregory VII, Gebuinus played an important role in the reform of the church in two councils held at Lyon in 1080 and 1082—particularly with regard to the widespread practice of simony (paying for the sacraments or for a position in the church hierarchy). Gebuinus suffered horribly from bladder stones, accounting for his patronage. He died of natural causes in 1087.

REFERENCES 16, 36

189
Genevieve

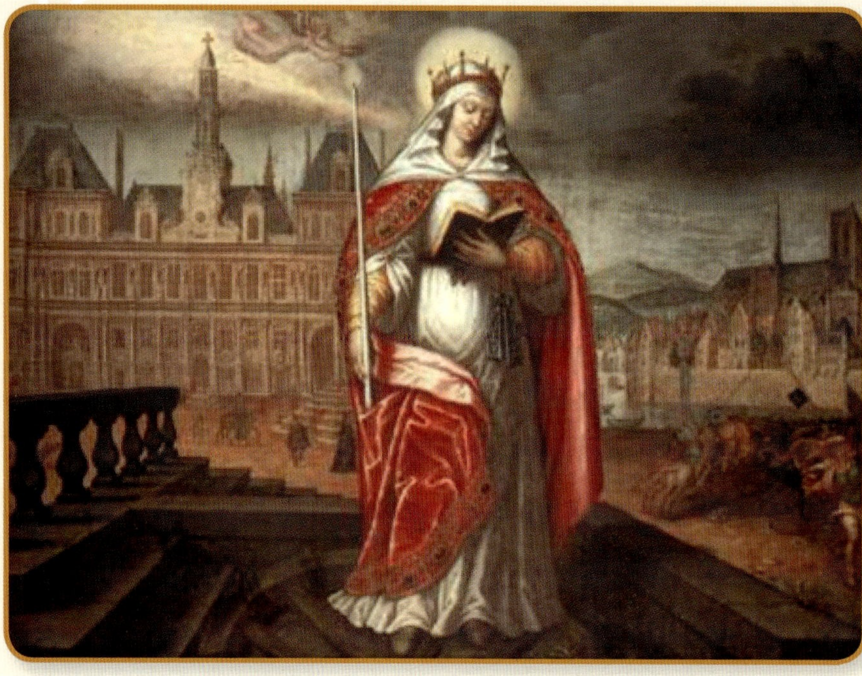

MEMORIAL DAY **January 3**

PATRONAGE **Fever, plague, ergot poisoning, Paris, Women's Army Corps**

LIFE & LEGEND

Genevieve was born at Nanterre near Paris in 422. The meaning of her name is uncertain, although it is known to have a Germanic origin. Perhaps it is derived from a word meaning "woman of the people." When she was 7 years old, Genevieve met Saint Germanus of Auxerre on his way to England, and she was stimulated to lead a life of piety.

She took the veil at age 15 and became noted for her prophesies related to events in Paris. In 451, when Attila and the Huns invaded Gaul, Genevieve persuaded the Parisians to remain and trust in God. The barbarians changed their course and proceeded to Orleans, leaving Paris unscathed. Years later, when Childeric laid siege to Paris, Genevieve successfully exerted her influence to gain clemency for the citizens. She catalyzed the building of a church in Paris to honor Saints Peter and Paul shortly before she died in 511. Her remains were preserved in that church, and it was purported that prayers to Genevieve saved Paris from severe flooding in 834.

In 1129, during an epidemic of plague or ergot poisoning, a procession in her honor resulted in the sudden cessation of the disaster. The event is still commemorated in several Parisian churches. A small church was built to honor her that stood until the middle of the eighteenth century, when it was torn down to build a foundling hospital. The Daughters of Saint Genevieve was established in Paris in 1636. After a merger with another group, the order was revived in 1806 and maintains its role of supervising schools and orphanages in France.

REFERENCES 6, 9, 42

190
Gengulf

MEMORIAL DAY **May 11**

PATRONAGE **Sick infants, unhappy marriage**

LIFE & LEGEND

Gengulf was a member of a noble family in Burgundy and a knight in the service of Pepin the Short. When Gengulf learned of his wife's infidelities, he provided for her maintenance and then withdrew to his estate at Avallon (between Auxerre and Autun). He lived there as a hermit, distributing his wealth to the poor. Stung by her husband's reproofs and his continued generosity to her, Gengulf's wife convinced her lover to murder her pious husband in 760.

REFERENCES 6, 14, 16, 36

191

Gens

MEMORIAL DAY **May 16**

PATRONAGE **Colic, fever**

LIFE & LEGEND

Gens is known solely in the department of Vaucluse and in some neighboring parishes in Provence, France. The saint is more popular and enjoys the greatest credit among peasants and agricultural workers. He was born in Monteux early in the twelfth century. At age 15, he withdrew into the countryside near Bausset (diocese of Avignon), where he lived a life of solitude and holiness, effecting several miracles. At age 22, sensing the approach of death, Gens dug his own grave in the solitude of Bausset and lay himself in it.

According to du Broc de Segange, "All those who are afflicted with colic or with fevers lay themselves upon this tomb and are immediately cured."

REFERENCES 16, 36

192

George

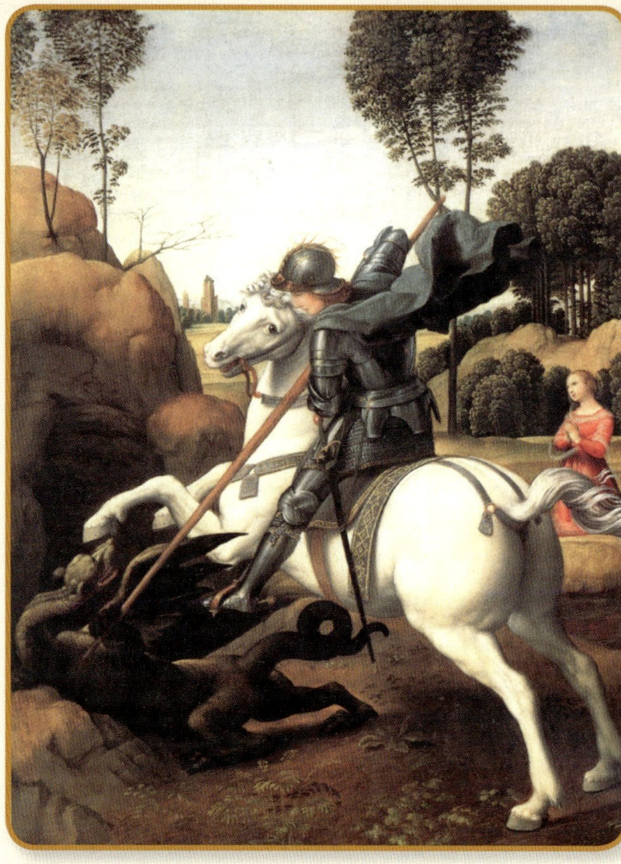

MEMORIAL DAY **April 23 (Russian Orthodox: November 3)**

PATRONAGE **Skin diseases, herpes, leprosy, syphilis, plague, butchers, farm workers, chivalry, horsemen, saddle makers, shepherds, Canada, England, Ethiopia, Germany, Greece, Malta, Palestine, Beirut, Constantinople (Istanbul), many German and Italian cities, Moscow, the Boy Scouts of America**

LIFE & LEGEND

The name George is derived from a Greek word that means "earth worker." He was born between 275 and 281 in Nicomedia, Bithynia, to a Christian family, and followed his father's example by becoming a soldier. George eventually gained the title of Tribune and later Count and served as a member of the personal guard of Emperor Diocletian. During the period of systematic persecution of the Christians, George was ordered to participate. He refused and confessed his religion, at which point he was tortured and eventually decapitated at Lydda, Palestine (now Lod, Israel) ca. 304.

The legends surrounding his death are numerous and dramatic, including tales that he was chopped into pieces, thrown into fire, and buried in the earth. Each time, he was brought back to life, thereby stimulating wholesale conversions, including the Empress Alexandra. The most notable legend associated with his name is the slaying of the dragon. The dragon resided near a city in Libya. On the occasion of a planned sacrifice of the local princess, George, who happened to be in the region, cut off the dragon's head and saved the princess.

The legend in which George saves the princess and slays or tames the dragon probably has an eastern European or Arabian origin and was brought to western Europe during the Crusades. It was popularized initially in the thirteenth century through *The Golden Legend,* written by Jacobus de Voragine, and was widely disseminated by the English version printed by William Caxton in the fifteenth century.

During the fourth century, veneration of George spread from Palestine throughout the Eastern Roman Empire. When it spread to the west, George was canonized in 494 by Pope Gelasius I. The cult of Saint George reached England in the twelfth century when he replaced Edward the Confessor as the patron saint of that country. Saint George is one of the Fourteen Holy Helpers.

REFERENCES 6, 9, 33, 42

193

Gerald of Mayo

MEMORIAL DAY March 13

PATRONAGE Plague

LIFE & LEGEND

Gerald, whose name has a Germanic derivation, meaning "spear ruler," was born in Northumbria in England and became a monk at Lindisfarne. After the Council of Whitby forbade the Celtic observance of Easter in Northumbria, Gerald, accompanied by many Irish and English monks and novices, withdrew to the island of Inishbofin off the coast of Mayo, where he established a new monastery. When the Irish and English monks fell to quarreling, Gerald founded another monastery for the English monks on the English mainland.

It is uncertain whether he lived in Mayo initially, although he later became abbot of this monastery in 670. He also founded the abbey of Elytheria in Connaught, Ireland, and a convent led by his sister, Segretia. Gerald, who died ca. 732, is invoked in time of plague on the basis of a legend that recounts the success of his prayers on behalf of Ireland during a murderous epidemic.

REFERENCES 6, 14, 16, 36

194

Gerard of Brogne

MEMORIAL DAY **October 3**

PATRONAGE **Fever, jaundice, scrofula**

LIFE & LEGEND

A native of Namur in present-day Belgium, Gerard, whose name has the same derivation as Gerald, was born of nobility ca. 895. He gave up a military career to pursue a monastic life. He spent 11 years in the monastery of Saint-Denis in Paris before founding a monastery on his own property at Brogne in 919. Gerard did not live in the monastery but as a recluse in a cell he built near Brogne.

Later Gerard was asked by the archbishop of Cambrai to undertake the reformation of the monastery of Saint Ghislain near Mons. He was so effective in this effort that Arnulf, count of Flanders, charged Gerard with the reformation of monasteries throughout Flanders, Lorraine, and Champagne. After 20 or more years of such work, Gerard retired to Brogne to prepare his soul for death; he died there of natural causes in 959. Kerler describes the waters of a fountain associated with Gerard in the cloister at Brogne that have been effective in miraculous cures.

REFERENCES 6, 14, 36, 42, 45, 46

195

Gerard (Gerbus, Gerio, Girio) of Lunel

MEMORIAL DAY **May 24**

PATRONAGE **Headache, epilepsy**

LIFE & LEGEND

Born into a baronial family of Lunel (between Nimes and Montpellier), Gerard, although still a minor, became a count when his family's ancestral holdings in Languedoc were ceded to the king of France in exchange for new holdings in Languedoc. When he came of age, however, Gerard renounced his worldly position and withdrew with his brother Effrenaud into the wilderness near the Pont du Gard.

When the fame of their holiness and attendant miracles attracted too many visitors, the brothers decided to make a pilgrimage to the Holy Land via Rome. After visiting the holy sites of Rome, the brothers set out for the port of Ancona. Gerard was prostrated, however, by a severe headache near present-day Potenza Picena (in the Marches, Italy), where he died in 1298. Although of French origin, the cult of San Girio was confined to the Marches and was unknown in France until the late eighteenth century.

REFERENCES 16, 36, 46

196

Gerard Majella

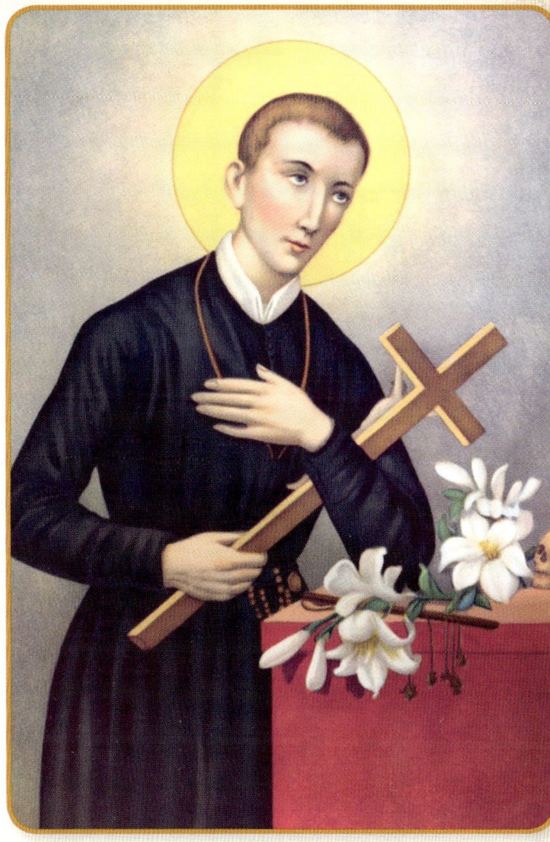

MEMORIAL DAY **October 16**

PATRONAGE **Pregnant women, unborn children, childbirth, pro-life movement, people accused falsely**

LIFE & LEGEND

Gerard, whose name has a Germanic origin and means "power of the spear," was born the son of a tailor in Muro, Italy, in April, 1725. His sister reported that, on the way to church as a young boy, he stopped in front of a statue of the Virgin Mary and the Child Jesus. The Child Jesus came down and played with Gerard, gave him a loaf of bread, and returned to the statue. Later, Gerard tried to join the Capuchin Order, but, because of poor health, he served instead as a lay brother of the Redemptorists. He was once falsely accused by a pregnant woman of being the father of her child, although she later recanted. Thus began his association with several aspects of pregnancy. He died of tuberculosis in 1755.

Gerard supposedly had the ability to be in two places at the same time (bilocation). Several miracles purportedly occurred during pregnancies in which women offered prayers to Gerard. He brought back to life a young boy who died after falling from a cliff. He blessed a small supply of wheat that consequently lasted until the next harvest, and he also walked across water to save a group of fishermen. Based on his many reported miracles, he was canonized by Pope Pius X in 1904. Saint Gerard Majella was featured on an Italian-Euro stamp in 2005.

REFERENCES 6, 10, 11

197

Gereon

MEMORIAL DAY **October 10**

PATRONAGE **Headache**

LIFE & LEGEND

In all likelihood, Gereon was the principal figure or leader of a group of martyrs who were decapitated ca. 287 for their Christian faith. Legend has long associated Gereon and his companions with the Theban Legion, a Roman legion of Egyptian origin composed largely of Christian soldiers who refused to sacrifice to the pagan gods and who were subsequently martyred en masse in the Swiss canton of Valais (see Defendens and Maurice). Some sources suggest that Gereon and his companions were a company of the Theban Legion that escaped the fate of the greater part of the legion, only to meet an identical end in Cologne. In their iconography, Gereon and his companions are always depicted in military dress. Gregory of Tours in the sixth century maintained that, in his day, there was a basilica at Cologne erected on the site where 50 martyrs of the Theban Legion met their end.

As is true of many decapitated martyrs, patronage for headache was assigned to Gereon. It is reported that the invocation of Saint Gereon cured a bishop of Cologne of this chronic malady as early as the fifth century.

REFERENCES 36, 46

198

Germanus of Auxerre

MEMORIAL DAY **July 31**

PATRONAGE **Diarrhea, mental illnesses, rabies**

LIFE & LEGEND

Germanus was born in Autesiodorum (modern Auxerre). His parents, Rusticus and Germanilla, may have belonged to the senatorial order. They were propertied and could afford to provide their son the best education available in Arles and Lyons, and were able to send Germanus to Rome to study civil law. It is uncertain how long Germanus practiced in Rome before returning to Autesiodorum and his native province as governor.

He initially led a worldly life that included hunting. He hung his trophies on a tree that had been the object of worship by pagans. This led the bishop, Amator, to cut down the tree and burn the trophies. Germanus intended to kill Amator, who, however, convinced Germanus to become a priest.

When Amator died in 418, the clergy, nobility, and people acclaimed Germanus as their choice for bishop. On his appointment to the episcopate, Germanus radically changed his manner of life. He distributed his wealth to the poor, embraced an ascetic life, and lived with his wife, Eustachia, as if she were his sister. Germanus greatly extended the monastic presence in Gaul, including the foundation of a monastery on the bank of the Yonne named in honor of Saints Cosmas and Damian.

Germanus converted and trained Saint Camilla. In 429, Germanus was sent to Britain with Saint Lupus, bishop of Troyes, by Pope Celestine I to combat the heresy of the British monk, Pelagius. He met Saint Genevieve en route when she was a young child. He was largely successful in his mission, although he had to return to Britain on a second occasion in 445. When he learned that the Roman general Aetius was threatening to send an army of barbarian Alani (a Germanic people who had crossed the Rhine into the border provinces of Gaul) to suppress a revolt in Armorica, Germanus hastened to Ravenna to dissuade Emperor Valentinian III from pursuing this course.

Germanus died in 448 while in Ravenna. His body was returned to Autesiodorum, where it was buried in the oratory of Saint Maurice. This oratory was later replaced by the church named in his honor (Saint Germain). The cult of Germanus spread well beyond the confines of his native province throughout France and England.

REFERENCES 14, 36, 42, 45, 46

199

Germanus (Germain) of Montfort

MEMORIAL DAY **October 29**

PATRONAGE **Sick children**

LIFE & LEGEND

An eleventh-century native of Montfort near Mechelen (Malines) in present-day Belgium, Germanus was educated in Paris and became tutor to the future Saint Bernard of Montjoux. Germanus was later elected prior of the monastic community at Talloires on Lake Annecy (Haute-Savoie), where he lived a life of exceptional holiness for 40 years.

REFERENCES 16, 36, 46

200

Germanus of Paris

MEMORIAL DAY **May 28**

PATRONAGE **Fever**

LIFE & LEGEND

Born in 496 to a noble family of Burgundy (in Autun), Germanus was raised and educated by an uncle because of the perfidy of the child's parents. He was ordained by Saint Agrippinus, the bishop of Autun, and 3 years later he was made abbot of the monastery of Saint Symphorien outside the city.

Germanus' reputation for holiness and for working miracles was the motive for King Childebert I to put the abbot's name forward for the vacated see of Paris. Germanus was consecrated bishop of Paris in 554. He was renowned for his great charity, for his evangelization of pagan unbelievers, and for his courage in making known to the court its many moral failings. Childebert was greatly taken with Germanus, especially after he was cured of a fatal illness through the saint's intercession. Germanus was unsuccessful, however, in his attempt to end the fratricidal struggles of the royal family.

After his death in 576, Germanus was buried in the monastery church of Saint Vincent founded by Childebert. This church was later renamed Saint-Germain-de-Prés, and for several generations was the burial place of the royal family.

REFERENCES 6, 16, 36, 46

201

Germanus of Scotland (Germain d'Ecosse)

MEMORIAL DAY **May 2**

PATRONAGE **Fever**

LIFE & LEGEND

The son of a Scottish nobleman, Germanus was converted and baptized (receiving a new name) during the fifth century by Saint Germanus of Auxerre, who had been sent to Britain by Pope Celestin I to combat the Pelagian heresy. The newly named Germanus renounced the position and honors of a noble birth to begin a life of missionary activity that took him to Gaul. On landing on its shores, Germanus is said to have confronted a seven-headed dragon that had been terrorizing the region. Germanus lassoed the beast with his stole and dragged it into a cistern. Hundreds of those who witnessed the event were immediately converted.

Germanus spent several months evangelizing in what is now Normandy before moving on to the city of Treves, where he was consecrated a bishop, but without a diocese. Germanus made a pilgrimage to Rome and returned to Scotland through Spain (where orthodox Christians were under persecution from the Arian Goths). He then returned to Gaul, evangelizing in Bayeux, Amiens, and Rouen. Near Rouen, a stronghold of paganism, Germanus was seized and beheaded for his faith. He was buried, and a church was erected in his honor where the village of Saint Germain sur Bresle (Somme) now stands.

REFERENCES 16, 36

202
Germer

MEMORIAL DAY **September 24**

PATRONAGE **Fever**

LIFE & LEGEND

Germer was a Frankish nobleman of Beauvais attached to the court of Dagobert I. He was married to a woman named Domana, by whom he had a son (Amalbert) and two daughters (who predeceased him). When Amalbert came of age, Germer and Domana agreed to separate and enter the religious life. Germer embraced the monastic life at Pentale on the Risle River, at a monastery he had established while still a layman.

After he was made abbot, there was dissatisfaction on the part of monks who objected to the strictness of Germer's rule, and an attempt was even made on his life. Germer left Pentale and withdrew into solitude along the banks of the river. When Germer was informed of the death of his son Amalbert (ca. 655), he took the wealth that reverted to him and founded the monastery at Flay, of which he was abbot and where he died ca. 658.

REFERENCES 6, 14, 36

203

Gertrude of Nivelles

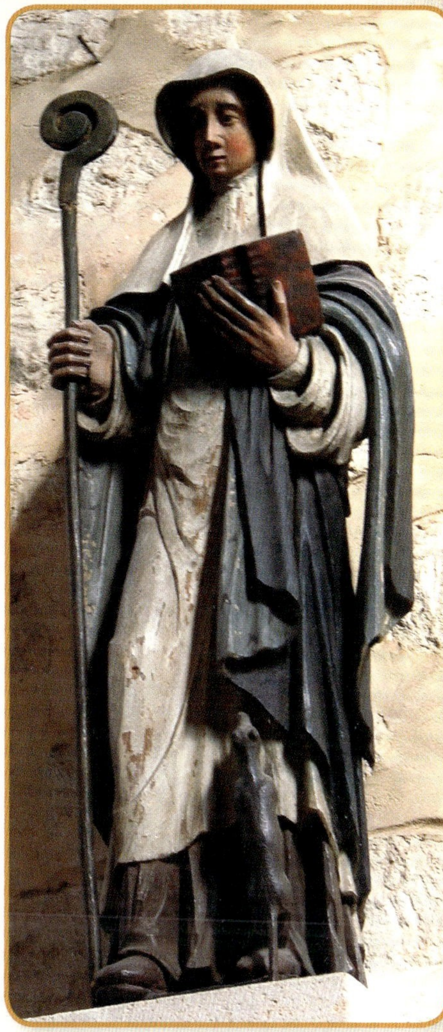

MEMORIAL DAY **March 17**

PATRONAGE **Fever**

LIFE & LEGEND

Gertrude, whose name has a Germanic derivation, meaning "strength of a spear," was born in 626, the younger daughter of Blessed Pepin of Landen, Prince of Brabant, and Blessed Itta (Ida or Iduberge). Gertrude's early dedication to the faith was made evident when King Dagobert requested that Pepin give Gertrude in marriage to the son of one of his nobles. On being asked by Dagobert what she thought of being engaged to such a handsome young man, Gertrude responded that she would have no lord or master other than Jesus Christ. The matter was not pursued.

After Pepin died in 639, Itta consulted the bishop of Maestricht to determine how she and her daughter could best serve God, and she was instructed to build a monastery at Nivelles. Itta placed her young daughter, already renowned for the strictness and holiness of her life, in the position of abbess. Itta died in the monastery she founded in 652. Gertrude remained abbess for 7 more years, resigning in 659 to devote herself wholely to prayer, an ascetic life, and the study of Scripture. She died at the age of 33.

Gertrude is best known as a patron saint of travelers, in part from her hospitality to travelers and pilgrims who passed through Nivelles. Water from the crypt in which Gertrude lay buried was regarded as effective for curing fever. The cult of Saint Gertrude spread throughout the Low Countries and England. Offerings at her shrine in Cologne continued into the nineteenth century.

She once protected some subjects against a threatening sea monster on a sea journey to distant lands. During the Middle Ages, sea travelers drank a toast that invoked her name, "Sainte Geerts Minne," before embarking.

REFERENCES 6, 14, 16, 36, 42, 45

204

Gervasius of Milan

MEMORIAL DAY **June 19**

PATRONAGE **Colic, epilepsy, hemorrhage, foot deformity, incontinence in children**

LIFE & LEGEND

In the calendar of the Roman Catholic Church, the feast of Gervasius is celebrated with that of his brother Protasius. The brothers entered the church calendar with the discovery of their remains in 386 by Saint Ambrose of Milan, who placed their relics under the altar of the cathedral he was building (later named in memory of Ambrose).

Although an anonymous legend dating from the late classical period provides many fictive details of the lives of Gervasius and Protasius, our actual knowledge of them is limited to their martyrdom during either the persecutions of the third century (under Decius or Valerian) or the persecution of Diocletian (early fourth century). Du Broc de Segange writes that there is "at Jarnages [in the Limousin region of France], a fountain known as the fountain of Saint Gervais. On the saint's feast day, a crowd of pilgrims drawn from all over—but principally from Berry—come devotedly to drink of and carry away this water endowed with the power of healing the colic and attacks of epilepsy."

REFERENCES 16, 36, 46

205 Gibrian

MEMORIAL DAY **May 7**

PATRONAGE **Lameness, children's diseases**

LIFE & LEGEND

Gibrian left his native Ireland with his six younger brothers and three younger sisters to seek a distant place in which to better serve God. The 10 siblings became solitaries in the forests of Châlons-sur-Marne. Solitude could not mask Gibrian's holiness, and an oratory was built over his grave after his death ca. 515. Many miracles occurred at this place until the oratory was destroyed by Norman marauders. His relics had earlier been moved to the cathedral at Reims, where they remained until scattered during the French Revolution. Many of his siblings also have been canonized.

REFERENCES 6, 14, 16, 36

206

Gilbert of Meaux

MEMORIAL DAY **February 13**

PATRONAGE **Dropsy**

LIFE & LEGEND

A native of Ham (Somme), Gilbert, whose name is derived from German, meaning "bright oath," began his ecclesiastic career as a canon in Saint Quintin. He was elevated to the position of archdeacon by Archanrad, bishop of Meaux, and succeeded him in that office in 995 after the latter's death. Gilbert died in 1015 and was buried in the cathedral at Meaux, where many miracles occurred at his tomb.

REFERENCES 16, 36

207

Gilbert of Neufontaines

MEMORIAL DAY **June 7**

PATRONAGE **Infertility, difficulty nursing**

LIFE & LEGEND

Born into a noble family of Brout-Vernet (Allier), Gilbert took up the cross and accompanied King Louis VII to the Holy Land ca. 1146. His experiences as a crusader left Gilbert thoroughly disillusioned with the world, and on his return to France he convinced his wife Petronille to separate so that they might both embrace the monastic life. Gilbert founded a convent at Brout-Vernet that his wife and daughter both entered and in which they successively served as abbesses. He then established a house for lepers and a monastery at Neufontaines (Auvergne), of which he was abbot. Gilbert died ca. 1152 and was buried at Neufontaines. His tomb was the site of pilgrimages.

REFERENCES 11, 16, 36

208
Gildas

MEMORIAL DAY **January 29**

PATRONAGE **Rabies**

LIFE & LEGEND

Born ca. 516 in the lower valley of the River Clyde in Scotland, Gildas, whose name is derived from Welsh, meaning "servant of God," lived the peripatetic life common to many Celtic monks of the period. Early in his career he lived as a hermit in Llanilltud (Wales). He moved to Ireland to study and devote himself to the faith. He founded churches there and evangelized in Britain.

He lived on an island in the Bristow Channel, where he may have written *De Excidio Britanniae,* a scathing denunciation of the moral evils prevalent among the British clergy and laity. Gildas spent the last years of his life in Brittany on the island of Rhuys in Morbihan Bay. He is among the earliest British historians, and his works were used by Bede. He died ca. 570 at Houat, Brittany.

REFERENCES 1, 6, 14, 16, 36

209
Giles

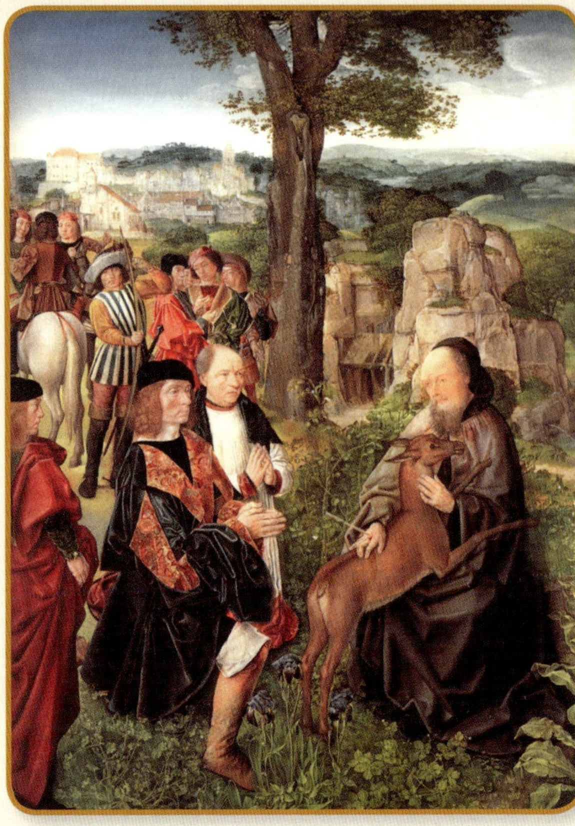

MEMORIAL DAY **September 1**

PATRONAGE **Disabled people, breastfeeding, breast cancer, epilepsy, leprosy, plague, noctiphobia, nightmares, panic, mental illness, beggars, blacksmiths, Edinburgh (Scotland)**

LIFE & LEGEND

Giles, whose name is derived from Greek, meaning "shield," was born into a wealthy Greek family during the seventh century. Some believe that he was the son of King Theodore and Queen Pelagia of Athens. He gained attention and a large following as a miracle worker. Because he sought a reclusive life, he left Greece for France, where he settled as a hermit in a cave near Nimes.

Legend indicates that God sent him a doe to nourish him with her milk. A member of a royal hunting party inadvertently hit Giles in the leg with an arrow, crippling him, but Giles continued to prophesy and perform miracles. The French king built a monastery near present-day Saint-Gilles-du-Gard for Giles' followers, and Giles was the first abbot. It was a destination of pilgrimages and later became a Benedictine house. Giles died ca. 710 in France and is the only one of the Fourteen Holy Helpers who was not a martyr. Saint Giles is the patron saint of Edinburgh, where the cathedral bears his name.

REFERENCES 6, 9, 33, 42, 45

210

Gislenus (Ghislain)

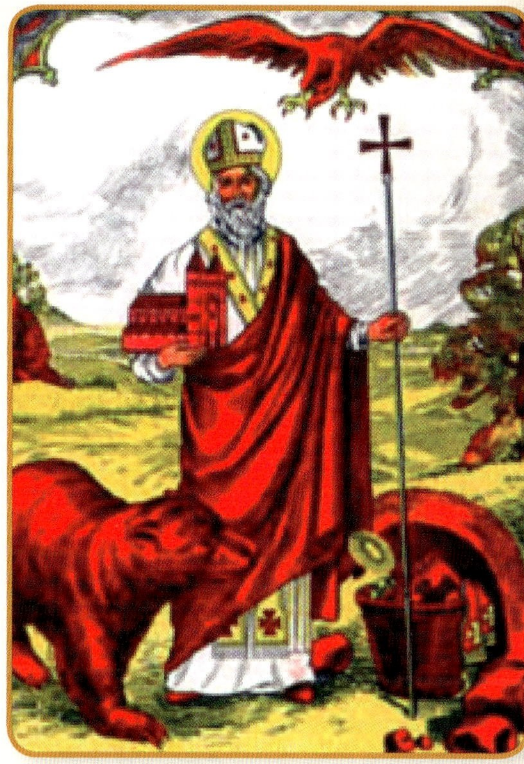

MEMORIAL DAY **October 9**

PATRONAGE **Pregnancy, childbirth, convulsive disorders, epilepsy, children's diseases**

LIFE & LEGEND

Gislenus was a Greek monk who had been bishop of Athens before resigning his see to venerate the tombs of the apostles Peter and Paul in Rome. While in the Eternal City, Gislenus was invited by the pope to journey with two companions to the Hainaut region of modern-day Belgium. Butler maintains that Gislenus was a Frank and that he lived in a forest of Hainaut before founding a monastery there in honor of Saints Peter and Paul (now known as Saint-Ghislain, near Mons). Gislenus also had a profound influence on several noblewomen of the region, each of whom subsequently founded a convent.

When Gislenus was a guest at a household in Roisin, his host's wife was suddenly seized with a difficult labor. When implored by his host for prayers, Gislenus handed the man his own belt and told him to put it around his wife. The delivery proceeded without further difficulty. Gislenus, who died ca. 680, was the spiritual teacher of Saint Waltrude.

REFERENCES 14, 36, 46

211

Giuseppe Moscati

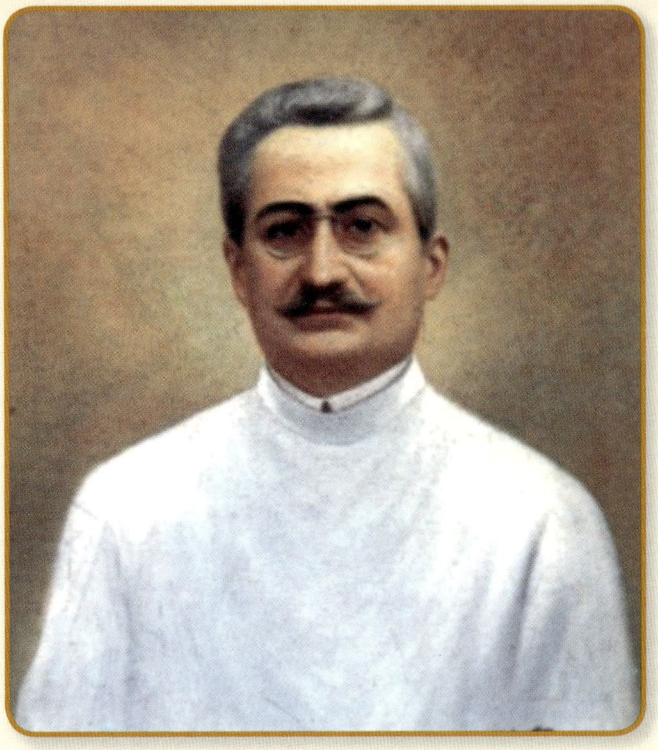

MEMORIAL DAY **November 16**

PATRONAGE **Leukemia, [physicians]***

LIFE & LEGEND

Giuseppe Moscati was born in 1880, the sixth of nine children in a noble Beneventene family near Avellino, Italy. He received his doctorate in medicine from the University of Naples in 1903. He practiced medicine at the Hospital for Incurables in Naples and taught medicine at the university. He became a hospital administrator while he continued to care for patients. He participated in the care of patients after Mount Vesuvius erupted in 1906 and during a cholera epidemic in 1911. He received a doctorate in physiological chemistry and conducted research at the Institute of Anatomical Pathology.

He remained true to his faith and attended mass daily. He was considered a miracle worker during his life, and this reputation continued after his death in 1927. He was beatified in 1975, and, after the invocation of his name was accepted as a miraculous cure in a case of leukemia, he was canonized by Pope John Paul II in 1987.

*Proposed patronage

REFERENCES 20, 38

212
Gobrianus

MEMORIAL DAY **November 3**

PATRONAGE **Gout**

LIFE & LEGEND

Gobrianus was a bishop of Vannes (Morbihan) early in the eighth century. He retired from that position when he was 87 and became a hermit. He died of natural causes ca. 725.

REFERENCE 36

213
Godeberta

MEMORIAL DAY **April 11**

PATRONAGE **Plague, epidemic diseases, contagious diseases**

LIFE & LEGEND

Although she was intended by her family for marriage, Godeberta, a native of Amiens, wanted to become a nun. She was eventually allowed to enter the religious life through the intervention of Saint Eligius, bishop of Noyon. After her parents acquiesced, King Clotaire III gave Godeberta a house in Noyon for the establishment of a convent under her direction.

The holiness of the lives led by Godeberta and her fellow nuns was influential in the Christianization of a region that still had a predominantly pagan population in the late seventh century. When an epidemic struck Noyon, Godeberta convinced the local clergy to proclaim 3 days of penitence and fasting; the plague subsided. Godeberta died ca. 700.

REFERENCES 6, 16, 36

214

Godehard (Gothard)

MEMORIAL DAY **May 4**

PATRONAGE **Urinary bladder stones, calculi**

LIFE & LEGEND

Born at Reichersdorf in Bavaria, Godehard received a clerical education and came to the attention of the local hierarchy. He was taken to Rome by Archbishop Frederick of Salzburg, who made him a canon at age 19. In 990, Godehard was made abbot of the recently restored Benedictine abbey at Niederaltaich. He performed with such zeal and efficiency that Henry, duke of Bavaria, charged Godehard with the reformation of other monasteries in his territories.

At the death of the bishop of Hildesheim in 1022, Henry, by then crowned emperor, nominated Godehard to the vacant episcopal throne. Despite his age and protestations, Godehard was consecrated. He built and restored churches, and did much to foster education, especially in the cathedral school. Godehard established such strict order in his chapter that it resembled a monastery. On a swampy piece of land that he reclaimed on the outskirts of Hildesheim, he built a hospice where the sick and poor were cared for. Godehard died of natural causes in 1038 and was canonized in 1131 by Pope Innocent II. The celebrated Pass of Saint Gothard takes its name from a chapel built on its summit by the dukes of Bavaria that was dedicated to the prelate of Hildesheim.

REFERENCES 14, 25, 36

215

Godeleva (Godelina)

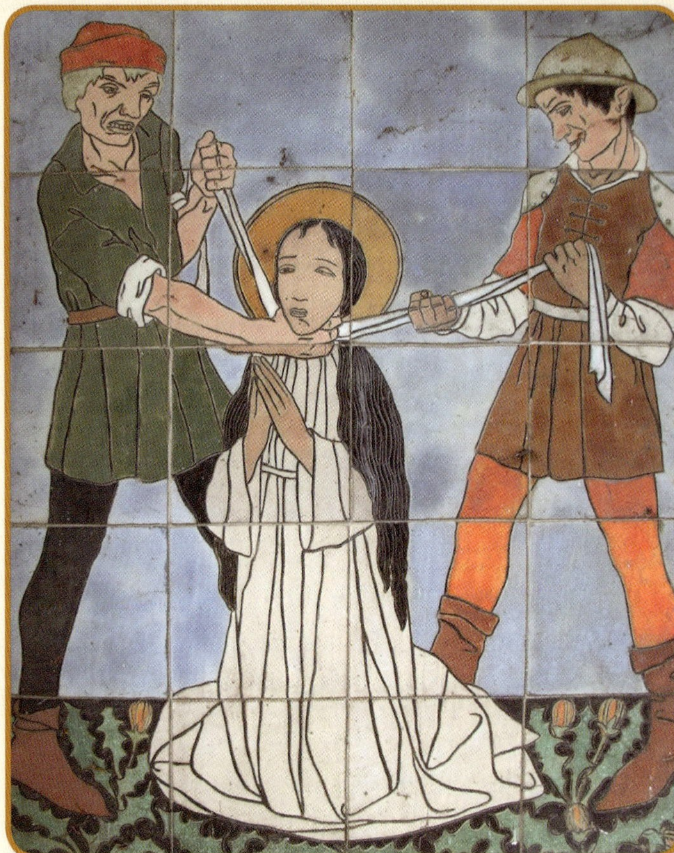

MEMORIAL DAY **July 6**

PATRONAGE **Sore throat, fever, blindness, unhappy marriage**

LIFE & LEGEND

Godeleva was born in 1049 at Londefort-lez-Boulogne, the daughter of Hemfried, a nobleman of Wierre-Effroy. She was married at 18 to a Flemish nobleman named Bertulf of Ghistelles. She was deserted by her husband on her wedding day or soon after and was left in the care of his mother, who treated her cruelly because she had other plans for her son's marriage and was furious that he had married a Londefort-lez-Boulogne woman. Godeleva was locked in a cell, starved, and subjected to assorted physical and mental abuse.

Godeleva eventually fled and returned to her parents, who complained about the treatment of their daughter to the count of Flanders and the bishop of Tournai. Bertulf was compelled to take Godeleva back but continued to alternately ignore her or treat her poorly. Ultimately, Bertulf ordered two servants to strangle Godeleva on July 6, 1070. Her body was dumped into a well, or, according to another account, it was made to appear that Godeleva had died of natural causes. In either case, Bertulf, who made certain that he was in Bruges at the time of the murder, was never publicly incriminated.

Although she was a pious and charitable young woman, Godeleva was never known for a life of unusual holiness, nor was she martyred for her faith. Nonetheless, miracles were soon reported at the place where she was buried. Among those cured by her intercession was one of Bertulf's daughters by his second marriage, who was born blind. Later repenting of the crime he had committed against Godeleva, Bertulf made a pilgrimage to Rome and then to the Holy Land. On his return he entered a monastery in Bergues.

In 1084, Godeleva's remains were exhumed and placed within the church. Many people were healed of sore throats and of fevers after drinking water from a nearby well. That well, according to some, was the well down which her body had been thrown after her murder.

REFERENCES 6, 14, 36, 45, 46

216

Godfrey of Le Mans

MEMORIAL DAY **August 3**

PATRONAGE **Fever**

LIFE & LEGEND

A native of Treves, Godfrey, whose name means "God's peace," was chosen bishop of Le Mans in 1254. A man of great charity, he completed construction of the cathedral at Le Mans and founded a Carthusian monastery at Parc d'Orques. Godfrey died at Anagni (Lazio), south of Rome, during a visit to Pope Alexander IV.

REFERENCE 36

217
Godo

MEMORIAL DAY **May 26**

PATRONAGE **Plague, epidemics**

LIFE & LEGEND

Godo belonged to a notable family of Verdun. He was the nephew of Saint Wandrille, who had fled the court of King Dagobert for a life of prayer in the monastery of Saint Romain in the Jura. Godo spent several years with his uncle before founding a monastery near Rouen, which grew rapidly. To accommodate the increasing number of men entering his monastery, Godo founded satellite hermitages near Sezanne (Sezaune en Brie). Soon after his arrival, the area was struck by an epidemic. Godo provided spiritual comfort to the afflicted, and through his prayers the epidemic ceased. He died ca. 690. His name was continually invoked, especially by the inhabitants of Langres, in times of plague and epidemic disease.

REFERENCES 16, 36

218
Gratus

MEMORIAL DAY **October 16**

PATRONAGE **Headache, mental disorders**

LIFE & LEGEND

Gratus was a Roman martyr who was sent with a companion to evangelize in Gaul—specifically in Rouergue, a former province of France bounded on the north and south by Auvergne and Languedoc. Gratus and his companion settled at Capdenac, where they were often visited by the sick who sought miraculous relief of their diseases. Eventually they were seized by angry peasants who beheaded both men ca. 316. Gratus is venerated particularly in the diocese of Rhodez.

REFERENCES 16, 36

219

Gregory of Armenia

MEMORIAL DAY **March 16**

PATRONAGE **Toothache**

LIFE & LEGEND

Gregory, whose name is derived from Greek, meaning "watcher," entered a monastery in Nicopolis in Armenia. There he attracted the attention of the bishop, who ordained Gregory into the priesthood and encouraged him to preach. When the bishop died, Gregory was chosen to take his place. In his episcopal role, Gregory was known for his eloquence, his holiness, and the miraculous healing of the sick. Gregory was anxious to escape the attention he had thus gained and left Nicopolis in secret with two Greek monks. They traveled to Italy and then to France.

Gregory finally settled at Pithiviers near Orleans, where he hoped to live a hermetic life. Even here, however, Gregory's manner of life attracted much attention. For the last 7 years of his life, Gregory combined the hermetic life with the provision of spiritual counsel to those who visited him, including those seeking relief from their physical infirmities. He died ca. 1021.

REFERENCES 6, 16, 36

220
Gregory the Great

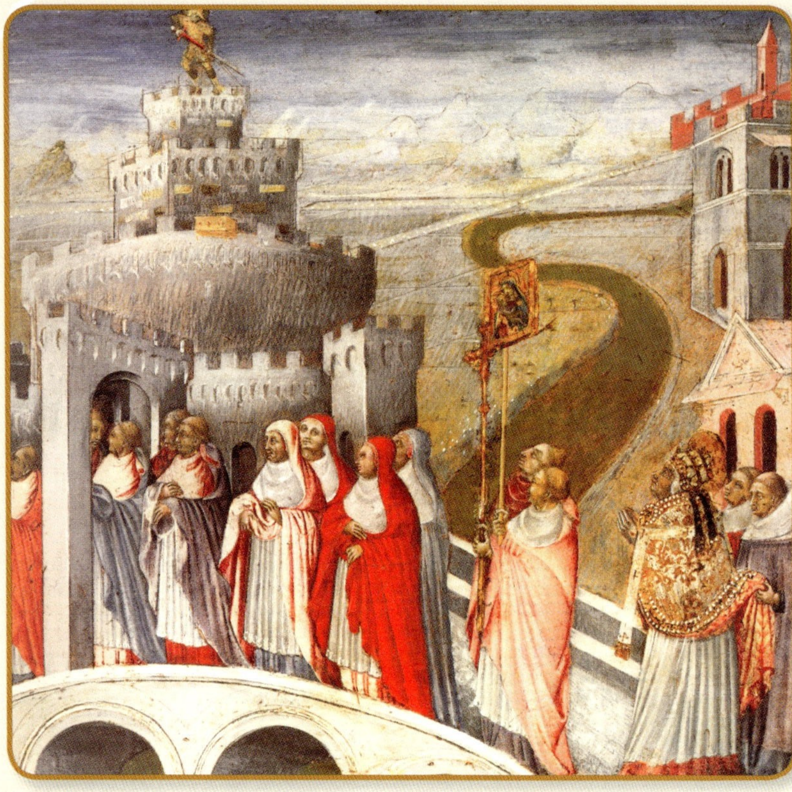

MEMORIAL DAY **September 3 (formerly March 12)**

PATRONAGE **Gout, plague, stomach disorders, popes, musicians, England**

LIFE & LEGEND

Gregory was born ca. 540 into a wealthy Roman family. His great-great grandfather had been Pope Felix III. Early in his life, Gregory was active in the political life of Rome and served as prefect, the highest civilian position. After his father died, he sold his estates and converted his suburban villa into a monastery and also built six monasteries in Sicily. He lived in the monastery in Rome for about

3 years and was elected abbot. He was drawn from a life of seclusion when he was appointed one of the seven deacons of Rome. In that capacity he was dispatched as permanent ambassador to the Court of Byzantium in Constantinople, where he served for 6 years.

He was elected pope in 590, the first pope to come from a monastic background. As pope, Gregory sent Saint Augustine of Canterbury to evangelize in England and sent other missionaries to France, Spain, and Africa. He introduced the edict of celibacy to the priesthood and is also noted for incorporating melodies and plainsong into the daily service—the so-called Gregorian chants.

Throughout his years as pope, he was afflicted with constant ill health, particularly gout, which accounts for his patronage. He was noted for his monastic personality and his charities. Gregory died on March 12, 604, and was almost immediately canonized. Artistic representations of Saint Gregory the Great often include a dove. It was said that he dictated to a secretary from behind a curtain. When the secretary would peek through the curtain, he saw that a dove had its beak between the pope's lips. The pope would only speak when the dove removed its beak.

Gregory is a Doctor of the Church and was one of the most influential popes during early medieval times. His feast day was originally March 12, the date of his death, but in 1969 it was transferred to the date of his consecration as pope (September 3) to move it out of Lent.

REFERENCES 6, 9, 33, 42, 45

221

Gregory of Utrecht

MEMORIAL DAY **August 25**

PATRONAGE **Paralysis**

LIFE & LEGEND

Born in the city of Trier ca. 707, Gregory became a disciple of Saint Boniface after hearing him expound on a passage of Scripture that he himself had just read in the convent where his grandmother was abbess. Gregory accompanied Boniface on his missionary travels through Austrasia until he was appointed abbot of the monastery of Saint Martin in Utrecht by Boniface.

Although he was never consecrated bishop, Gregory administered the diocese of Utrecht for 20 years after the martyrdom of its bishop, Eoban, in 755. Gregory was known for the zeal of his missionary work, his charity, and his spirit of forgiveness—notably in pardoning the murderers of his two half brothers. Gregory lay paralyzed on one side during the last 3 years of his life. He died ca. 775.

REFERENCES 6, 14, 36, 46

222

Guenole (Guignolet, Wennole)

MEMORIAL DAY **March 3**

PATRONAGE **Infertility**

LIFE & LEGEND

Guenole was born in Brittany of Fracan and Gwen, who had emigrated from Britain. Because he was their third son, Guenole's parents dedicated him to God. He was taken to a monastery on the small island of Laure, which was under the direction of Abbot Budoc. Guenole progressed in the monastic life and entertained the thought of continuing the missionary work of Saint Patrick in Ireland, until dissuaded in a vision by the saint himself. Instead, Budoc sent Guenole with 11 other monks to found a monastery in Brittany. For several years the community settled on an island in the mouth of the river Aulne. It later moved to Landevennec near Brest, where Guenole served as abbot until his death ca. 550.

A number of sterile couples conceived children by invoking the saint and by drinking water from his skull. In the place where his tomb once was, in a church now demolished, a spring rose. The sick came to the site over the years to seek health.

REFERENCES 6, 16, 36

223

Guibert (Wibert)

MEMORIAL DAY **May 23**

PATRONAGE **Croup**

LIFE & LEGEND

Born into an aristocratic family of Lorraine, Guibert retired from a distinguished military career to establish a hermitage on his own estates at Gembloux in Brabant in 936. Guibert did not profess monasticism at Gembloux, but left his foundation in the hands of a monk named Herluin so that he could enter the Benedictine monastery at Gorze near Metz. He took this step to avoid the respect with which he was regarded at Gembloux and the complacency he might feel in his own foundation.

Guibert's monastic serenity was soon interrupted by Emperor Otto I, who challenged Guibert's right to transfer the title of an imperial fief to the new monastery at Gembloux. Guibert was confirmed in this right, but later had to contend with his brother-in-law, the count of Namur, who had seized the revenues of Gembloux under the pretext that the estate now belonged to his wife. Once again Guibert successfully defended the rights of the monastery at Gembloux. Guibert remained at Gorze until he died in 962. Many miracles were worked at his tomb.

REFERENCES 6, 14, 36

224
Guimerra

MEMORIAL DAYS **February 13, May 15**

PATRONAGE **Eye diseases**

LIFE & LEGEND

Of humble origin, Guimerra was educated by the priests of the church of Saint Nazaire in his native Carcassonne (Aude), where he was consecrated the thirteenth bishop of Carcassonne. He died ca. 932. His cult was very popular in Carcassonne, especially in the suburb of Barbacane, where his family lived. Diseases of the eye were once common among the tanners who inhabited this district, and the name of Guimerra was often invoked for the healing of ocular disorders.

REFERENCES 16, 36

225

Gummarus (Gomer)

MEMORIAL DAY **October 11**

PATRONAGE **Fractures, hernia, impotence, unhappy marriage**

LIFE & LEGEND

Gummarus was the son of the lord of Emblem, near Lierre in Brabant. An unlettered man, he served at the court of King Pepin the Younger, who arranged a marriage for Gummarus with a well-born woman named Guinimaria. This marriage was a continuous trial for Gummarus, who did his best to reform his wife and make peace with her. After an absence of 8 years while on military service in Italy, Germany, and France, Gummarus returned to find that Guinimaria had entirely mismanaged his estate and had alienated everyone associated with its operation. Gummarus managed to settle his disordered affairs, but finding his wife as difficult as ever, determined to separate from her. He found peace as a holy recluse and founded a monastery at Lierre with the Irish monk and future saint, Rumold. He died of natural causes ca. 774.

REFERENCES 6, 14, 36

226

Gunsaldus (Goussaud)

MEMORIAL DAY **November 5**

PATRONAGE **Asthma, sore throat, goiter**

LIFE & LEGEND

Nothing is known of the early life of Gunsaldus. He became a disciple of Saint Priest, bishop of Clermont, ca. 666. After the martyrdom of Priest in 674, Gunsaldus withdrew from the world and founded a hermitage in the mountains of Limousin. He died of natural causes in 689. The village of Saint Goussaud (Creuse) took its name from this foundation.

REFERENCES 16, 36

227

Gurloes (Urlo)

MEMORIAL DAY **Unknown**

PATRONAGE **Headache, kidney diseases**

LIFE & LEGEND

In 1029, Gurloes was made the abbot of the newly founded monastery of Sainte-Croix de Quimperlé by Orscand, bishop of Nantes. Gurloes remained abbot until his death 28 years later. In his article on Breton saints, Guyotjeannin notes, "The central nave of the crypt beneath the church of Sainte-Croix de Quimperlé shelters the gothic effigy of Saint Gurloes. The very first abbot of this church, the saint was once regarded by Bretons as a healer. They would crawl on all fours through the passage beneath the tomb to obtain the cure of their kidney disorders; or, hoping to relieve their headaches, would place their heads in a cavity to be found at one end of the base."

REFERENCE 32

228

Guy of Anderlecht

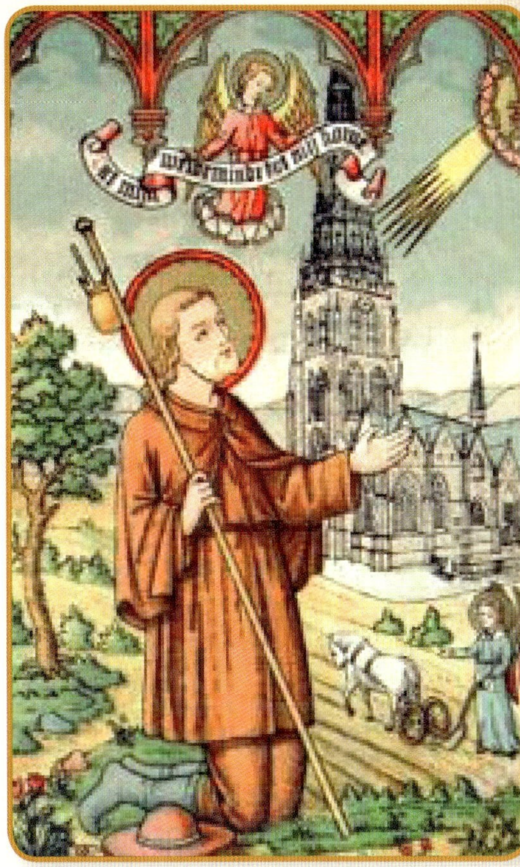

MEMORIAL DAY **September 12**

PATRONAGE **Epilepsy, rabies, dysentery, hydrophobia, workhorses, horned animals**

LIFE & LEGEND

Guy was born into poverty ca. 950 at Anderlecht, Belgium, and was known as the "poor man of Anderlecht." He worked the field while caring for the sick and poor, although he was aided in his labor by an angel. After he lost money in a get-rich-quick oceanic expedition, he took it as a sign to return to his piety and poverty. He walked to Rome as penance and on to Jerusalem, where he served as a guide for pilgrims before returning to Belgium. He died in 1012, and his grave was forgotten until it was uncovered when a workhorse kicked it. Many miracles were attributed to him after his death, and an annual festival was established around his grave.

REFERENCES 6, 9, 42

H

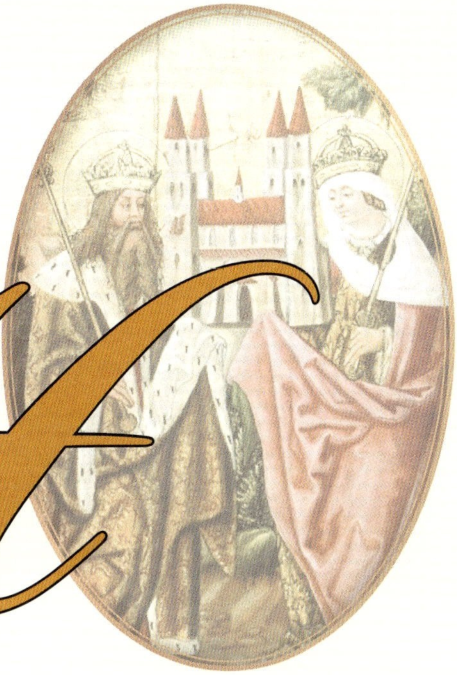

229 Haberilla

MEMORIAL DAY **January 30**

PATRONAGE **Sick children**

LIFE & LEGEND

Haberilla was a disciple of Saint Gall, who gave her the veil and who placed her in charge of a community of nuns at Bregentz on Lake Constance. After her death in the seventh century, Haberilla's remains were placed in the church of Saint Peter in Constance. Miracles were reported to have taken place at her tomb almost immediately. The parents of sick children commonly took their ailing offspring to Haberilla's tomb to pray for a cure, passing three times beneath the sepulchre that was elevated on columns.

REFERENCES 16, 18, 36

230

Hadeloga (Halloie)

MEMORIAL DAY **February 2**

PATRONAGE **Fever**

LIFE & LEGEND

Hadeloga was born into a prominent family of Schwanberg in Franconia. (Some sources make her the daughter of Charles Martel, others of King Pippin.) Hadeloga was noted for her beauty and piety. She attracted noble suitors from across Europe, but she refused them all, preferring instead a life of celibacy and prayer. Her father was angered at her obstinacy, and ordered her from his presence. With her chaplain and a handful of followers, Hadeloga built cells in a clearing in the forest, where the tiny community followed the Rule of Saint Benedict. Hearing of her manner of life in the wilderness, her father regretted his harshness and gave her lands and formally recognized the community that she headed at Kitzingen.

Immediately after her death ca. 750, Hadeloga was buried in a cave where she had often gone alone to pray. Later her remains were placed in a tomb near an altar dedicated to the Virgin. Du Broc de Segange notes, "Her first coffin having been distributed to her followers as a precious relic, those who drank water in which pieces of this coffin had been soaked . . . were healed of their fevers."

REFERENCES 16, 18, 36

231
Hartman of Brixen

MEMORIAL DAY **December 23**

PATRONAGE **Pregnancy**

LIFE & LEGEND

Hartman, whose name has a Germanic derivation, meaning "powerful hero," was born at Polling in Austria and was educated at the monastery of Saint Nicolas in Passau. His intelligence and talents resulted in his appointment to a series of ecclesiastical posts, culminating in his consecration in 1140 as bishop of Brixen (or Bressanone, Italy). He held this office for 24 years and came to be much respected by Emperors Conrad III and Alexander I, and he was always the intermediary for settling differences between the emperors and the papacy. He died in 1164.

REFERENCES 6, 14, 36

232

Henry II (Good King Henry)

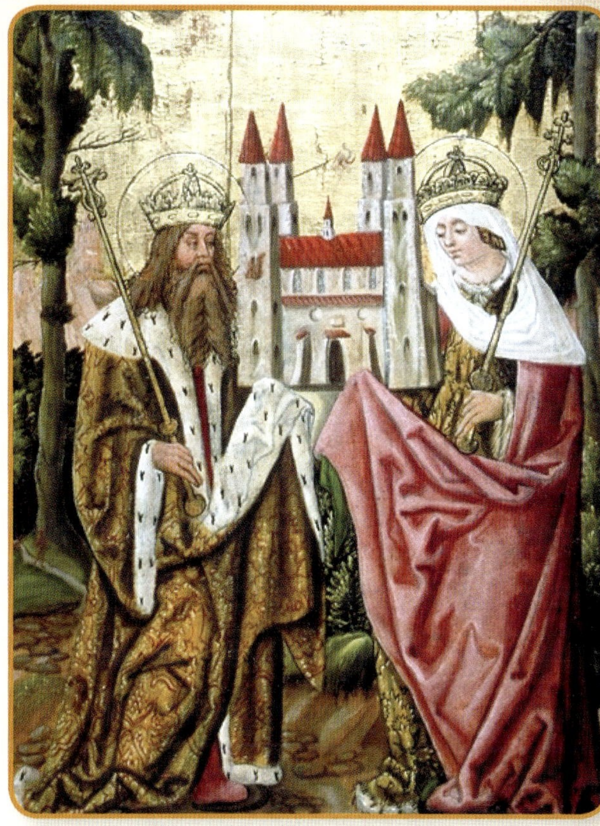

MEMORIAL DAY **July 13**

PATRONAGE **Stability, handicapped or disabled people, Basel (Switzerland)**

LIFE & LEGEND

Henry, whose name has a Germanic derivation, meaning "home ruler," was born in Bavaria in 972. He was the son of the duke of Bavaria, who was known as "the Quarrelsome," and he was educated by the bishop of Regensburg. Henry's plans to become a priest were aborted when his father died, and he became duke of Bavaria. He married Saint Cunegunda; they had no children. He eventually ascended to the throne of Germany in 1002 and was crowned Holy Roman Emperor by Pope Benedict VIII in 1014. He was the last of the Saxon emperors. He founded many schools and acted to both stabilize and reform the Church. He established Bamberg as the center for missions to Slavic countries, accounting for his statue at the entrance of the Bamberg cathedral. He also initiated the construction of the cathedral at Basel, Switzerland, and became that city's patron saint.

He was allegedly cured of an illness by the laying on of hands by Saint Benedict at Monte Cassino. Henry became lame during the latter part of his life, and this accounts for his patronage of disabled people. He died in Saxony in 1024 and was canonized in 1146 by Pope Eugene III.

REFERENCES 6, 9, 42, 45

233

Hervé (Harvey)

MEMORIAL DAY **June 17**

PATRONAGE **Eye diseases, depression**

LIFE & LEGEND

One of the most popular of the Breton saints, Hervé, whose name is derived from Old English, meaning "battle ready," was the son of a British bard named Hyvarnion, who had been attached to the court of Childebert I in Paris. Hervé was born blind at Guimiliau in Brittany, or, as contended by others, at the manor of Lanrioul near Plouzevede. Abandoned by his father in infancy, Hervé was raised until age 7 by his mother, Rivanon, who then decided to become a hermit.

Hervé was entrusted to a holy man named Arthian and later to an uncle, Urfol, who maintained a small monastic school and farmed at Plouvien. It was here that one of the most popular stories of Saint Hervé's legend is told. One day while he was plowing with the boy who had been made his guide, a wolf appeared and killed the donkey that pulled the plow. While his young guide cried out in distress, Hervé prayed to God. The wolf returned, repented, and put his neck into the harness to finish the day's plowing. Hervé is often portrayed with a wolf and used to be invoked by those threatened by wolves.

Hervé succeeded his uncle as abbot of the small monastic community at Plouvien. He later moved to Lanhouarneau, where he founded a new monastery and where he remained until his death in the sixth century. It does not appear that he was ever ordained to the priesthood, although he was often called on as an exorcist.

REFERENCES 6, 14, 16, 32

234
Hidulf

MEMORIAL DAY **July 11**

PATRONAGE **Mental disorders, plague, contagious diseases, epidemics**

LIFE & LEGEND

Hidulf was born at Regensburg in Bavaria. He entered the monastic life at Trier and was later consecrated auxiliary bishop of that city. He eventually left Trier to pursue a secluded life in the Vosges Mountains, where he founded the monastery at Moyenmoutier ca. 671-676 and served as abbot. He died ca. 707.

REFERENCES 6, 14, 36

235
Hildegund

MEMORIAL DAY **February 6**

PATRONAGE **Headache, childbirth**

LIFE & LEGEND

Hildegund was the daughter of Count Herman of Lidtberg and Countess Hedwig. She was married to Count Lothair of Meer and had three children. After his death, and following the examples of her mother and her sister, Gertrude, Hildegund entered the religious life. She made a pilgrimage to Rome in 1178, then returned to her property at Meer, north of Cologne, and converted it to a convent with the help of her son, Herman, who was a monk. She was joined at Meer by her daughter, Hedwig, and in time by many other women. She died in 1183.

REFERENCES 6, 14, 16, 36

236
Hildevert

MEMORIAL DAY **May 27**

PATRONAGE **Madness, epilepsy, scrofula, worms**

LIFE & LEGEND

The deeds of Hildevert are very obscure and much disputed. It is believed that he was born at Vers-Hébécourt in the diocese of Amiens, and that after losing his parents, he was entrusted to Saint Faro, the bishop of Meaux. The bishop was witness to Hildevert's virtues and development, and conferred on him the sacred orders of the diaconate and priesthood. After Faro's death, Hildevert was proclaimed by the clergy and the faithful to succeed him as bishop. Hildevert died ca. 680.

Whatever he may have been, the memory of his virtues and his miracles remained alive in the hearts of the people, and when his relics were transferred to Gournay, his cult spread to Paris, Rouen, Reims, Beauvais, and other locales. In all these places Saint Hildevert was invoked against folly, madness, and epilepsy. The origin of this invocation is unknown. The Bollandists are inclined to think that it may be from the similarity of the name Hildevert to the word "vertigo," a similitude that often exists between the names of saints and the maladies for which they are invoked.

REFERENCES 16, 36

237
Hiltrude

MEMORIAL DAY **September 27**

PATRONAGE **Fever**

LIFE & LEGEND

After Hiltrude refused a marriage to the count of Burgundy that had been arranged by her family, she fled her paternal home. During the flight from her father's house, Hiltrude stopped at a spring that afterward possessed the power to cure fevers. She took the veil from the bishop of Cambrai and lived as a recluse in close proximity to the Benedictine monastery founded at Liessies by her father, Wilbert, a Poitevin nobleman. Her brother was the abbot at the Liessies monastery, where Hiltrude lived for 17 years. She died in 785.

REFERENCES 16, 36, 46

238

Honoratus of Toulouse

MEMORIAL DAY **December 21**

PATRONAGE **Pregnancy, childbirth**

LIFE & LEGEND

Honoratus, who lived during the third century, succeeded Saturninus as bishop of Toulouse. Honoratus converted and consecrated Saint Firminus into the episcopate.

REFERENCES 16, 36, 46

239

Honorina of Conflans

MEMORIAL DAY **February 27**

PATRONAGE **Pregnancy, prisoners**

LIFE & LEGEND

Honorina was martyred during the reign of Diocletian at the juncture of the third and fourth centuries. One source maintains that she was martyred at Juliobona (present-day Lillebonne), another that she was martyred at Graville, and yet another that she was martyred at Coulonces. One source maintains that Honorina was burned to death and that her bones were placed in the church at present-day Graville in Normandy. Other sources indicate that after she was martyred, her body was thrown into the Seine and retrieved at Graville, where her tomb was built. During the Norman invasions in the ninth century, her remains were transferred to Conflans-Sainte-Honorine at the confluence of the Oise and Seine rivers to ensure their safety.

REFERENCES 16, 18, 36, 46

240

Hubert of Liège (Apostle of the Ardennes)

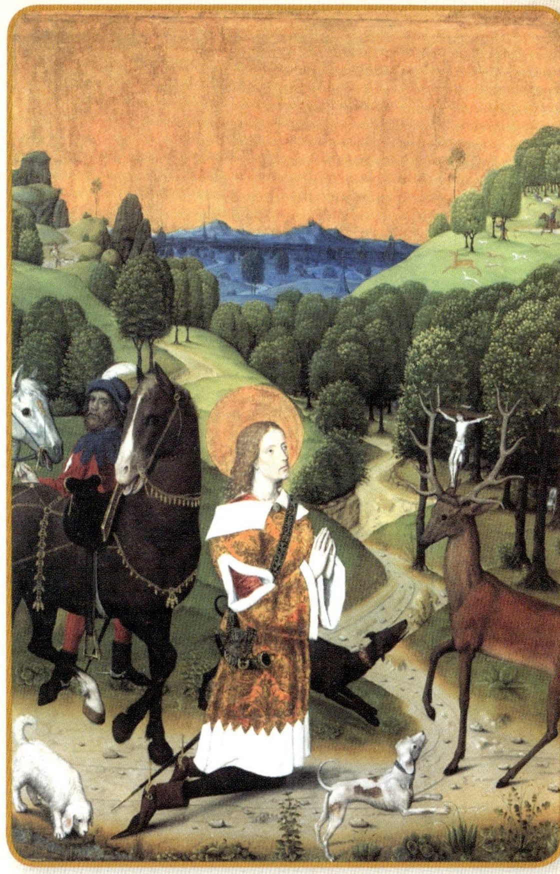

MEMORIAL DAY **November 3**

PATRONAGE **Dog bites, rabies, hydrophobia, huntsmen, forest workers, machinists, mathematicians, opticians**

LIFE & LEGEND

Hubert, whose name means "bright mind," was born ca. 656 at Maastricht, Holland, the eldest son of the Duke of Aquitaine. He emigrated to a border area between Germany and France. He withdrew from the court when his wife died in childbirth, and he devoted himself to hunting in Ardennes. While hunting on a Good Friday morning, he had a vision of a crucifix between the antlers of a deer he was pursuing and took it for a sign. A voice told him to seek out Lambert, the bishop of Maastricht, as a spiritual mentor. Hubert complied, gave up his birthright in Aquitaine, distributed his wealth to the poor, and was ordained as priest.

Early in the eighth century, Lambert was assassinated and Hubert was made bishop at Maastricht. In 720, in response to a vision, Hubert removed Saint Lambert's remains to Liège, which was a small village at the time. This act served as a foundation for its growth. Saint Lambert is honored as its patron saint, and

Saint Hubert is honored as its founder and first bishop. Hubert's son, Floribert, also later became the bishop of Liège. Hubert is particularly noted for his successful evangelism of the pagans in the Ardennes forest. He died in 727 in Brabant, Belgium, of natural causes after he had predicted the date of his death.

REFERENCES 6, 9, 42

241
Hugh (Hugo) of Cluny

MEMORIAL DAY April 29

PATRONAGE Fever

LIFE & LEGEND

Hugh, whose name has a German derivation meaning "mind, heart, spirit," was born in 1024 at Brionnais in the diocese of Autun, France. He was the eldest of the eight sons of Count Dalmatius of Semur. Against the wishes of his father, who wanted him to become a knight and assume a station befitting his noble birth, Hugh entered the monastery at Cluny, in Burgundy, at age 15 under Saint Odilo. He was ordained at 20, and in 1049 succeeded Saint Odilo as abbot.

Hugh was abbot there for 60 years, during which period Cluny attained the height of its prosperity, reputation, and influence. During Hugh's abbacy, Cluniac institutions multiplied from Italy to England and from Germany to Spain.

Hugh's influence was not confined to the monasteries under his jurisdiction. He vigorously supported Pope Leo X in his reforms against simony and clerical laxity. In 1057, he served as papal legate seeking peace between the Emperor Henry IV and King Andrew of Hungary. When the Cluniac monk, Hildebrand, was elected Pope Gregory VII, Hugh worked closely with him to continue the reforms of his predecessors. At the behest of the pope, Hugh mediated the difficulties between Gregory VII and Henry IV. He was also a principal figure in organizing the first Crusade at the Council of Clermont in 1065.

Despite his acquaintance and influence with nine popes and most of the sovereigns of Europe, Hugh remained a man of modesty, austerity, and prayer. He was a guide to both highly placed men who sought his advice and intervention in matters purely worldly, and to those who had left the world behind. Hugh is also supposed to have worked miracles during his lifetime. Several accounts survive of his healing persons suffering from febrile disease. So esteemed was Hugh by his contemporaries that he was canonized by Pope Callistus III in 1120, only 11 years after his death; he is often called Saint Hugh the Great. His relics were destroyed by Huguenots in 1575.

REFERENCES 14, 16, 36, 42, 45, 46

242
Hugh of Grenoble

MEMORIAL DAY **April 1**

PATRONAGE **Headache**

LIFE & LEGEND

A native of Chateauneuf-d'Isere, Hugh was the son of a soldier, Odilio, who became a Cistercian monk. Hugh was well educated, and while still a layman, was made a canon of the cathedral at nearby Valence at age 25. He attracted the attention of the bishop of Die, who attached the young man to his household. In 1080, Hugh accompanied the bishop to the synod held at Avignon, where disorders troubling the diocese of Grenoble were discussed. The virtues and abilities of the young canon attracted much attention, and Hugh found himself elected bishop of Grenoble at age 27, an office that he accepted with great reluctance. He was thereupon ordained to the priesthood by the papal legate, who took Hugh with him to Rome, where he was consecrated bishop by Pope Gregory VII.

Hugh served as bishop for 52 years, during which time he struggled against the problems that afflicted his diocese—specifically simony and a clerical indifference to celibacy. He tried to restore discipline among clergy and laity alike and to get the diocese back on sound financial ground. Discouraged by a seeming lacking of progress, Hugh blamed himself and withdrew to the Benedictine monastery of Chaise-Dieu until ordered to return to his bishopric by the pope.

Hugh welcomed Saint Bruno and his disciples to Grenoble and gave them the property north of the city on which the Grande Chartreuse monastery was built. Hugh often sought spiritual refuge there from the demands of his episcopal duties, while repeatedly asking the pope to relieve him of these burdens—a request that was repeatedly refused.

Hugh suffered from headaches most of his adult life and is therefore a patron saint of those similarly afflicted. He died of natural causes in 1132 and was interred in Saint Mary's Cathedral, Grenoble. His relics were destroyed by the Huguenots. So obvious was his patience, humility, obedience, and holiness that Hugh was canonized by Pope Innocent II only 2 years after his death.

REFERENCES 6, 14, 36, 46

243
Hyacinth

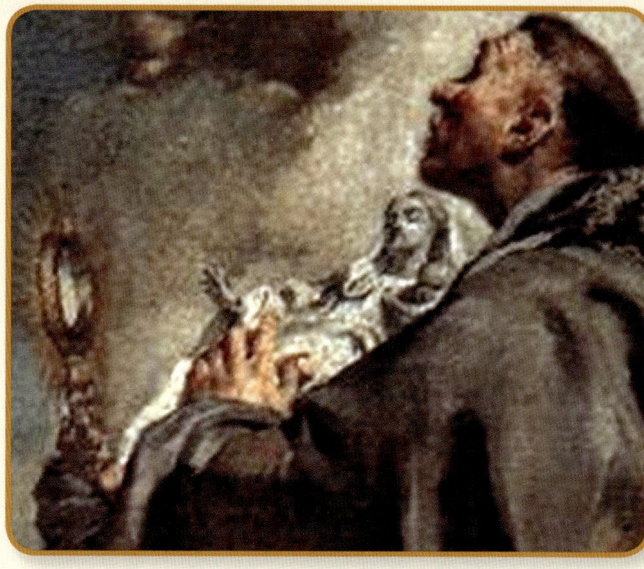

MEMORIAL DAY **August 17**

PATRONAGE **Infertility, labor**

LIFE & LEGEND

Hyacinth, whose name is derived from Greek, meaning "purple," was born into a noble family near Opole, Silesia (modern Poland), in 1185. He was educated at Krakow, Prague, Paris, and Bologna, and he received a Doctorate of Canon Law and Divinity. As a priest, he accompanied his uncle, Bishop Ivo Konski of Krakow, to Rome, where he joined the nascent Dominican Order after witnessing a miracle performed there by Saint Dominic de Guzman. Hyacinth was then dispatched to Silesia, from where he evangelized those in a geographic area that included Scandinavia, Poland, Lithuania, and Muscovy.

Hyacinth was the first Polish Dominican and brought the order to Poland. A legend indicates that during a Tartarian attack on a monastery in Kiev, he saved a crucifix and a statue of Mary despite the excessive weight of the statue. Hyacinth died of natural causes in Krakow in 1257, and his relics were translated to Paris. He was canonized by Pope Clement VIII in 1594.

REFERENCES 14, 16, 36, 42, 45

I

244

Ida of Nivelle

MEMORIAL DAY **December 16**

PATRONAGE **Toothache**

LIFE & LEGEND

Ida, whose name is derived from German, meaning "work," probably was born at Nivelle and entered the Cistercian convent of Ramey in Brabant, Belgium, at an early age. She was noted for her extraordinary asceticism and mystical gifts, and she is said to have received the five wounds of Christ. She died at age 32 of natural causes in 652. One of her teeth is enclosed in a container and preserved at her convent. It provides cures for maladies of the teeth by contact with it. Du Broc de Segange and Kerler place her in the thirteenth century.

REFERENCES 16, 18, 36, 45

245

Ignatius of Antioch

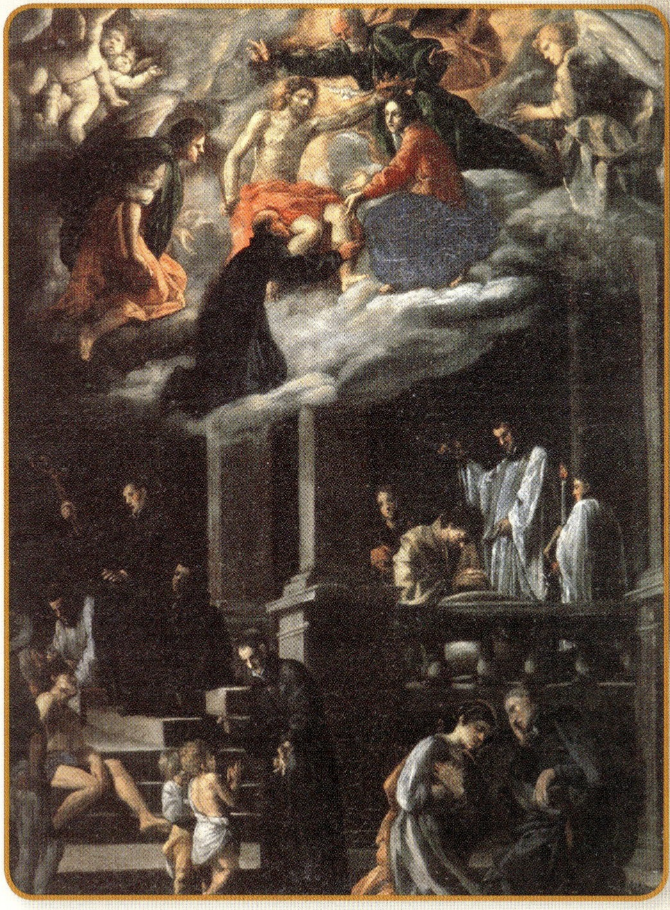

MEMORIAL DAY **October 17 (formerly February 1)**

PATRONAGE **Throat diseases, tinea**

LIFE & LEGEND

Ignatius, whose name is derived from Latin, meaning "fiery," converted from paganism to Christianity and succeeded Saint Peter the Apostle as bishop of Antioch in Syria. He was ordered to Rome during the persecution of Trajan, and on the way he wrote a series of letters to the churches for which he had responsibility. Those writings contain the first use of the term "Catholic Church." He was thrown to the lions in the arena at Rome ca. 107. His relics are preserved at Saint Peter's Basilica in Rome.

REFERENCES 6, 33, 42, 45

246

Inventus (Trouvé, Trobat)

MEMORIAL DAY **January 22**

PATRONAGE **Fever (malarial/quartan)**

LIFE & LEGEND

Inventus was martyred with 360 other Christians at Gerunda (present-day Girona in northeastern Spain) during the persecutions of Diocletian and Maximian during the late fourth or early fifth century.

REFERENCES 16, 36

247

Isberga (Giselle)

MEMORIAL DAY **May 21**

PATRONAGE **Fever, skin diseases, deformity**

LIFE & LEGEND

Isberga was a daughter of Pepin the Short and sister of Charlemagne. Under the spiritual direction of the hermit and future saint, Venant, Isberga developed an early inclination for a life of solitude and prayer. Because she was an attractive young woman from a notable family, both the emperor in Constantinople and the son of the English king sought to marry her, the second of whom came to the court of her father in person to win her hand. She prayed that God would remove her physical charms and was ravaged by a fever and skin disease that completely disfigured her face. The English prince departed and was imputed in the later murder of Venant. Isberga was healed of her malady, including its deforming effects, and after the death of her father was sought in marriage by the king of the Lombards. To put an end to these proposals, Isberga founded a convent at Aire into which she withdrew and where she lived for 30 years and died ca. 806.

REFERENCES 16, 36

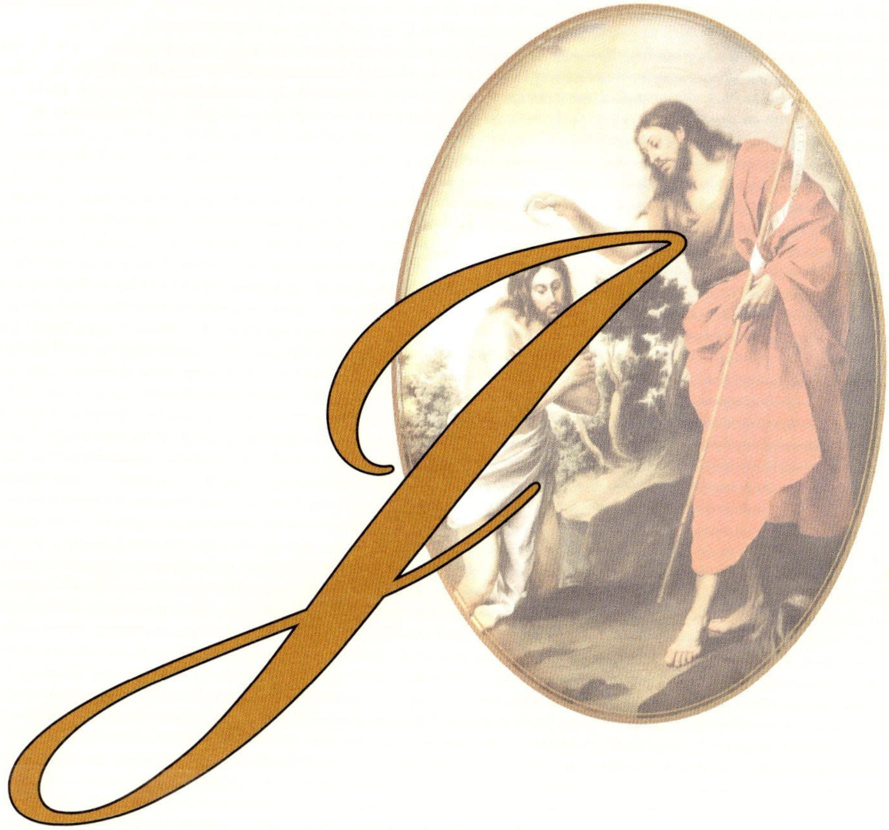

248

James the Greater

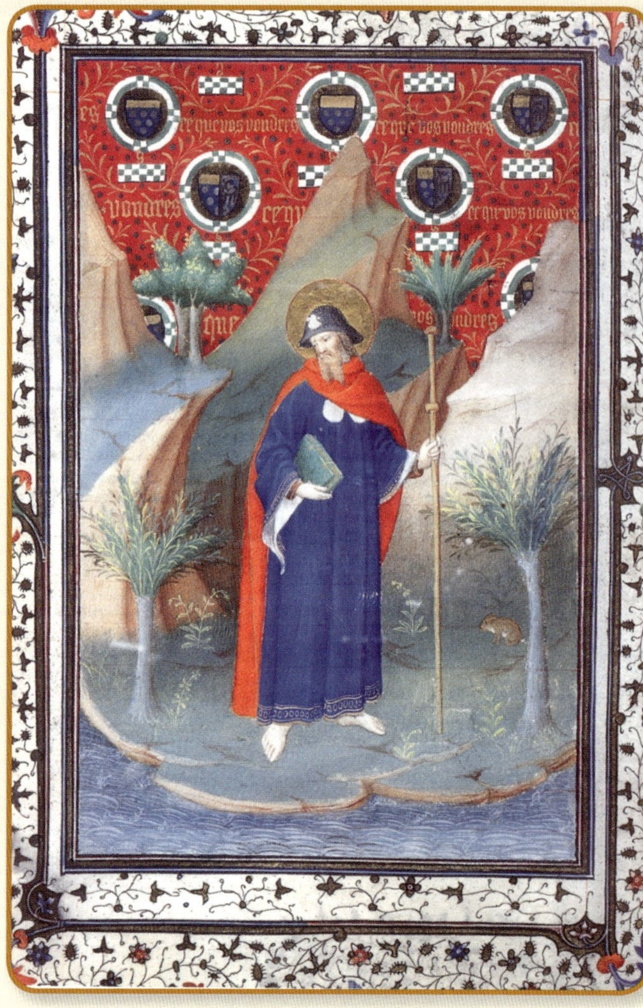

MEMORIAL DAY **July 25 (formerly August 5)**

PATRONAGE **Arthritis, rheumatism, pharmacists, Spain, Guatemala, Nicaragua, many cities**

LIFE & LEGEND

The name James has a Hebrew derivation, meaning "supplanter." James the Greater is distinguished from James the Lesser, because the former became an Apostle before the latter. James the Greater was the son of Zebedee and Salome, and the brother of Saint John the Apostle. He witnessed most of Christ's recorded miracles and preached in Sumaria, Judea, and Spain. He was the first Apostle to be martyred when he was stabbed by King Herod Agrippa I in 44 at Jerusalem.

James is particularly revered in Spain, where he was known as Santiago. One of the many legends associated with him is that he brought back to life a boy who had been dead for 5 weeks. When the boy's father was informed at the dinner table, he said that his returned son was no more alive than the fowl on the table—at which point, the cooked bird sprouted feathers and flew away. James the Greater's relics are preserved at Compostela, Spain.

REFERENCES 9, 33, 45

249

Jean François Régis

MEMORIAL DAY **June 6**

PATRONAGE **Infertility, fractured legs, medical social workers, lacemakers**

LIFE & LEGEND

Born in 1597 at Fontcouverte in the Aude to a recently ennobled family of Languedoc, Jean François received his education at the Jesuit college of Beziers. He entered the Jesuit novitiate at Toulouse in 1616 and subsequently taught at several Jesuit colleges while continuing his studies in philosophy. Jean François began his theological studies at Toulouse in 1628 and was ordained to the priesthood in 1630. His great desire was to save souls and to preach salvation to the most endangered elements of society. He faithfully attended those afflicted by the plague that visited Toulouse in 1632, and, from 1632 to 1634, he lived in Montpellier where he preached, taught, established a home for former prostitutes, and set up workshops where young women could make their living in lacemaking. From 1633 until his death, Jean François traveled, preached, and worked tirelessly with the poor of the Vivarais, Forez, and Velay regions of France. He died at Louvesc, a village in the mountains of Ardèche in December, 1640.

REFERENCES 16, 36

250

Jeanne Françoise de Chantal

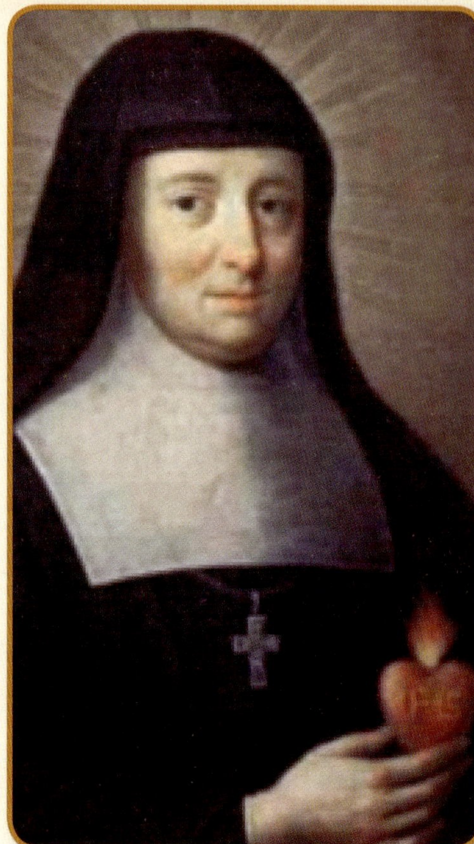

MEMORIAL DAY **August 21**

PATRONAGE **Childbirth**

LIFE & LEGEND

Jeanne was born in 1572, the daughter of Bénigne Frémyot, president of the parliament of Burgundy. She was married at age 20 to Christophe de Rabutin, the Baron de Chantal and an officer in the French army. For 9 years she lived with her husband on their estate at Bourbilly, where she bore seven children; the first three died soon after birth. Jeanne was widowed when her husband died of injuries from a hunting accident. Much grieved by her loss, Jeanne sought a spiritual advisor who might direct her in her life. At this time she went to live with her rather difficult father-in-law at his chateau near Autun. While visiting her own father in Dijon during Lent of 1604, Jeanne heard the famous preacher and future saint, Francis de Sales. Although she had never met him before, Jeanne immediately recognized Francis as the director promised her in an earlier vision. Although Francis was a frequent dinner guest in her father's house, Jeanne was initially reluctant to seek his advice. Eventually she came under his spiritual direction, learning to accommodate a life of strict prayer and extensive charity to her responsibilities in the world as a mother and the daughter of an aging father.

She became attracted to the life of the Carmelite nuns in Dijon, but in 1607 was made privy to the plans of Francis for a women's religious order to be called the Visitation of the Virgin Mary. When her son and three daughters were older and preparing to enter the world, she overcame her final reservations about leaving her family and in 1610 entered the religious house established at Annecy by Francis, and she was appointed its director. In 1619, she went to Paris to take charge of the Visitation convent that had just been founded there. After the death of Francis de Sales in 1622, the number of convents of the Visitation increased to 65, of which Jeanne, the order's spiritual director, made a tour in 1635-1636. She died after a brief illness in her sixty-ninth year at Moulins.

REFERENCES 6, 16, 36

251

Joachim of Siena

MEMORIAL DAY **April 16**

PATRONAGE **Epilepsy**

LIFE & LEGEND

Joachim of Siena, whose name is derived from Hebrew, meaning "God will establish," was born in Siena in 1258 with the forename Chiaramonte. He was formerly thought to have been a member of either the Pelacani or Piccolomini families, but this genealogy has been discredited. Chiaramonte's name was changed to Gioacchino (or Joachim) when he entered the Ordine dei Servi (Servites) in his native city at age 14. He spent his entire life at the monastery of Santa Maria dei Servi in Siena, except for a year's residence at the Servite house in Arezzo. During his stay in Arezzo, Joachim was so moved by the sufferings of an epileptic that he prayed to God that the man might be healed by transferring the malady to himself. His prayer was heard, and Joachim was thenceforth an epileptic. Joachim was noted for his extraordinary humility, obedience, prayerfulness, and ability to effect miracles. Not many years after his death in 1306, numerous miracles were recorded through Joachim's intercession. These events were testified by the numerous ex-votos placed at an altar where his remains had been transferred.

REFERENCES 6, 16, 36, 46

252
Job

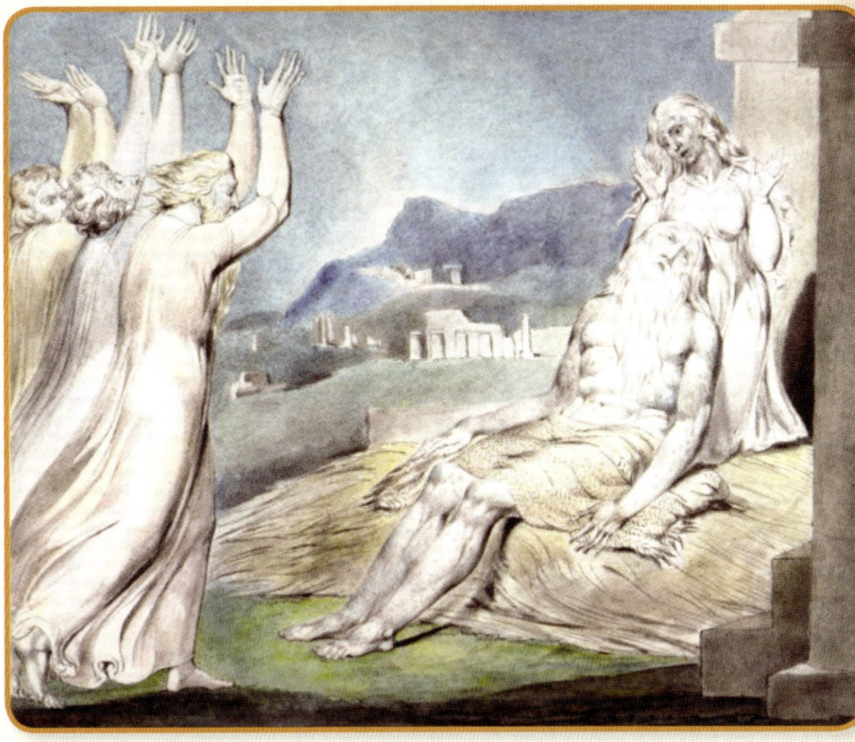

MEMORIAL DAY **May 10**

PATRONAGE **Skin diseases, including leprosy, acne, scabies, ulcers, and the cutaneous manifestations of sexually transmitted diseases; plague, melancholy, hospital workers**

LIFE & LEGEND

According to the Old Testament, "There was a man in the land of Uz, whose name was Job; and that man was blameless and upright, one who feared God, and turned away from evil. There were born to him seven sons and three daughters. He had seven thousand sheep, three thousand camels, five hundred yoke of oxen, and five hundred she-asses, and very many servants; so that this man was the greatest of all the people of the east" (Job 1:1-3). But Satan was jealous of Job, and challenged God, "Does Job fear God for nought? Hast Thou not put a hedge about him and his house and all that he has, on every side? Thou hast blessed the work of his hands, and his possessions have increased in the land. But put forth Thy hand now, and touch all that he has, and he will curse Thee to Thy face" (Job 1:10-11).

To prove the faithfulness of his servant Job, God allowed Satan to take away his sons and daughters, his herds and flocks, his oxen and servants. Still Job remained faithful, exclaiming, "Naked I came from my mother's womb, and naked shall I return; the Lord gave, and the Lord has taken away; blessed be the name of the Lord" (Job 1:21). Again Satan challenged God, "Skin for skin! All that a man has he will give for his life. But put forth Thy hand now, and touch his bone and flesh, and he will curse Thee to Thy face" (Job 2:4-5). Again Job was placed within the power of Satan, who "afflicted Job with loathsome sores from the sole of his foot to the crown of his head. And he took a potsherd with which to scrape himself, and sat among the ashes" (Job 2:7-8).

Even Job's wife could say to him only, "Do you still hold fast to your integrity? Curse God, and die" (Job 2:9). Yet Job remained faithful—a model of faithfulness amid the instability and transitory nature of everything pertaining to human existence. In Venice, the church of San Giobbe (Saint Job) is one of the city's four plague churches.

The story of Job, "a man in the land of Uz," (probably located between Idumea and northern Arabia), circulated orally in the Middle East during the second millennium BC. It was recorded in Hebrew between 1000 and 800 BC, and probably existed in an early version of its present form from the time of the Exile in the sixth century BC.

REFERENCES 12, 16, 36, 46

253

John of Arras

MEMORIAL DAY **June 24**

PATRONAGE **Hernia**

LIFE & LEGEND

John, whose name is derived from Hebrew, meaning "God is gracious," was a fifteenth-century shepherd who tended the flocks at Monchy-le-Preux, a village two leagues from Arras. We know neither the date of his birth nor of his death.
The only evidence we have concerning him is the testimony publicly given by Pierre de Ranchicourt, the bishop of Arras from 1463 to 1499. His secretary visited Monchy-le-Preux at the time of Jean's death. "All the faithful of Jesus Christ," according to this prelate, "know that in the village of Monchy-le-Preux in the diocese of Arras, there lived a man named Jean who was a simple layman faithful to Jesus Christ, and lived his entire life in the manner of a saint. By the gift of God he rose to the highest levels of contemplation, ignored impure desires, and to the moment of his death avoided everything that might tarnish the purity of his soul." Even during his lifetime Jean effected miraculous healings—among these the cure of hernia, for which he was invoked after his death.

REFERENCES 16, 36

254

John the Baptist (John the Forerunner)

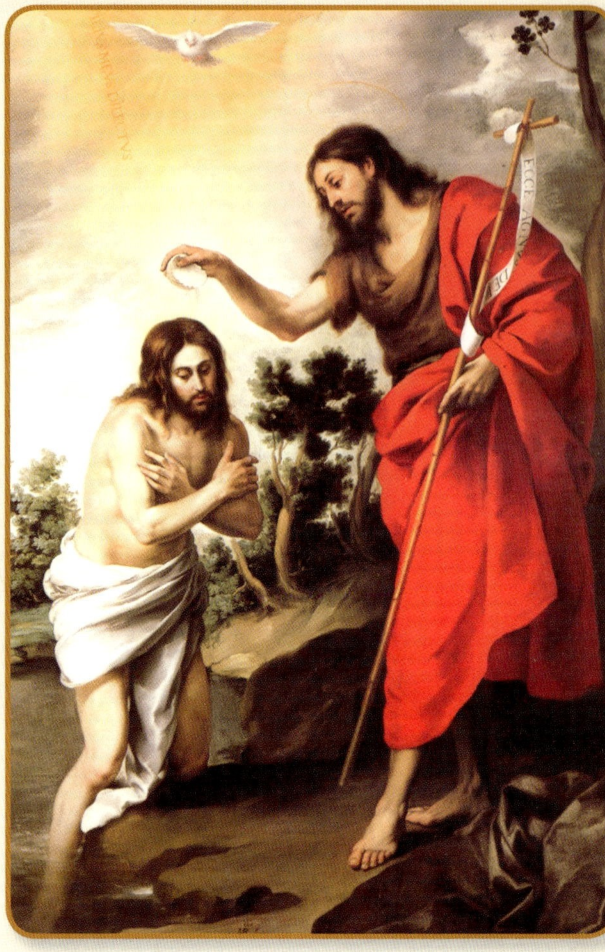

MEMORIAL DAY **August 29**

PATRONAGE **Epilepsy, spasms, children's diseases, vertigo, farriers, tailors, bird dealers, many cities**

LIFE & LEGEND

John was a cousin of Jesus Christ and 6 months older. He baptized Jesus and instructed his own disciples to follow Jesus. John was imprisoned by Herod during an uprising of Christians. Perhaps because of John's condemnation of Herod's marriage to Herodias, he was beheaded ca. 36, and his head was presented to Herodias on a platter. His relics are maintained in Saint Sylvester's church in Rome and at Amiens, France.

REFERENCES 9, 45

255

John Chrysostom

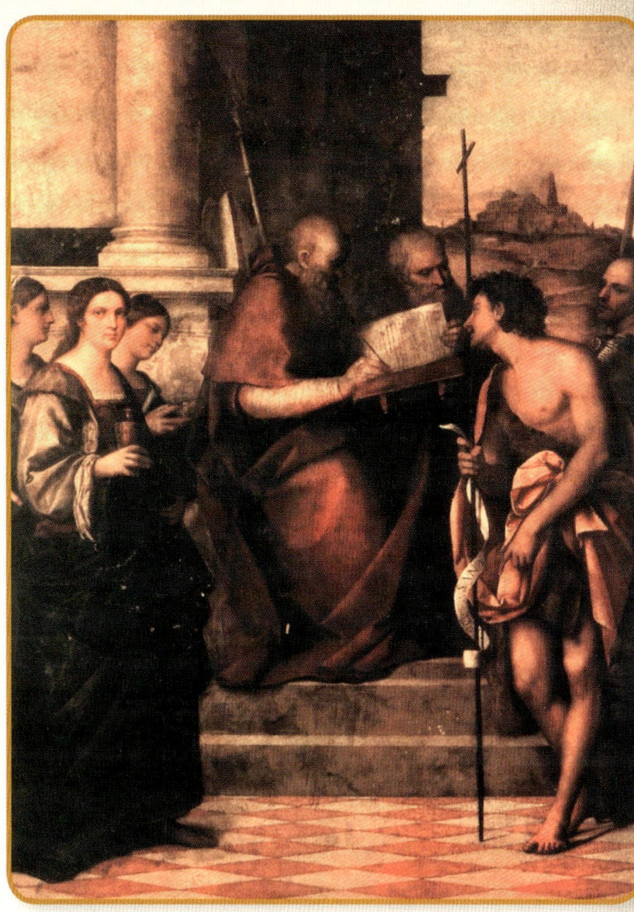

MEMORIAL DAY **September 13 (Eastern Orthodox Church: November 13)**

PATRONAGE **Epilepsy, orators, Constantinople, Istanbul**

LIFE & LEGEND

After he died, John was given the name Chrysostom, meaning "golden mouth," because of his oratorical skills. He was born in Antioch, Asia Minor, ca. 349. His father died shortly after his birth, and John's mother arranged for his education under the pagan teacher, Libanius. John became a scholar and, at the same time, committed to Christianity. In his early years he was as an ascetic and hermit. He was ordained as priest in 386 in Antioch where his oratorical skills became manifest.

John has been referred to as the greatest preacher of the early church. He is noted for the anti-Semitic theme of several of his sermons. John held the Jews responsible for the crucifixion of Jesus and considered synagogues to be analogous to pagan temples. In 398, he became the Patriarch of Constantinople, where he converted many pagans to Christianity and founded a series of hospitals to care for the poor. Eventually, John was exiled because he was tactless and denounced several influential people. He died in 407 on his journey of departure from Constantinople.

The Eastern Orthodox Church honors John as one of the Three Holy Hierarchs, with Saint Basil the Great and Saint Gregory the Theologian. The Divine Liturgy of Saint John Chrysostom is still celebrated by the Eastern Orthodox Church. His relics were looted from Constantinople by Crusaders in 1204 and taken to Rome, but they were returned to their original site in 2004 by Pope John Paul II.

REFERENCES 9, 20, 21

256

John of God

MEMORIAL DAY **March 8**

PATRONAGE **Alcoholism, heart diseases, nurses, hospitals**

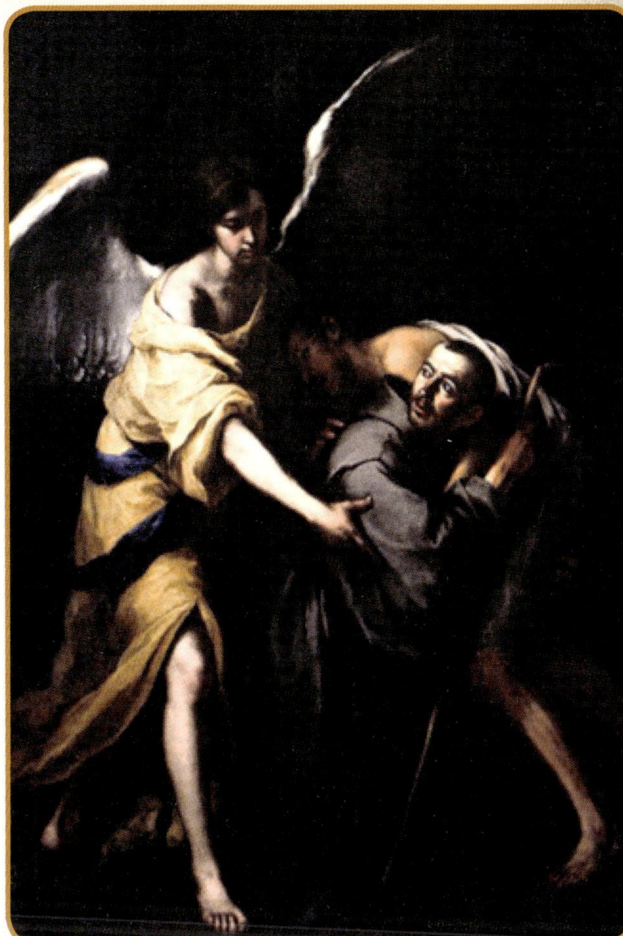

LIFE & LEGEND

John Ciudad was born in 1495 in Montemor-o-novo, Portugal, and led a varied and unsettled life. He left home while still a child and migrated to Spain, where he labored as a peasant shepherd near Oropesa in Castile. In 1522, he enrolled in a company of soldiers raised by the Count of Oropesa in the service of Charles V. He saw combat first in the wars between Spain and France and later against the Turks in Hungary. When his company was disbanded, John returned to Seville and to shepherding.

John had a change of heart at age 40 and decided to atone for his past profligacy's by providing relief to Christian slaves in North Africa and nurturing the hope of martyrdom. Instead he became attached to the family of an exiled Portuguese gentleman bound for Cueta in Barbary. John returned to Spain where he peddled holy pictures and religious books. By 1538 he was able to open his own bookshop in Gibraltar. That same year, a sermon by Saint John of Avila induced such an overwhelming sense of remorse in him for his past that John ran through the streets of Grenada behaving as a madman. He was committed to a lunatic asylum, received succor and spiritual advice from John of Avila, and was released the following year. John immediately embarked on a lifestyle devoted to the care of the sick and the poor. His work attracted the attention and monetary support of the bishop and various wealthy patrons. John continued this work until his death in 1550. Six years later, John's followers were organized into the Order of Brothers Hospitalers.

REFERENCES 6, 14, 50

257

John the Great Sinner (Juan Grande, Juan Grande Pecador)

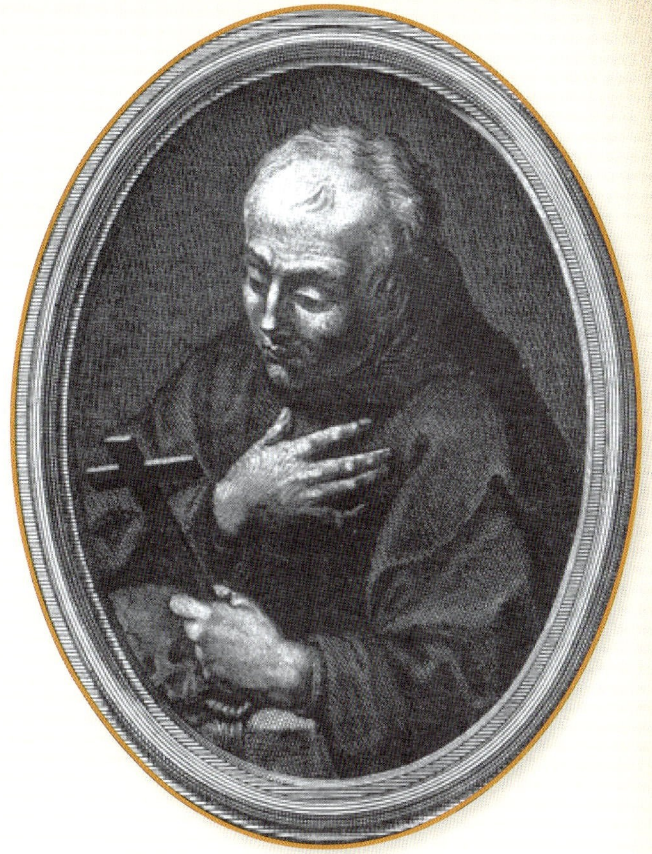

MEMORIAL DAY **June 3**

PATRONAGE **Plague, epilepsy, insanity**

LIFE & LEGEND

Born at Carmona in Andalusia in 1546, John went to live with a relative at Seville after the death of his father, and he became an apprentice in the linen trade. John returned to Carmona and started his own business. At age 22, he turned his back on the world and joined a hermitage near Marcena. It was at this time that John substituted for his surname the title El Grande Pecador, by which he is commonly known.

John did not long remain in seclusion. He abandoned the hermetic life and moved to Jerez de la Frontera, where he devoted himself for 3 years to the care of prisoners who lived there in appalling conditions. He later transferred his energies to the care of the sick in the city's inadequately run hospital. His efforts so impressed a wealthy family of the city that they provided funds for the construction of a new hospital where they placed John in charge. His efforts soon attracted a corps of young men who joined him in the care of the sick. John eventually affiliated this institution with the Order of Brothers Hospitalers founded by John of God. John extended his charitable efforts beyond the care of prisoners and the sick to include the care of orphans and the provision of dowries to poor, marriageable young women. He is supposed to have been blessed with mystical gifts, including the gift of prophecy. It is said that he predicted the loss of the Armada that sailed against England in 1588. John died of the plague, an illness he contracted while caring for victims of the epidemic that broke out at Jerez de la Frontera in 1600.

REFERENCES 6, 16, 36, 42, 45

258
John Licci

MEMORIAL DAY **November 14**

PATRONAGE **Head injuries, paralysis**

LIFE & LEGEND

John Licci is referred to as Blessed rather than Saint, because he was beatified but never canonized. His life, which extended more than 111 years, was replete with miracles.

His mother died in childbirth when he was born in Sicily in 1400, and his father, a poor farmer, left him home alone. On one occasion, a neighbor woman took the child home to feed him. When she placed him on the bed next to her paralyzed husband, the paralysis disappeared. When the child was removed from the house by the father, the paralysis recurred, only to be cured again when the child was returned.

John joined the Dominicans in 1415, and remained a member for 96 years, the longest known tenure. He founded the convent of Saint Zita in Caccamo, Sicily. While the convent was being built, construction material mysteriously appeared, as did bread and wine to feed the workers. One mason died after a fall at the site, but John prayed over him and his life was restored. John also cured the withered and paralyzed hand of a young boy who had assailed him.

John was a noted healer throughout his long life. His patronage of head injuries is based on his curing at least three individuals who had sustained critical crush injuries. He died in 1511 and was beatified in 1753 by Pope Benedict XIV.

REFERENCES 6, 45

259

John of Ortica (Ortega, Oca)

MEMORIAL DAY **June 3**

PATRONAGE **Infertility**

LIFE & LEGEND

John was the only offspring of parents who, during the 20 years before his birth, had prayed for the conception and birth of a child, which accounts for his patronage. After his ordination to the priesthood, John made a pilgrimage to the Holy Land. On his return he became a hermit in the inhospitable mountains of Ortica, where he eventually established a monastery. He died in 1143.

REFERENCES 16, 36

260

Joseph (José)

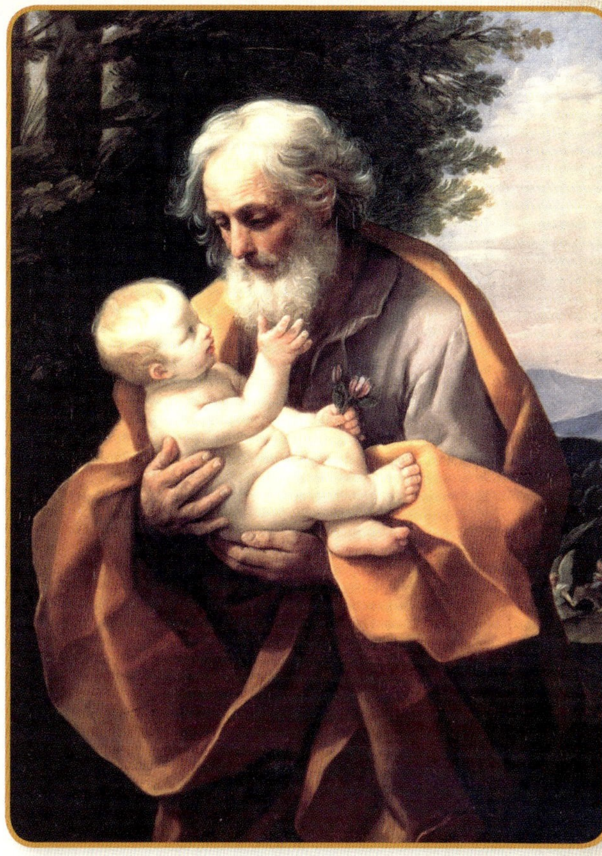

MEMORIAL DAYS **March 19, May 1 (Saint Joseph the Worker)**

PATRONAGE **Eye diseases, pregnant women, dying people, many communities, geographic features, hospitals, universities, churches, Universal Church**

LIFE & LEGEND

The only reliable sources for the life of Joseph, whose name is derived from Hebrew, meaning "he will enlarge," are the Gospels of Matthew and Luke. His genealogy is not defined, but it is believed that he was born in Bethlehem. According to the beginning Gospel history, a few months before the Annunciation (announcement of the incarnation of Jesus made to the Virgin Mary by the Archangel Gabriel), Joseph settled in Nazareth, where he worked as a mechanic or carpenter. In apocryphal writings, he is said to have married at age 40, lived with his wife (Melcha or Escha) for 49 years, and sired six children. A year after his wife died, he was chosen by priests under the direction of God to marry Mary, then 12 to 14 years of age.

At Nazareth, Joseph and Mary were betrothed and married. The couple went to Bethlehem in response to a decree by Caesar Augustus to be enrolled. A few years after Jesus was born, the Holy Family returned to Nazareth and settled there. The last mention of Joseph is associated with the family's Passover visit to the Temple in Jerusalem when Jesus was about 12 years old.

The sainthood of Joseph was first celebrated by the Copts at the beginning of the fourth century. His feast day was not compulsory for the whole Catholic Church until 1621. His name was inserted into the Litany of Saints in 1726. He was proclaimed patron of the Universal Church in 1870. The Feast of Saint Joseph the Worker (May 1) was introduced by Pope Pius XII to counteract May Day as a union, worker, and socialist holiday.

REFERENCES 9, 42, 45

261

Josse (Huec, Jodok, Joos)

MEMORIAL DAY **December 13**

PATRONAGE **Fever, snakebite**

LIFE & LEGEND

Josse was the son of Juthaël, king of Armorica (present-day Brittany). About 636, he renounced the crown that he might have worn, sought tonsure as a monk, and decided to make a pilgrimage to Rome. Whether he actually completed his pilgrimage is uncertain. Josse was befriended by the duke of Ponthieu and was ordained a priest by the bishop of Amiens at the duke's request. It was also through the latter's agency that Josse was able to enter the hermetic life, settling finally at a place called Runiacum near the mouth of the river Canche. The monastery of Saint Josse was later built on the site of this retreat. The cult of Saint Josse was carried across the English Channel by monks fleeing Norman raiders early in the tenth century. The cult later spread through the Low Countries, Germany, and Scandinavia.

REFERENCES 6, 36, 46

262
Julia of Troyes

MEMORIAL DAY **July 21**

PATRONAGE **Fever, plague**

LIFE & LEGEND

Julia, whose name is derived from Latin, meaning "down-bearded youth" (the feminine form of Julius), was a nun when taken captive by a barbarian chieftain named Claudius, who intended to make the pretty young woman one of his wives. Julia warned Claudius that she was protected by a powerful lord to whom she was espoused by her vows. Claudius asked her the name of this lord and protector. Claudius, who was cognizant of the Christians, treated Julia with respect and separated her from the other women of his household. Julia was able to resume her life of devotion, and prayed for Claudius in his affairs. Claudius himself believed that he was protected by Julia's intervention with her Lord, particularly against the Romans with whom his tribe was often engaged in the eastern reaches of Gaul.

Julia had been captive 28 years when she was told in a vision that she must return to her native place and ready herself for martyrdom. Claudius not only let her go, but accompanied her to the city of Troyes (Augustobona Tricassium), where the emperor Aurelian happened to be at that time. When she was identified as a Christian, Julia was arrested and tortured on the emperor's orders. When, after this ordeal, she still refused to sacrifice to the Roman deities, Aurelian ordered her to be executed. Although not baptized, Claudius himself came forward and demanded to be executed as a Christian by his Roman enemies. Twenty other Christians were martyred at Troyes with Julia and Claudius ca. 275. A spring appeared at the place where Julia was beheaded that was associated with cure of fevers.

REFERENCES 18, 36

263

Julian of Alexandria

MEMORIAL DAY **February 27**

PATRONAGE **Gout**

LIFE & LEGEND

Julian was a wealthy and elderly citizen of Alexandria who was so badly crippled with gout that he was unable to walk. Nevertheless, Julian was denounced for his faith and arrested during Decius' persecution of the Christians in Alexandria. Julian was scourged and burned to death with one of his litter bearers, named Cronion, ca. 250. At this same time, a soldier named Besas was beheaded for defending Julian and Cronion from the insults of the crowd while they were being paraded through the city.

REFERENCES 6, 14, 16, 36

264

Julian of Brioude

MEMORIAL DAY **August 28**

PATRONAGE **Fever, epidemic**

LIFE & LEGEND

A native of Vienne, Julian served in one of the Roman legions stationed in Gaul. When Crispinus, governor of the province of Vienne, launched a persecution of the Christians, Julian initially withdrew to Auvergne, but eventually surrendered to the authorities. He was immediately beheaded at Brioude (near Clermont-Ferrand) ca. 304. A church was later built in his honor in that region. This church became a place of pilgrimage in the fourth century, and many miracles occurred at a fountain associated with the saint. Gregory of Tours maintained that water mixed with dust from the tomb of Julian cured fevers.

REFERENCES 6, 14, 16, 36, 46

265

Julian the Hospitaler

MEMORIAL DAY **February 12**

PATRONAGE **Leprosy, scabies, skin diseases, innkeepers, travelers, boatmen, wandering musicians, minstrels, showmen, jugglers**

LIFE & LEGEND

The story of Julian the Hospitaler was one of the most popular legends of the Middle Ages, although it has little foundation. It is related by du Broc de Segange: "Julian, born of a noble family, was pursuing a stag one day during the hunt, when the beast turned upon him and said, 'Why do you pursue me, you who will take the lives of those who gave you life?' Julian was stunned, and in order to prevent such a crime fled far from his native land. A noble foreigner, having taken Julian into his service, was so taken with the young man's good qualities that he set about marrying him to a wealthy widow.

"Desolated by the absence of their son, Julian's parents set about to find him. One day, having wandered long, they unknowingly sought hospitality at the house of their son. Julian was away, but his wife realized from their accents that the couple were her husband's parents and accorded them the honor of occupying her own bedroom. The next day, while the elderly couple was still asleep, Julian's wife rose early to hear mass. Julian returned in her absence, and on entering her bedroom and drawing back the bed curtains, was shocked to see two persons asleep in her bed. Believing that he had caught his wife in the act of adultery, Julian plunged his sword through both bodies. On leaving the bedroom, the first person he encountered was his wife returning from mass. The horrible secret was quickly revealed. To expiate this crime, Julian resolved to thenceforth place himself in the service of the poor—a service that his wife decided to share. They sold all their possessions and retired to the banks of a river where the crossing was very dangerous. There they built a hospice in which Julian's wife cared for the poor and the pilgrims who Julian had ferried in his boat—often at great risk to his own life.

"One intensely cold and completely dark winter night, they heard the lamentable cries of a poor man asking for passage. In spite of the weather, Julian set off in search of the man on the opposite bank. He was a leper, covered with sores and horrible to look at. As the man was half frozen and unable to warm himself, Julian put the man in his own bed between his wife and himself. Then the leper, now healthy and white as brilliant snow, told Julian that his crime had been pardoned on account of his love for the poor and that both he and his wife would soon receive eternal life as their recompense. The messenger then disappeared. A short time later, both Julian and his wife died."

REFERENCES 6, 14, 16

266

Juliana of Collalto

MEMORIAL DAY **September 1**

PATRONAGE **Headache, migraine**

LIFE & LEGEND

Juliana was born in 1186 at Collalto in the province of Treviso, Italy. She was the daughter of Count Rambaldo VI and Countess Giovanna di Sant'Angelo of Mantua. At age 12, Juliana took the veil among the Benedictines of Santa Margherita di Salarola in the Eugean hills to the west of Padua. Juliana was later transferred to Venice, where she directed a community of nuns attached to the church of Saints Biagio and Cataldo on the sparsely occupied western end of the Giudecca (where the Molino Stucky now stands). Juliana was noted for her charitable work among the poor of Venice. During the final years of her life, she was afflicted with chronic headaches. She died in 1262.

REFERENCES 36, 46

267

Juliana Falconieri

MEMORIAL DAY **June 19**

PATRONAGE **Nausea, vomiting, stomach disorders**

LIFE & LEGEND

Juliana was the daughter of Chiarissimo and Riguardata Falconieri, who were members of the wealthy family that built the church of the Annunziata in Florence with their own funds. Juliana was born to this pious couple in 1270 when they were well along in years—an answer to their prayers for a child. Even as a young girl, Juliana preferred prayer and attending church services to the games that interested other children. When at age 15 she learned that her family was arranging a marriage for her, Juliana decided to become a nun. She was guided in this ambition by her uncle, the future Saint Alessio Falconieri, one of the founders of the Servite Order, and she was received as a tertiary among the Servites the following year. As such, Juliana was able to live at home with her widowed mother. After the death of her mother in 1304, Juliana lived with a community of like-minded Florentine women who devoted themselves to prayer and acts of mercy. In 1316, she was made superior of this community, and formulated the rule by which the women of the Servite Order would long be directed.

The community combined the contemplative life with a very active life of charity: relieving the poor, caring for the sick, and, in the contentious and often violent political climate of late fourteenth century Florence, reconciling enemies among contending parties and families. Later in life, Juliana developed gastric problems with frequent nausea and vomiting. These incidents became so severe that she was eventually unable to receive communion for fear of not being able to retain the consecrated elements, accounting for her patronage. She died in 1341.

REFERENCES 6, 16, 36, 46

268

Juliana of Nicomedia

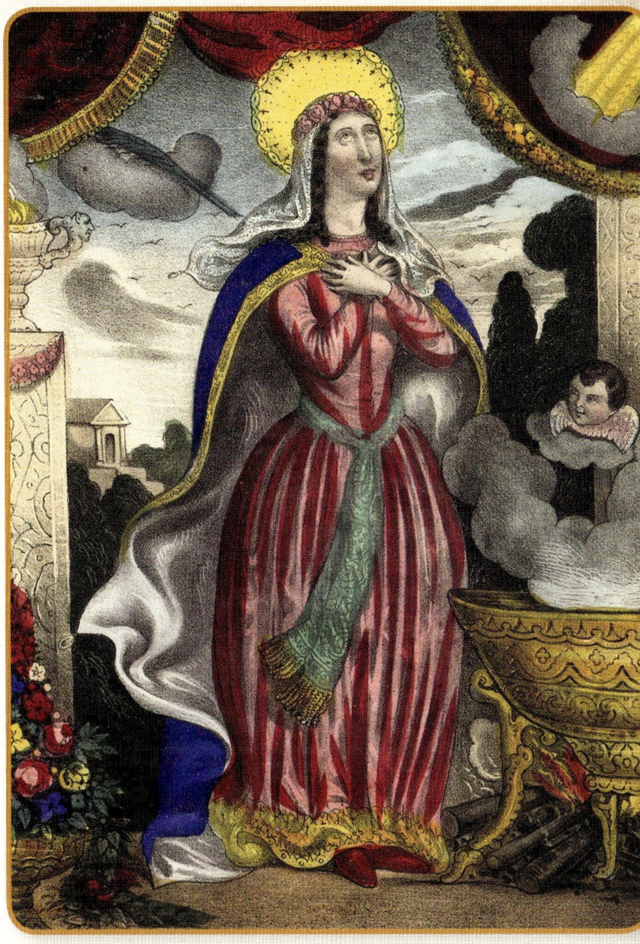

MEMORIAL DAY **February 16**

PATRONAGE **Contagious diseases, childbirth**

LIFE & LEGEND

Juliana is supposed to have been scourged by her pagan father, Africanus, for persisting in her Christian faith. She was then tortured by the city prefect, Evilasius, whom she refused to marry. Her tormenters exposed her body to fire and immersed her in boiling oil. While in prison, she triumphed in a struggle with Satan. After surviving these ordeals, Juliana was beheaded ca. 305.

At one time, there was some question whether Juliana was martyred at Nicomedia during the persecution of the emperor Maximian or at Cumae near Naples. Although her cult in the West originated around Naples, it seems likely that she was martyred at Nicomedia and that her relics were later transferred to Pozzuoli, then to Cumae, and finally to Naples. The veneration of Juliana was widespread throughout Campania. Her relics were later distributed throughout Europe. Thousands of pilgrims visited the church of Sainte-Julienne in Val Saint-Germain (Ile de France) to heal contagious diseases or to pray for a successful childbirth.

REFERENCES 6, 14, 16, 36, 46

K

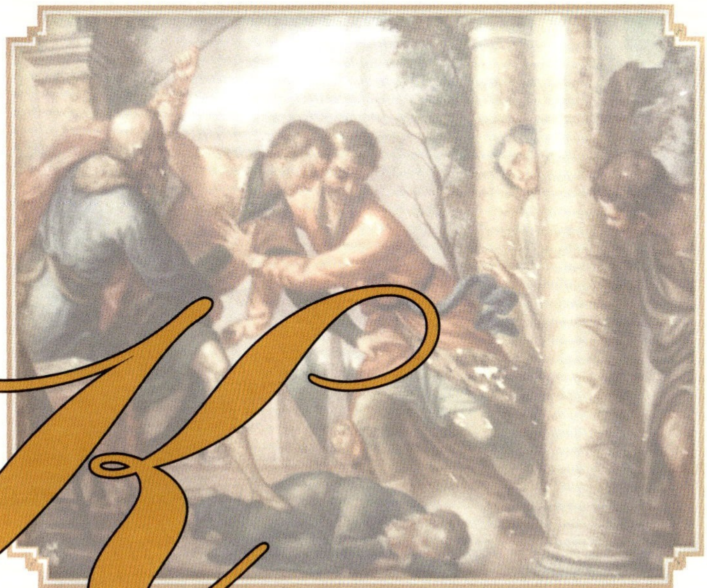

269
Kilian

MEMORIAL DAY **July 8**

PATRONAGE **Gout, rheumatism, Würzburg**

LIFE & LEGEND

There are two accounts of the Irish monk, Kilian. One relates that he was born in Ireland ca. 640, left home and traveled through France and then to Rome, where he was consecrated bishop with a charge to evangelize the Germanic tribes on the east bank of the Rhine (Franconia). The other account maintains that Kilian had been made a bishop before he left Ireland, and that, after a brief residence in Rome, he was sent by Pope John V to evangelize the Franconians.

Kilian is said to have converted Gosbert, the duke of Franconia, requiring him to separate from his brother's widow—a marriage regarded as unlawful by the Church. In revenge, the soon-to-be former countess, Geilana, took advantage of Gosbert's absence from Würzburg to have Kilian and his companions murdered outside the city in 689. Gosbert may have conspired with Geilana in removing the meddlesome Irishmen.

When Saint Boniface learned of Kilian's influence in Germany, Saint Burchard had Kilian's remains exhumed and transferred in 788 to a vault in the newly erected Cathedral of the Savior in Würzburg in the presence of Charlemagne.

REFERENCES 6, 14, 36, 46

L

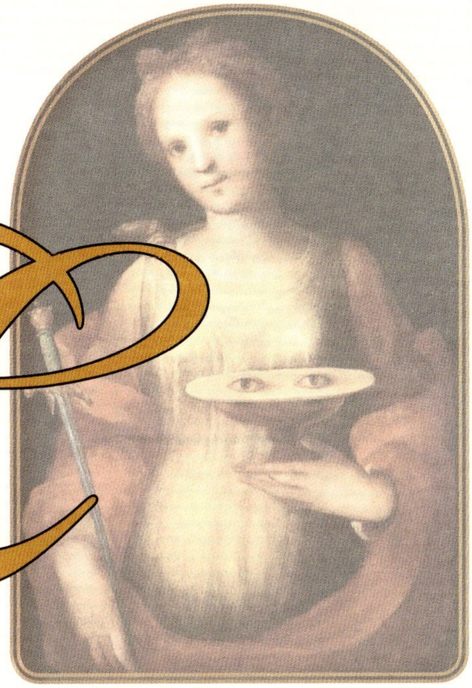

270

Lambert (Landebert) of Maastricht

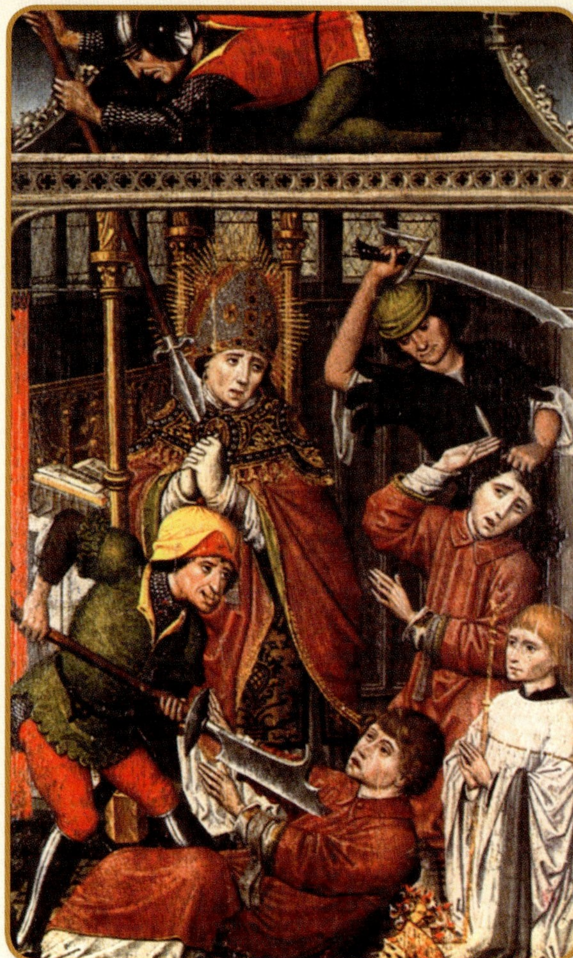

MEMORIAL DAY **September 17**

PATRONAGE **Hernia, biliary calculi, epilepsy, kidney diseases, wet nurses, surgeons, dentists**

LIFE & LEGEND

Lambert was born into a noble Christian family of Maastricht ca. 635. He was educated in the court of the bishop and future saint, Theodard. When Theodard was murdered ca. 670, Lambert succeeded him on the episcopal throne. Four years later, Lambert was expelled from his see by Ebroin, mayor of the palace, for political reasons, namely his support of the recently murdered King Childeric II. Lambert retired to the Stavelot monastery where, for 7 years, he lived as a simple monk. He was reinstated in his see by Pepin of Herstal after the assassination of Ebroin. Lambert resumed his duties with zeal—particularly evangelizing the many pagans who still lived in the surrounding region. Lambert denounced Pepin for an adulterous affair he was having with his sister-in-law, Alpais (Alpaida), the mother of Charles Martel.

There are three versions of Lambert's death. In one, he was murdered by Alpais' brother, Dodo, while kneeling before the altar in the church of Saints Cosmas and Damian in Liège, because Lambert was so forceful in his defense of the sanctity of marriage. In another version, he was killed by one of Dodo's men, who had climbed through a window in Lambert's house and cast a spear at the praying bishop. A third version maintains that his opposition to the taxation of Church property may have been a motive for his assassination. In any case, after his death, ca. 700, the martyred bishop's remains were brought back to Maastricht, but were later transferred to a church built over the house where he was murdered. The remains were exhumed and translated to Liege by Saint Hubert ca. 720.

REFERENCES 6, 14, 36, 45, 46

271

Landericus (Landry)

MEMORIAL DAY **June 10**

PATRONAGE **Incurable diseases**

LIFE & LEGEND

Nothing is known of the early years of Landericus. While still a young man, he was chosen by the clergy and King Clovis II to be bishop of Paris in 650. Landericus was noted for his attention to the poor. He sold his own and even Church property for their maintenance, and erected the first true hospital at Paris, which Landericus dedicated to Saint Christopher. This establishment later evolved into the Hôtel-Dieu. After his death ca. 660, Landericus' remains were interred at Saint-Germain-des-Prés. Many miracles were recorded at his tomb, including the healing of diseases that had been declared incurable. A church was later erected in Paris in his honor.

REFERENCES 6, 16, 36

272

Lando (Lanno)

MEMORIAL DAY **May 5**

PATRONAGE **Headache**

LIFE & LEGEND

Born into a Christianized and Romanized Germanic family near Cologne, Lando enlisted in the Roman army at Treves (Augusta Treverorum) in 292 while still in his adolescence. The XIII Legion (Gemina), in which Lando was enrolled, was under the command of the emperor Maximian, who brought the legion with him when he returned to Italy and Rome. Lando was billeted at Falerii Novi on the via Flaminia (31 miles north of Rome), where he was active in promoting his faith. When Diocletian, the senior figure in the imperial tetrarchy, renewed the persecution of Christians at the beginning of the fourth century, Lando was arrested and ordered to acknowledge the traditional Roman deities. When Lando refused to sacrifice to the martial deity, part of the temple of Mars at Rome collapsed and killed several pagan priests. Lando was tortured and beheaded at Rome. Du Broc de Segange does not acknowledge Lando's German origins, stating that he came to Italy from Greece and that he was martyred in the north of Italy.

REFERENCES 16, 36, 46

273

Lawrence

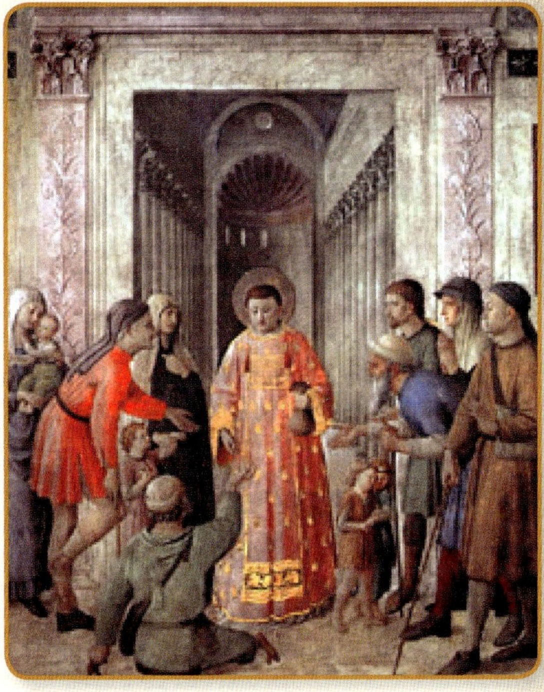

MEMORIAL DAY **August 10**

PATRONAGE **Lumbago, librarians, cooks, Sri Lanka, many cities throughout the world**

LIFE & LEGEND

Lawrence, whose name is derived from French, meaning "bearing laurels," was born at Huesca, Spain, and became one of the seven deacons of the Church in the third century. He had responsibility for the early archives, hence his patronage for librarians. During the persecutions by Emperor Valerian, Pope Sixtus II and the six other deacons were beheaded on August 6, 258. When Lawrence was told to produce the wealth of the Church 2 days later, he presented 287 diseased, orphaned, or crippled Christians and indicated that they represent the treasures of the Church. Lawrence was killed on August 10.

Although he was probably also beheaded, legend states that he was slowly roasted on a grill, accounting for his patronage of cooks. Lawrence is one of the revered martyrs of the Church, and the basilica of San Lorenzo in Rome was built in his honor. The reliquary of Saint Lawrence's head is in the Vatican library. The annual Perseid meteor shower is referred to as "The tears of Saint Lawrence" because it occurs near his feast day. The Gulf of Saint Lawrence was so named because it was entered by Jacques Cartier on the saint's feast day in 1534.

REFERENCES 9, 42, 45

274

Lazarus of Bethany

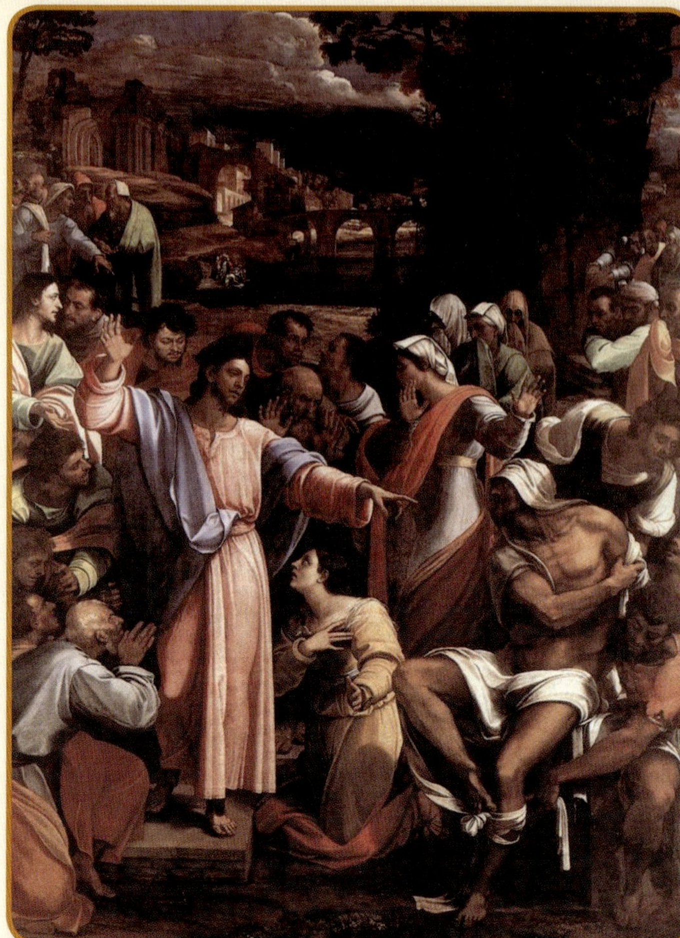

MEMORIAL DAY **July 29**

PATRONAGE **Leprosy**

LIFE & LEGEND

The name of Lazarus is derived from Hebrew, meaning "God is my help." The eleventh chapter of John provides the only account of Lazarus, his illness, and his return from death. According to John, Lazarus lived with his sisters Mary and Martha in Bethany, a village two miles east of Jerusalem. Jesus was notified by Lazarus' sisters that their brother was seriously ill, but he delayed his arrival, telling his disciples, "Our friend Lazarus has fallen asleep, but I go to waken him out of sleep." By the time Jesus arrived at Bethany, Lazarus had been in the tomb 4 days. He was met on the way by Martha, who reproached him, "Lord, if you had been here, my brother would not have died." This charge was repeated by Mary when she encountered Jesus on her way to Lazarus' tomb. When he came to the place, Jesus ordered that the stone covering the tomb be removed and commanded, "Lazarus, come out." Lazarus did so, "his hands and feet bound with bandages, and his face wrapped with a cloth." (John 11:44). John adds that Lazarus was "at table" with Jesus when he next visited Bethany, 6 days before his final Passover; and that "the chief priests planned to put Lazarus also to death, because on account of him many of the Jews were going away and believing in Jesus" (John 12:10).

According to tradition, Lazarus did not die at the hands of the chief priests but at the hands of the Romans. The accepted tradition is that Lazarus went to Cyrpus where, for 30 years, he was bishop of Kition (modern-day Larnaka), where he died—probably as a martyr. Additional evidence for this tradition is provided by ancient frescos that testify to Lazarus' presence on the island and by the removal of his relics from Kition to Constantinople in 900. Less reliable sources relate that Lazarus and his sisters were placed in a boat with neither oars nor rudder and cast adrift. They are supposed to have come ashore on the coast of Provence, where Lazarus became the first bishop of Marseilles and a martyr during the persecution by Nero.

REFERENCES 14, 36, 46

275
Lazarus the Poor Man

MEMORIAL DAY **June 21**

PATRONAGE **Leprosy**

LIFE & LEGEND

The sixteenth chapter of Luke relates the parable of Lazarus and an unnamed rich man (Luke 16:19-31). The latter was "clothed in purple and fine linen" and "feasted sumptuously every day." Lazarus lay at the rich man's door, "a poor man . . . full of sores, who desired to be fed with what fell from the rich man's table; moreover the dogs came and licked his sores." When Lazarus died he "was carried by the angels to Abraham's bosom." When the rich man died, he was cast into Hades and cried out, "Father Abraham, have mercy upon me, and send Lazarus to dip the end of his finger in water and cool my tongue; for I am in anguish in this flame."

Although related as a figure in a parable, Lazarus later assumed a historical persona and became the object of veneration, symbolizing patience during suffering and hope in the mercy of God. Lazarus' name gave rise to the words "lazaretto" (initially an isolation hospital for lepers), and, in the Neapolitan dialect, "lazzarone" (street beggars). He was also the inspiration for the Order of Saint Lazarus of Jerusalem, which was established in the twelfth century and cared for lepers.

REFERENCES 14, 46

276
Leander

MEMORIAL DAY **February 27**

PATRONAGE **Gout, rheumatism**

LIFE & LEGEND

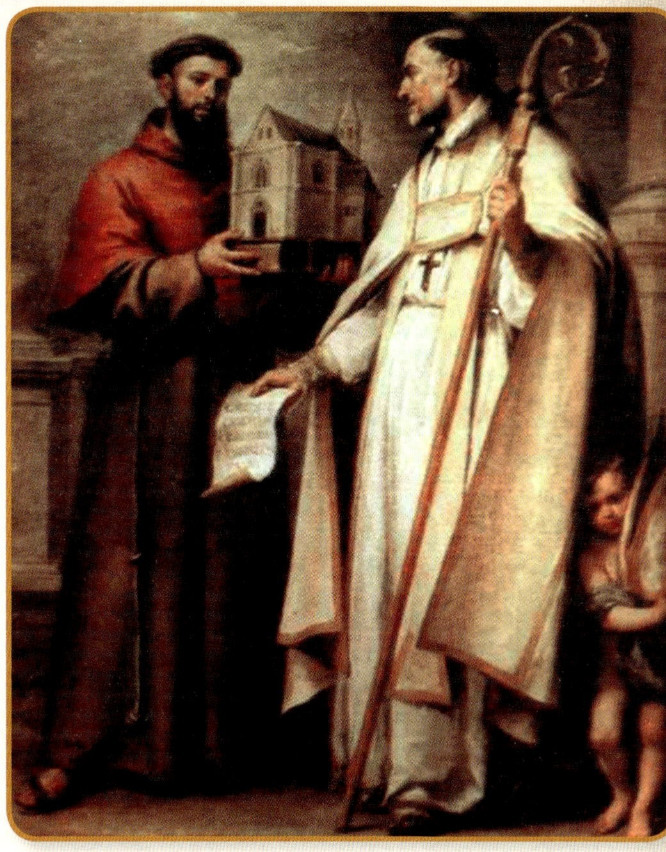

Leander, whose name is derived from Greek, meaning "lion man," was descended on his father's side from an ancient and influential Romano-Hispanic family. His mother was a daughter of the Ostrogothic king, Theodoric. Leander was born at Cartagena, the elder brother of the future Saint Fulgentius and Saint Isidore, the noted encyclopedist who succeeded Leander in his see. Leander entered the monastic life at Seville, Spain, which had been under Visigoth rule from the late fifth century, was divided into contending factions of Arian and orthodox Christians. The Visigoth king, Leovigild, was an Arian, and it was his intent to unify Spain in matters of faith as well as administration. Nevertheless, he approved the elevation of the orthodox monk Leander to the episcopal throne of Seville. Through his writings and preaching, Leander was determined to convert the Arians to orthodox teaching concerning the equality of the first two persons of the Trinity (the Father and the Son).

Leander was successful to the point of converting one of the king's sons, Hermenegild, to orthodoxy. The political consequences of this event were unfortunate, because Hermenegild led a revolt against his father and was subsequently put to death. Sources differ on what happened next. Some maintain that Leander was sent by Leovigild on a diplomatic mission to the emperor in Constantinople; it seems likely, however, that Leander was exiled from Spain among those who had been among Hermenegild's supporters.

While in Constantinople, Leander established a lifelong friendship with the future Roman pope, Gregory the Great. His sojourn in Byzantium did not last long, because Leovigild soon recalled those whom he had exiled. The king restored Leander to his see and made him a counselor to his son, Reccared, who assumed the royal throne on Leovigild's death in 586. Leander was subsequently able to convert many of the Arian bishops to the orthodox position and brought much of the Visigoth population into the Catholic fold. In 589, Leander convened a Church council at Toledo, a decisive moment in the triumph of orthodoxy. He introduced the recitation of the Nicene Creed during the mass as was done in the Eastern churches—a decided symbol of the Spanish Church's orthodoxy and a practice adopted by other Western churches. Leander suffered terribly from gout, accounting for his patronage. He died ca. 600.

REFERENCES 6, 14, 16, 36, 46

277

Leo (Léon) of Rouen

MEMORIAL DAY **March 1**

PATRONAGE **Pregnancy, childbirth, sailors**

LIFE & LEGEND

Leo, whose name is the Latin for "lion," was born in the village of Carentan in Normandy. Leo studied theology in Paris, where he was noted as much for the sanctity of his life as for his intellectual gifts and attainments. Leo was a young man when he was made archbishop of Rouen by Pope Stephen V. It was Leo's desire to evangelize the yet unconverted peoples of southwestern France and northern Spain. Therefore, he left his diocese in the care of vicars and journeyed to Bayonne with two monks to convert the pagan population.

When Leo was seized at Bayonne and dragged before a statue of Mars, the idol was reduced to dust by Leo's prayers. This miracle resulted in the conversion of the city. Leo left Bayonne to continue his evangelical mission in the Basque provinces of Spain.

There are two versions of Leo's martyrdom. According to one tradition, Leo was seized and beheaded by Saracen raiders while he was preaching among the coastal villages of northern Spain. The other tradition relates that, after a long absence among the Basques, Leo returned to Bayonne. He was preceded by the return of a pirate fleet that operated out of that city. When the pirates learned that their fellow citizens had converted to Christianity and were now ill-disposed to their continued use of the harbor as a base, the pirates seized Leo and beheaded him ca. 900. Because they feared popular retaliation, the pirate fleet left the city, during which voyage it was destroyed by a tempest.

REFERENCES 16, 36

278
Leobonus

MEMORIAL DAY **October 13**

PATRONAGE **Fever, epilepsy, contagious diseases, epidemics**

LIFE & LEGEND

Born into a noble family at Saint-Étienne-Fursac (Creuse), Leobonus withdrew from the world as a very young man to dedicate his life to solitary prayer on a forested mountain. The young hermit's chastity and sobriety inspired some young profligates to hire a prostitute to seduce him. One night she was led through the forest and instructed to knock at the hermit's door, tearfully pretending to be lost and to be afraid of wild beasts. Leobonus opened his door to the seemingly distraught young woman, whose tears suddenly dried as she made her intentions clear. Leobonus immediately pulled the brazier with which he warmed his cell into the middle of the room and invited the young woman to share this "bed" with the words, "Come along, my poor friend, so that you may begin to feel in this life the eternal flames of hell, if you do not repent of your sin."

The young woman ran out of the cell and through the forest to the young men who had hired her. "Get out of here," she cried, "get out of here if you do not want the earth to open and swallow you. This hermit you are pursuing is a saint. If you do not believe me, go take a look for yourselves." The young men did so, and as they entered the cell were astonished to see Leobonus curled up on the brazier, but unharmed by its coals. The hermit then got up and exhorted his guests to change their way of life. Whether they did is not related. This incident was not the end of Leobonus' difficulties with his neighbors. He eventually left this place and built another cell at what is now the village of Salignac. The miracle of the burning coals inspired the inhabitants of Salignac to call on the saint for the cure of their fevers. Leobonus died ca. 530.

REFERENCES 16, 36, 45

279

Leocadia (Legadia)

MEMORIAL DAY **December 9**

PATRONAGE **Plague, Toledo**

LIFE & LEGEND

There are two distinct legends about Leocadia. According to one, she was born into a noble family of Toledo, Spain, and was imprisoned because of her faith by the governor Dacian during the persecution of Diocletian. She died in prison as a result of the tortures to which she had been subjected.

The other tradition indicates that she was a slave who was beaten for refusing to denounce her faith. She was scheduled for torture when she learned of the abuse suffered by a 13-year-old girl, later to become Saint Eulia. Leocadia prayed to be removed from a world with such evil, and she died before her proposed torture could be carried out ca. 303.

REFERENCES 6, 14, 18, 36, 45

280

Leodegar (Legér)

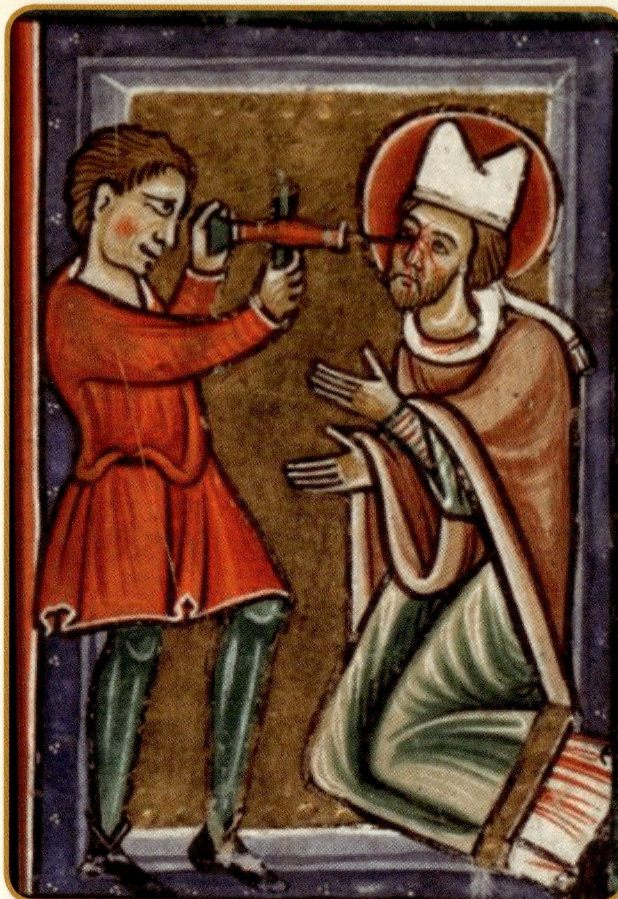

MEMORIAL DAY **October 2**

PATRONAGE **Blindness, eye problems, millers**

LIFE & LEGEND

Leodegar was born ca. 615 near Somme, France, into the Frankish nobility, the son of Bobilio and Saint Sigarda. He was educated in Paris at the court of Clotaire II, and he went on to Potiers to study under the guidance of his uncle, Desiderius (Dido), who was the bishop and who ordained Leodegar about 650. He entered the monastery at Saint Maxentius and was elected abbot. In that capacity, he introduced the Rule of Saint Benedict. Leodegar was engaged by the widowed Queen Bathildis to assist her in the governance of the kingdom and in the education of her children. As a consequence he was made bishop of Autun in Burgundy.

On the death of Clotaire III, king of the Franks, Leodegar backed Childeric II, whereas Ebroin, the mayor of Neustria, favored Theodoric III (Thierry). Childeric ascended to the throne in 670 and Ebroin was exiled. Three years later Childeric was murdered and Theodoric became king of Neustria. Ebroin returned from exile and stimulated an attack on Autun. To save the town, Leodegar surrendered. He had both eyes burned with hot irons (accounting for his patronage); his lips were cut and his tongue removed. He survived only to be murdered a few years later in 678, whereupon he became venerated as a martyr. His relics, which had been at the abbey of Saint Maxentius in Potiers, were translocated to Ebreuil, which was renamed Saint-Legér.

REFERENCES 6, 9, 45

281

Leonard of Noblac

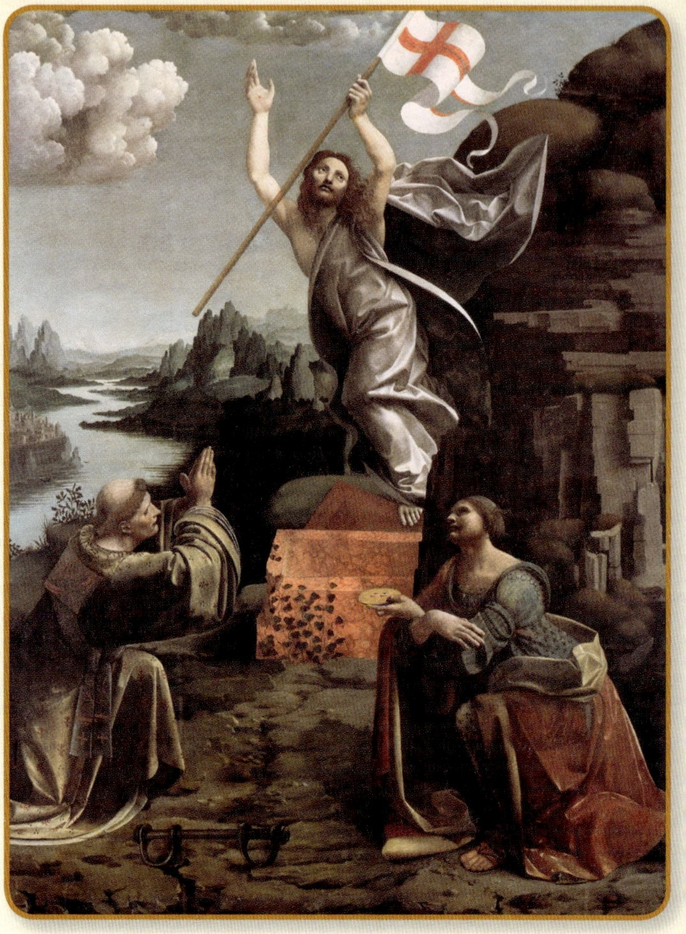

MEMORIAL DAY **November 6**

PATRONAGE **Women in labor, sick children, headache, syphilis, obesity, prisoners, prisoners of war**

LIFE & LEGEND

The earliest written accounts of the life of Saint Leonard, who lived during the sixth century, date from the eleventh century, making the veracity of his reported acts uncertain. Leonard is supposed to have been born into an influential Frankish family, and to have been the godson of Clovis, king of the Franks. While Leonard was at court, the Queen suggested that he pray to God for help in repelling an invading army. The army was repelled, and Remigius, archbishop of Reims, used the miracle to convert the king, Leonard, and many others to Christianity.

Leonard was disinterested in taking up the profession of arms, and he became a disciple of Remigius and an evangelizer of the Frankish people. The holiness of Leonard's life induced Clovis to offer him a bishopric, which Leonard refused so he could become a simple monk in the monastery at Micy. Because he sought a more secluded life, Leonard withdrew into the wilderness near Limoges. When

Queen Clotilde was in the throes of a difficult labor, Clovis had Leonard intercede for her through his prayers. The queen was safely delivered of a male child and Clovis rewarded Leonard by granting him as much land as he could circumscribe on the back of a donkey in a day. On this land Leonard founded the monastery of Noblac, around which later evolved the town of Saint-Leonard.

During his lifetime, Leonard was sought out by those who had heard of the healing power of his prayer. In emulation of his spiritual father Saint Remigius, Leonard devoted himself to the liberation of prisoners taken in the war-ravaged Gaul of his era. He died ca. 559. By the eleventh century the saint's cult had spread throughout Europe. Bohemund (1050-1111), the self-proclaimed Prince of Antioch, claimed that he was liberated after being taken prisoner during the First Crusade through the intercession of Leonard of Noblac.

REFERENCES 6, 14, 36, 45, 46

282

Leonard of Vandoeuvre

MEMORIAL DAY **October 15**

PATRONAGE **Deafness**

LIFE & LEGEND

Leonard entered the hermetic life at Vandoeuvre on the river Maine near Le Mans. The village of Saint Léonard-des-Bois presently stands near this site. Leonard attracted numerous disciples, whom he organized into a monastery of which he was abbot. Even though King Clotaire I considered that the renunciation of the world by able-bodied men was subversive and counterproductive to the development of military manpower, he was favorably disposed to Leonard and a supporter of his work. Leonard died of natural causes ca. 570.

REFERENCES 6, 14, 36, 46

283

Leontius (Liesne)

MEMORIAL DAY **February 1**

PATRONAGE **Fever, gout, scrofula**

LIFE & LEGEND

Leontius, who lived during the fourth century, was a priest and a disciple of Saint Hilaire. He was active in combatting the Arian heresy and died suddenly of a fever. On that account Leontius is invoked by those suffering from febrile diseases. Du Broc de Segange relates that a chapel at Moûtiers dedicated to Saint Leontius (since destroyed) was commonly visited by those suffering from scrofula.

REFERENCES 16, 36

284
Léothade

MEMORIAL DAY **October 23**

PATRONAGE **Epilepsy**

LIFE & LEGEND

A Frankish nobleman, Léothade renounced the world to become a Benedictine monk during the second half of the seventh century. He was later elected abbot of the monastery at Moissac and bishop of Auch (Gers). He died of natural causes ca. 718.

REFERENCES 16, 36

285

Leudomer (Lomer)

MEMORIAL DAY **October 3**

PATRONAGE **Blindness, eye diseases**

LIFE & LEGEND

A native of Limoges, Leudomer succeeded his brother, Saint Elaphius, as bishop of Châlons-sur-Marne after the latter's death in 580. When Queen Brunhilde summoned the reputedly handsome Leudomer, he returned her warm greeting with an icy stare. An eye has remained the symbol of Leudomer, and is related perhaps to his patronage of those suffering from blindness and eye diseases. Kerler states that Leudomer restored the sight of a blind woman by making the sign of the cross over her eyes.

REFERENCES 2, 36

286

Leutfridus (Leufroy)

MEMORIAL DAY **June 21**

PATRONAGE **Diseases of children**

LIFE & LEGEND

Leutfridus was born into a noble family of Evreux. After completing his studies at Chartres, he returned to Evreux where he devoted himself to the education of boys. Later he decided to test himself as a hermit in the monastery at Cailly. Leutfridus took the monastic habit at Rouen where he was under the spiritual direction of the Irish monk and future saint, Sidonius (or Saens). At the behest of the Ansbert, archbishop of Rouen, Leutfridus returned to Evreux, where he established the monastery of La Croix on the banks of the Eure ca. 690 (later La Croix-Saint-Leufroy). Leutfridus remained its abbot for 48 years until he died ca. 748.

On one occasion, Leutfridus was summoned by Charles Martel to intercede with prayers for the healing of his young son. Leutfridus rubbed the child's limbs with water he had blessed and restored the boy to complete health, accounting for his patronage and the portrayal of him surrounded by children.

REFERENCES 6, 14, 16, 36

287

Libaria (Leobaria)

MEMORIAL DAY **October 12**

PATRONAGE **Eye diseases, Conde-sur-Marne**

LIFE & LEGEND

The virgin martyr Libaria was executed with her siblings during the reign of the emperor Julian (the Apostate) in the fourth century.

REFERENCES 16, 18, 36

288

Liborius of Le Mans

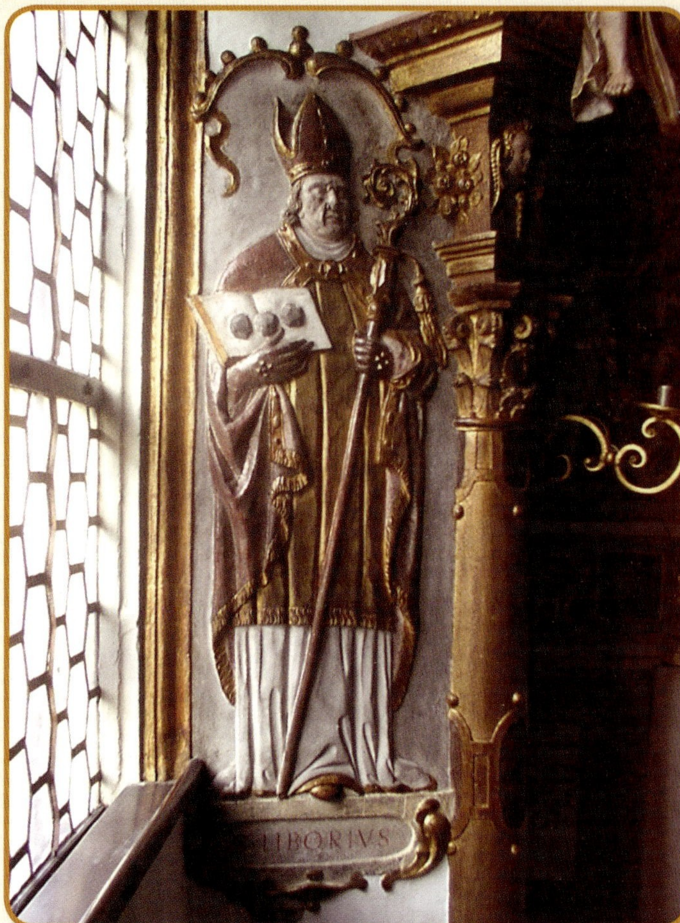

MEMORIAL DAY **July 23**

PATRONAGE **Urinary calculi, colic, [urology],* Paderborn (Germany)**

LIFE & LEGEND

Liborius was born of a noble family in Gaul in 348. He was ordained as the second or third bishop of Le Mans. During the 45 years of his episcopacy, he built many churches and became the patron of Paderborn, Germany. He died in 397 at a time when barbarian hordes were ravaging the Roman Empire. His relics were translocated from Le Mans to Paderborn in 836.

In the history of urinary lithiasis, Liborius's name is mentioned only sporadically. He is usually depicted as an aged bishop with a staff and an open book, with several small stones on the book. In the eighteenth century, Pope Clement XI was cured of calculi symptoms by prayers to Saint Liborius. Toward the end of the twentieth century, an oil on canvas painting at the Varazdin Monastery of Friars Minors Capuchins in Croatia provided support for his patronage. The text below the picture reads "Saint Liborius Bishop, a great patron against calculi."

*Proposed patronage

REFERENCES 6, 22

289

Licinius (Lésin)

MEMORIAL DAY **February 13**

PATRONAGE **Childbirth**

LIFE & LEGEND

Licinius was born into a prominent family of Burgundy, and at 20 he became a courtier to his cousin, Clotaire II. A favorite at court, Licinius was made count of Angers. The king also made certain that a young woman suitable to Licinius' station was found for him to marry. When the unfortunate girl was discovered to be afflicted with leprosy on the eve of her marriage, Licinius decided to renounce his place at court and become a monk, retiring to a monastery near Angers.

In 586, Licinius was chosen by the people of Angers to replace the recently deceased Audouin as their bishop. Their choice was confirmed by the clergy and the king. Licinius was widely known for the austerity of his life, for his charity to the poor, and for working miracles. In August 616, he was afflicted with an illness of which he died in November.

Licinius was buried in the church of Saint-Jean-Baptiste, which he had constructed. There, among his relics, was a belt that, as late as the seventeenth century, women would wrap around their bodies while invoking Licinius for the safe delivery of their children.

REFERENCES 14, 16, 36

290

Loup of Chalon

MEMORIAL DAY **February 19**

PATRONAGE **Fever, pain**

LIFE & LEGEND

Loup is French for "wolf." Loup of Chalon may have been bishop of Chalon-sur-Saône at the end of the sixth century. He died ca. 610. Du Broc de Segange relates the story of a fountain associated with the saint in the nearby village of Boyer: "This fountain was possessed of such power that those who drank of it, imploring God's aid through the intercession of Saint Loup, were often found to be relieved of their fevers."

REFERENCES 16, 36

291

Loup of Limoges

MEMORIAL DAY **May 22**

PATRONAGE **Fever, diarrhea, intestinal disorders**

LIFE & LEGEND

When the bishop of Limoges died, those charged with finding his successor decided to send two priests to King Clotaire II to ask him to select the new bishop. Although he possessed none of the qualities that would have made him stand out at court, Loup was one of two priests dispatched to Paris. He was a humble cleric, neither well born nor imposing in manner or appearance. At the time of Loup's arrival, Clotaire's son lay dying of a "malignant fever." One night in a dream, the queen saw a priest of humble appearance saying mass in her son's room and giving the boy communion. When he received the sacrament, the young prince immediately became well. Acting on her dream, the queen had numerous priests paraded before her. At last she recognized Loup de Limoges as the priest she had seen in her dream and begged him to say mass in her son's room. Loup complied, and the prince was cured of his fever on receiving communion. After inquiring the reason for Loup's presence at court, the queen arranged an audience for him with the king. On learning of his mission, Clotaire, without hesitation, chose Loup to fill the vacant see of Limoges. Loup died ca. 637.

REFERENCES 16, 36

292

Loup of Lyon

MEMORIAL DAY **September 25**

PATRONAGE **Sick children**

LIFE & LEGEND

Loup entered the monastic life at the monastery of Ile Sainte-Barbe on the Saône. He was abbot of this foundation when selected in 523 to succeed Saint Viventiol as bishop of Lyon. Loup presided at the third Council of Orleans in 538, which was summoned to restore discipline to the Church in France. He died about 4 years later.

REFERENCES 16, 27, 36

293

Loup of Sens

MEMORIAL DAY **September 1**

PATRONAGE **Epilepsy, convulsive disorders, dysentery**

LIFE & LEGEND

According to one account of his life written in the eighth century, Loup was the son of Betton and a member of a noble family of Orleans. He was guided into an ecclesiastic career by his two uncles, Austrenius, bishop of Orleans, and Aunacarius, bishop of Auxerre. When Artemius, the bishop of Sens, died in 600, Loup succeeded him on the episcopal throne. In spite of the purity of his manners and his charity toward all, Loup was exiled by Clotaire II to a village in the Vimeu—apparently for political reasons. The king later repented of his decision and restored Loup to his see. After the death of Loup in 623, miraculous cures were reported among those who visited his tomb.

REFERENCES 27, 36, 46

294
Loup of Troyes

MEMORIAL DAY **July 29**

PATRONAGE **Leprosy**

LIFE & LEGEND

Born in 383, in or near the city of Toul (Meurthe-et-Moselle), Loup was married to the sister of the future Saint Hilaire, archbishop of Arles. After a time the couple agreed to separate, and Loup entered the monastery at Lérins. In 426, he succeeded Ours as bishop of Troyes. Loup was active in combatting the Arian heresy and in defending his city against the incursions of the Huns. In 446, Loup was sent to Britain with Germanus of Auxerre to combat the Pelagian heresy on that island. Loup died in 479. Fay maintains that Loup de Troyes was invoked in parts of France by those afflicted with leprosy. The lepers of Navailles in the Basses-Pyrénées, for example, commonly passed beneath a sculpture of Saint Loup fixed over one of the portals of their church in the hope of being cured. "Their choice of this saint is founded perhaps on little more than his name," according to Fay, because his name, or a derivative (that is, lupus, leprosy) is applied to almost any ulcerative skin disease. Fay cites the fourteenth-century physician Guy de Chauliac's reference to leprosy as the mal du loup, "because just as the wolf, it devours all the body's members."

REFERENCES 23, 27

295

Lubin (Leobinus) of Chartres

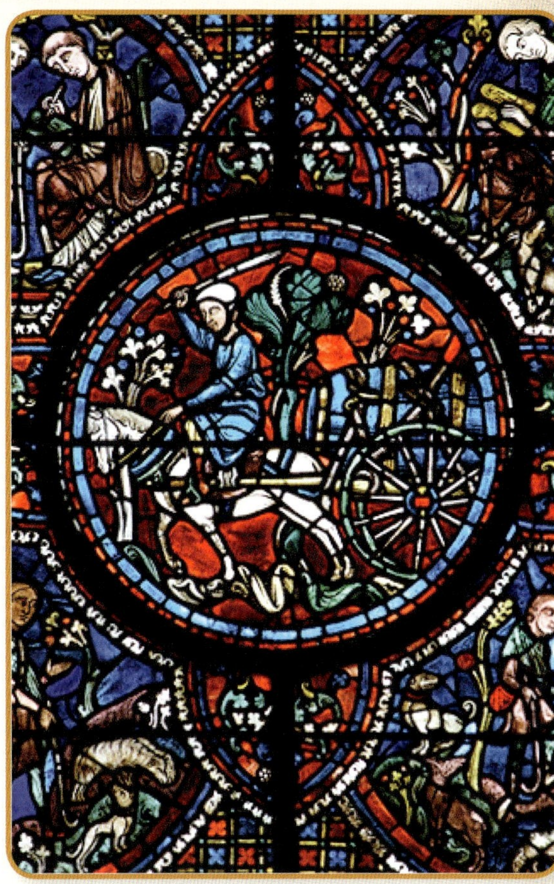

MEMORIAL DAY **March 14**

PATRONAGE **Dropsy (edema), eye diseases, rheumatism**

LIFE & LEGEND

Lubin was born into a peasant family near Poitiers. As a boy, he was eager to learn. Du Broc de Segange relates that one day, while tending a herd, the boy Lubin encountered a monk from the monastery at Noailles. He asked the monk to trace the letters of the alphabet on his belt so that he might learn to read from them. Eventually Lubin himself entered the monastery at Noailles, where he devoted his days to the menial tasks assigned to him and his nights to study. Lubin spent 8 years at Noailles before leaving to consult the hermit Avitus in the solitude of Le Perche. Avitus advised Lubin to delay his plan to withdraw into the wilderness and to spend more time in a cenobitic community.

Lubin lived 5 years in a monastery near Lyon, before that establishment was caught up in the fighting between Franks and Burgundians. Lubin and an old man were the only men who had remained at the monastery. He was captured and tortured by soldiers who wanted Lubin to reveal where the monastery's treasure was hidden. Lubin revealed nothing, perhaps because there was nothing to reveal. Eventually the raiders departed, leaving Lubin for dead.

Lubin recovered from his injuries and returned to Avitus at Le Perche, where he was temporarily able to fulfill his desire for the hermetic life until summoned by Aetherius, the bishop of Chartres, who ordained Lubin to the priesthood and made him abbot of the monastery at Brou. Lubin reluctantly assumed his new duties and sought opportunities to resign. When Aetherius died, Lubin was appointed to the vacant see of Chartres, and Lubin devoted himself to his episcopal duties. In this public role, his gifts as a wonder-worker became evident. He continued to work miracles, including the healing of a man with a particularly pronounced swelling from hydrops. Lubin died in 558 after a lengthy illness.

REFERENCES 6, 14, 16, 32, 36

296

Lucian of Beauvais

MEMORIAL DAY **January 8**

PATRONAGE **Leprosy (in children)**

LIFE & LEGEND

Lucian was a missionary, who, toward the end of the third century, was sent from Rome to evangelize the inhabitants of Gaul. He was martyred during the persecution of Diocletian at Beauvais, where his remains and those of his companions, Messien and Julian, were discovered in the seventh century. These relics were famous for the miracles that were associated with them. According to some sources, Lucian was the first bishop of Beauvais. Du Broc de Segange dates Lucian to the first century, maintaining that he was a member of a prominent Roman family and that he was converted to Christianity by Saint Peter.

REFERENCES 6, 16, 36, 46

297

Lucius (Lucio, Luguzzone, Uguzo) of Cavargna

MEMORIAL DAY **July 12**

PATRONAGE **Eye diseases**

LIFE & LEGEND

The cult of Saint Lucius originated in the Val di Cavargna (between Lago di Lugano and Lago di Como), in Italy. He was a pious shepherd in the twelfth or thirteenth century who was accused of theft by his employer for giving small sums from his property to the Church and to the poor. Lucius then went to work for another man, whose fortunes rose during Lucius' tenure as those of his former employer declined. Out of anger and envy, the latter killed Lucius. A spring rose on the spot where the shepherd was murdered, the waters from which were believed to be effective in healing diseases of the eye. His cult is common throughout northern Italy and the Swiss canton of Ticino.

REFERENCES 36, 46

298

Lucy (Lucia) of Syracuse

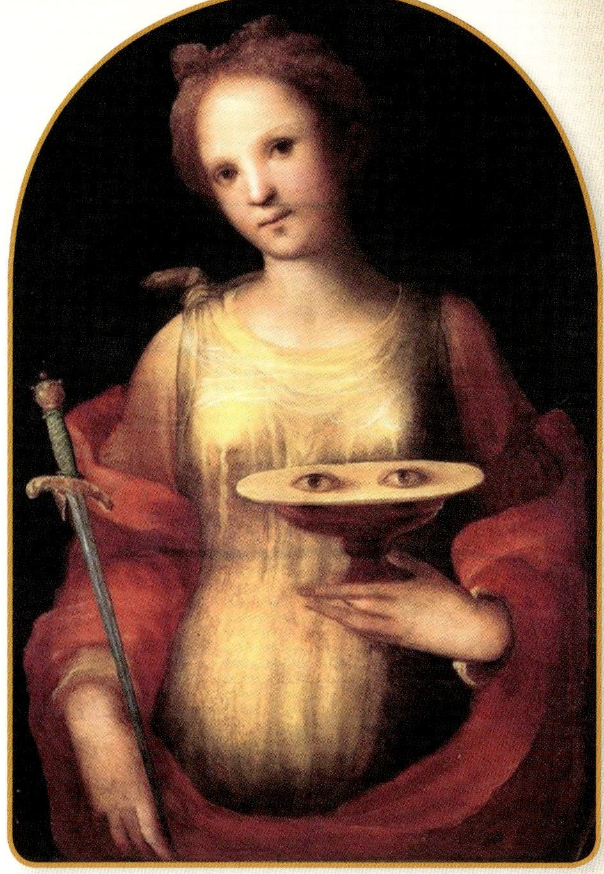

MEMORIAL DAY **December 13**

PATRONAGE **Eye diseases, blindness, [ophthalmology],* dysentery, hemorrhage, sore throat, contagious diseases, stained glass workers, Syracuse (Sicily), Perugia (Italy), Mtarfa (Malta)**

LIFE & LEGEND

Lucy was born of wealthy parents in Sicily ca. 283. Her father died when she was young, and her mother betrothed her to a pagan. Lucy was determined to devote herself to Christianity and consecrate her virginity to God. She convinced her mother, Eutychia, who was suffering from bloody dysentery ("bloody flux") to journey to Catania, about 50 miles from Syracuse, to pray at the relics of Saint Agatha. Her mother was cured and allowed Lucy to call off her betrothal and follow her calling.

Her rejected suitor denounced Lucy as a Christian to Paschasius, the governor of Sicily, during the Diocletian persecutions of 304. She was first sentenced to prostitution, but when the guards tried to carry her away, she was so heavy (filled

*Proposed patronage

with the Lord) that she could not be moved even when hitched to a team of oxen. As part of her torture, her eyes were gouged out, but her vision was miraculously restored. That miracle and the fact that her name means "light" account for the patronage of diseases of the eyes. She was also saved from being burned on a pyre when the fire went out, but she eventually met her death when a dagger pierced her throat. As she was dying, she predicted the punishment of the governor of Sicily who had arranged for her torture and that Diocletian's reign would come to an end soon. This came true.

Her relics purportedly remained in Sicily for 400 years and were then transferred to Corfinium, Italy. They were removed to Metz, Germany, toward the end of the first millennium. Some relics were found in Constantinople at the beginning of the thirteenth century and translated to Venice. In 1513, the Venetians presented Louis XII with the saint's head, which he deposited in the cathedral at Bourges.

Saint Lucy is one of seven women, excluding the Blessed Virgin Mary, commemorated by name in the Canon of the Mass. She is one of the few saints celebrated by the Lutheran Swedes, Finns, Danes, and Norwegians. Her celebration takes place on December 13, the longest night on the unreformed Julian calendar. Dante mentions Lucy in his *Inferno,* and also places her opposite Adam within the Mystic Rose in his *Paradiso.*

REFERENCES 6, 9, 33, 45

299

Ludan

MEMORIAL DAY **February 12**

PATRONAGE **Foot and leg problems**

LIFE & LEGEND

The son of a Scottish prince named Hiltebold, Ludan is said to have dispersed his inheritance in building churches, oratories, and a hospice for pilgrims and the poor. Butler relates that, while resting on his return from a pilgrimage to Jerusalem ca. 1202 (or to Rome, according to some sources), Ludan dreamt of his own death, was given communion by an angel on waking, and then died—whereupon the bells of all the surrounding churches began to peal. Du Broc de Segange, by contrast, indicates that Ludan died near Strasbourg while resting beneath a tree, worn out from "the austerities of his penitence and the length of his journey," accounting for his patronage.

REFERENCES 14, 16

300

Luglius and Luglianus

MEMORIAL DAY **October 23**

PATRONAGE **Fever, plague, cholera, Lillers, Montdidier**

LIFE & LEGEND

The two brothers, Luglius and Luglianus, were members of a royal Irish family. It is uncertain whether Luglius was elevated to the episcopate or whether he refused the episcopate to pursue a monastic life. His younger brother is supposed to have succeeded their father as ruler or king. The brothers decided to make a pilgrimage to the Holy Land (or perhaps Rome). They came ashore at Boulogne-sur-Mer, where the ship on which they were traveling had sought refuge during a storm. They continued their journey on land, traveling through the valley of Scyrendale, an area noted for its brigands. The brothers were captured and murdered by a gang of thieves ca. 700. Soon after the crime, their remains were gathered and taken to nearby Lillers. Some of their relics were later deposited at Montdidier.

REFERENCES 7, 36

301

Luke the Evangelist

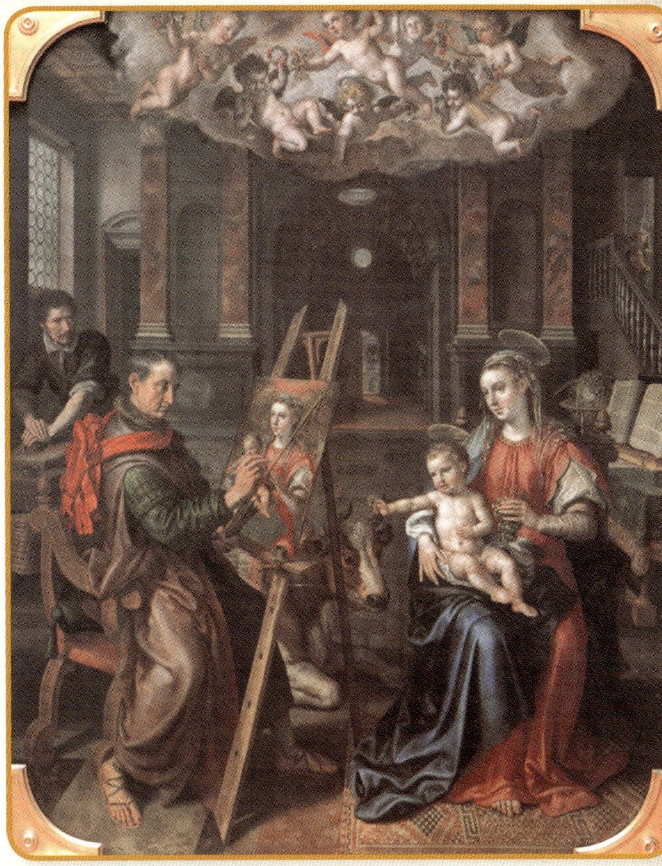

MEMORIAL DAY **October 18**

PATRONAGE **[Medicine],* doctors, physicians, surgeons, artists, painters, sculptors, stained glass workers, bookbinders, brewers, glass makers, goldsmiths, lace workers, notaries, bachelors, Hermersdorf (Germany)**

LIFE & LEGEND

Luke, whose name is derived from Latin, meaning "bringer of light," probably was born to pagan Greek parents in Antioch, the metropolis in ancient Syria. He studied medicine in Antioch and Tarsus. Saint Jerome indicates that Luke was an eminent physician, and Saint Paul refers to him as his "most dear physician," which accounts for his patronage in the field of medicine. No medical miracles are ascribed to him.

*Proposed patronage

He was also a painter, and he is thought by some to have done portraits of Mary and Jesus, but this has not been authenticated. Nevertheless, as a painter and as the author of a Gospel that gave inspiration to artists, he gained patronage in several aspects of art—painting, sculpture, and stained glass making.

Luke was one of the early proselytes to Christianity and is generally thought of as the only non-Jewish New Testament writer. His Gospel is unique in that it includes accounts of Christ's birth, infancy, and childhood. It is also notable for the parable of The Good Samaritan and that of The Prodigal Son, and three of the sayings of Christ on the cross; "Father forgive them," "Thou shalt be with me in Paradise," and " Father, into Thy hands I commend my spirit."

Luke's Gospel, which takes up more pages in the New Testament that the writings of any other author, emphasizes Christ's compassion for sinners, unhappy individuals, outcasts, tax collectors, lepers, poorly regarded shepherds, and the poor. A role for women in Christ's ministry is also emphasized. His writings focus on Jerusalem and the Temple.

Luke became the traveling companion of Paul and went with him to Macedonia and the cities of Greece. Luke was the faithful attendant of Paul during the latter's confinement in Rome that ended in 63 AD, the year that Luke finished his Acts of the Apostles. Luke died ca. 74 in Greece. It is said that Luke was crucified on an olive tree at Elaea in Peloponnesus near Achaia. But it is written in *Martyrologies* that he died very old in Bithynia. The bones of Saint Luke were taken from Patras in Achaia in 357 by order of Emperor Constantius and placed in the church of the Apostles at Constantinople. Some of the relics were later sent to a church in Brescia, to Saint Felix's church in Nola, and to a church at the monastery in Rome. Some of the relics reside in the monastery at Mount Athos in Greece.

REFERENCES 9, 42, 45

302
Lutgardis

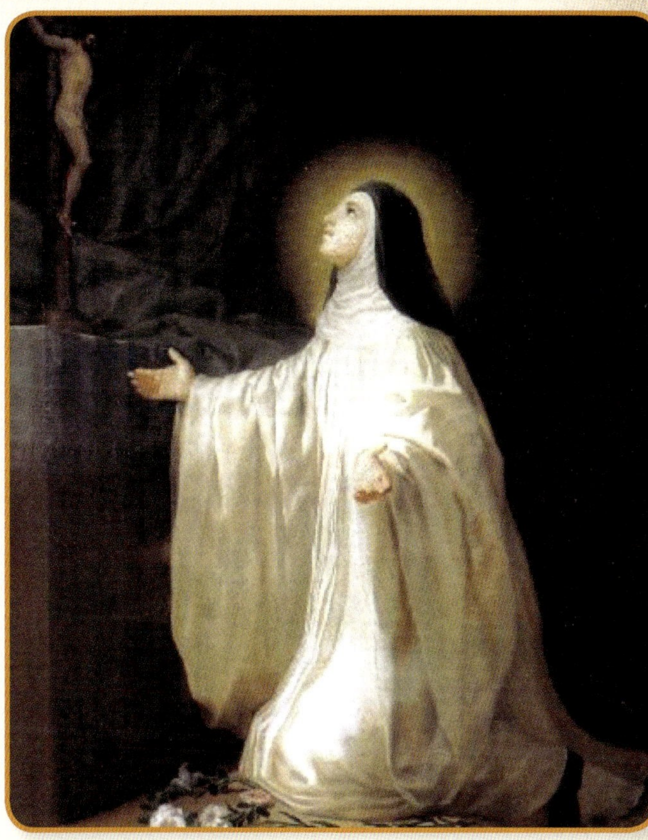

MEMORIAL DAY **June 16**

PATRONAGE **Blindness, physical handicaps, childbirth**

LIFE & LEGEND

Lutgardis was born in 1182, at Tongres, in the Netherlands (now Belgium), and was sent to a Benedictine convent when she was 12 years old, because her family became impoverished when their business failed. While in her teens, she had a vision of Christ showing her his wounds. Shortly thereafter, she became a Benedictine nun and continued to have visions and experience ecstasies, stigmata, and levitation. In 1208, she left the Benedictines for the stricter Order of Cistercians. She continued to demonstrate her healing powers, prophecy, and wisdom.

She was blind for the last 11 years of her life. She regarded the affliction as a gift to reduce the distraction of the material world. She died as she had predicted, after the feast of the Holy Trinity, at Aywieres, near Liege, in 1246. She is regarded as one of the leading mystics of the thirteenth century.

REFERENCES 6, 42, 45

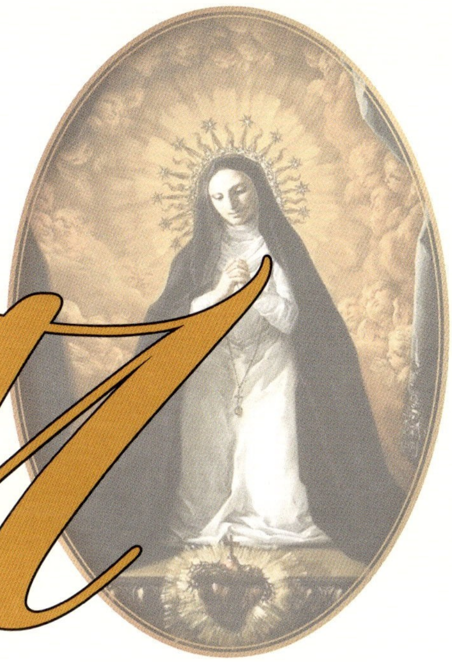

303

Macarius of Antioch

MEMORIAL DAY **April 10**

PATRONAGE **Plague, epidemic diseases, Ghent**

LIFE & LEGEND

Macarius was born in Antioch and was of noble Armenian descent. He was appointed archbishop of Antioch in Pisidia by an older Macarius who occupied that see and wished the younger Macarius to succeed him. To relieve himself of the honors of an office he never sought, the younger Macarius appointed a successor, gave all his possessions to the poor, and departed on a pilgrimage to Jerusalem. In the Holy City he was imprisoned and tortured by the Saracens, from whom he eventually escaped. Making his way to Europe, Macarius journeyed up the Rhine through Mainz and Cologne, and then west into Flanders. He is said to have worked miracles all along the way. When Macarius reached Ghent, he was received as a pilgrim by the monks of the monastery of Saint-Bavon.

Macarius was on the point of returning to Armenia when the plague appeared in Ghent. According to Kerler, "The saintly bishop offered himself to God for the health of these poor people." His prayer was accepted, and Macarius contracted the plague, of which he died. He was the epidemic's last victim, and the plague abated immediately on his death in 1012. The name of Macarius was long invoked in Flanders during outbreaks of plague and other epidemic diseases. He is represented with his mitre and crozier on the ground, symbolic of his resignation of the bishopric.

REFERENCES 6, 16, 36, 45

304
Macra

MEMORIAL DAY **June 11**

PATRONAGE **Breast diseases**

LIFE & LEGEND

The legend of Macra is strikingly similar to that of Saint Agatha. Macra was a pious virgin of the diocese of Reims who was a victim of the persecution of Christians under the emperors Diocletian and Maximian. After refusing to renounce her faith and sacrifice to the Roman gods, she was arrested and tortured. Her sufferings included the removal of her breasts. One night she was visited in her prison cell by a luminous figure who healed all her wounds. When she was discovered next morning to be perfectly sound, the imperial delegate ordered her to be roasted over live coals. Macra died ca. 303 during this final ordeal, which is supposed to have taken place at or near the present-day village of Fismes.

REFERENCES 16, 36

305

Madelbertha

MEMORIAL DAY **September 7**

PATRONAGE **Pregnancy**

LIFE & LEGEND

Madelbertha was the daughter of Saint Vincent Madelgarius, count of Hainault, and Saint Waldetrudis. All four children born to this couple were canonized. At a very young age, Madelbertha entered the convent founded by her aunt at Mauberge. She became its abbess in 697 and remained in that position until she died in 708.

REFERENCES 2, 36

306

Maginus of Tarragona

MEMORIAL DAY **August 25**

PATRONAGE **Pregnancy, infertility, smallpox, measles**

LIFE & LEGEND

Maginus lived as a hermit in the vicinity of Tarragona, Spain. He was beheaded for his faith during the persecution of Maximian, ca. 304.

REFERENCES 16, 36

307

Magnobodus (Mainbeuf)

MEMORIAL DAY **October 16**

PATRONAGE **Skin diseases, leprosy, boils, scabies**

LIFE & LEGEND

Magnobodus was born into a noble Frankish family that was closely associated with the royal house. His education was supervised by Licinius (Lezin), bishop of Angers, who also tonsured Magnobodus and ordained him to the priesthood. Licinius dispatched Magnobodus to Rome to solicit relics of Saint John the Baptist for the church that the bishop was building. On his return to Angers he was made abbot of Colonet. Magnobodus was proclaimed bishop of Angers in 606, and he remained in that office until his death in 654.

REFERENCES 7, 16, 36

308

Magnus of Füssen

MEMORIAL DAY **September 6**

PATRONAGE **Eye diseases**

LIFE & LEGEND

A history of the life of Magnus, written by the monks of Saint Gall in the ninth century, makes Magnus a contemporary of both Saint Gall and Saint Wichtbert. Magnus, who lived during the eighth century, was the first recorded bishop of Augsburg, and was entrusted by Bishop Wichtbert with the Christianization of the eastern Allgäu (the mountainous district between Bavaria and the Tirol). Magnus established a cell in the wilderness of the region that evolved into the monastery of Füssen. He is credited with the miraculous healing of a blind person, accounting for his patronage.

REFERENCE 36

309

Malo (Maclou, Macuto)

MEMORIAL DAY **November 15**

PATRONAGE **Dropsy, lameness**

LIFE & LEGEND

Malo, who lived during the seventh century, was born near Llancarfan in Wales and educated at the local monastery. He might have been a disciple of Saint Brendan at Llancarfan and later in Brittany, where he had gone as a missionary following his ordination to the priesthood. Malo centered his missionary activity in the area of Aleth (present-day Saint-Servan), enjoying success both through his preaching and the miracles he is said to have worked there. Malo became Aleth's first bishop (a see that was later transferred to nearby Saint-Malo), but local opposition forced him to withdraw for several years to Saintes (Saintonge provence). Malo returned to Aleth to miraculously relieve a drought, but he died in Saintonge on his way back to Saintes.

REFERENCES 6, 14, 27, 36

310

Mamas

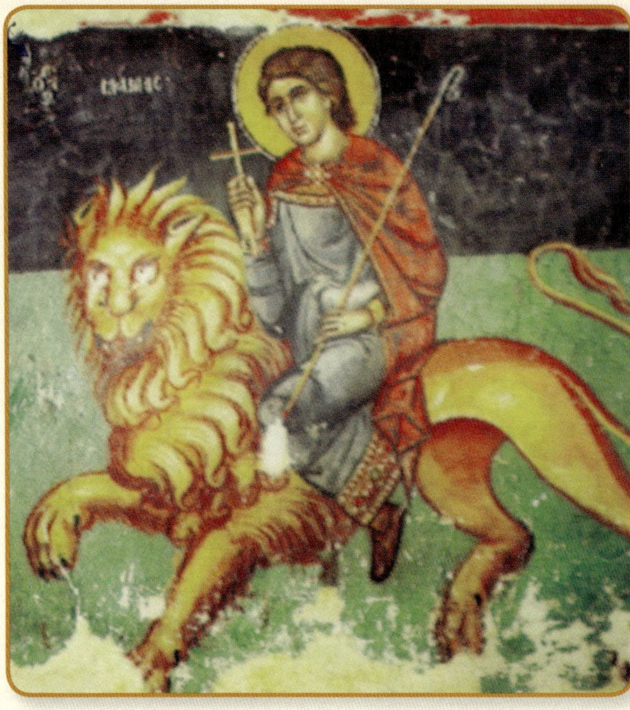

MEMORIAL DAY **August 17**

PATRONAGE **Colicky children, wet nurses**

LIFE & LEGEND

Mamas was a shepherd near Caesarea in Cappadocia. According to some sources, he was the son of saints Theodotus and Rufina. One version of Mamas' martyrdom maintains that the pious shepherd was stoned to death as a youth during the reign of Emperor Aurelian ca. 275. Another version maintains that, at the command of a voice that he alone heard, Mamas withdrew into the wilderness during this persecution, where he lived in solitude surrounded by birds and beasts, to whom he would preach and read the gospels. He was accompanied by a lion as a protector. When his whereabouts were discovered, Mamas converted the soldiers sent to arrest him. All of them returned to the city where they were tortured and beheaded. Yet another version maintains that Mamas was executed in his old age after a prolonged persecution. The cult of Mamas originated in Cappadocia, but eventually spread to France and Italy. Because he was nourished by the milk of wild animals during his exile in the wilderness, Mamas is regarded as a patron saint of wet nurses.

REFERENCES 6, 14, 36, 45, 46

311

Manechildis (Ménéhoud)

MEMORIAL DAY **October 14**

PATRONAGE **Plague**

LIFE & LEGEND

Manechildis was born at Perthois, one of the seven daughters of count Sigmarus—all of whom are venerated as saints. All the sisters took the veil from Alpinus, bishop of Châlons. Manechildis was known for her personal piety and for her devotion to the sick and the poor. After the death of her parents, Manechildis lived as a recluse near Bienville (Marne), where she died in the sixth century. She is the patron saint of the village of Saint Ménéhoud in the Champagne-Ardenne region, where she was invoked in times of pestilence.

REFERENCES 6, 14, 36

312
Marciana

MEMORIAL DAY **January 9 (Tortosa, Spain: July 12)**

PATRONAGE **Injury, Tortosa**

LIFE & LEGEND

The virgin martyr, Marciana, was a native of Rusuccus (present-day Dellys, Algeria). Marciana was arrested for having vandalized a statue of the goddess Diana in the streets of Caesarea (Mauritania). She was scourged and handed over to gladiators to be raped. She was miraculously saved from this outrage. Marciana persisted in her faith and was exposed to wild beasts in the amphitheater. She was ignored by a lion but gored by a bull and finally mauled to death by a leopard ca. 303.

REFERENCES 2, 36, 46

313

Marcuf (Marcoul)

MEMORIAL DAY **May 1**

PATRONAGE **Scrofula, skin diseases, rashes**

LIFE & LEGEND

Marculf, whose name derives from the Saxon, "marc" meaning "horse," or "border," and "culf," meaning "wolf," was born at Bayeux, France, into nobility toward the end of the fifth century, and he became a priest at age 30. He served as a successful missionary to the pagans of Gaul, and he sent Saint Helier to Jersey to convert the inhabitants there to Christianity. Although Marculf eschewed public life and became a hermit, he founded a monastery at Nanteuil, France. He died in 558, and his relics, which had been preserved at Corbigny and Leon, France, were used to cure scrofula and enlarged or draining lymph nodes in the neck, which was usually caused by bovine tuberculosis and was known as "The King's Evil" (see Saint Edward the Confessor). His relics were invoked by Louis IX and were brought to Reims for the coronation of Louis XIV. They were destroyed after having been used in the coronation of several of his successors.

REFERENCES 6, 42

314

Margaret of Antioch

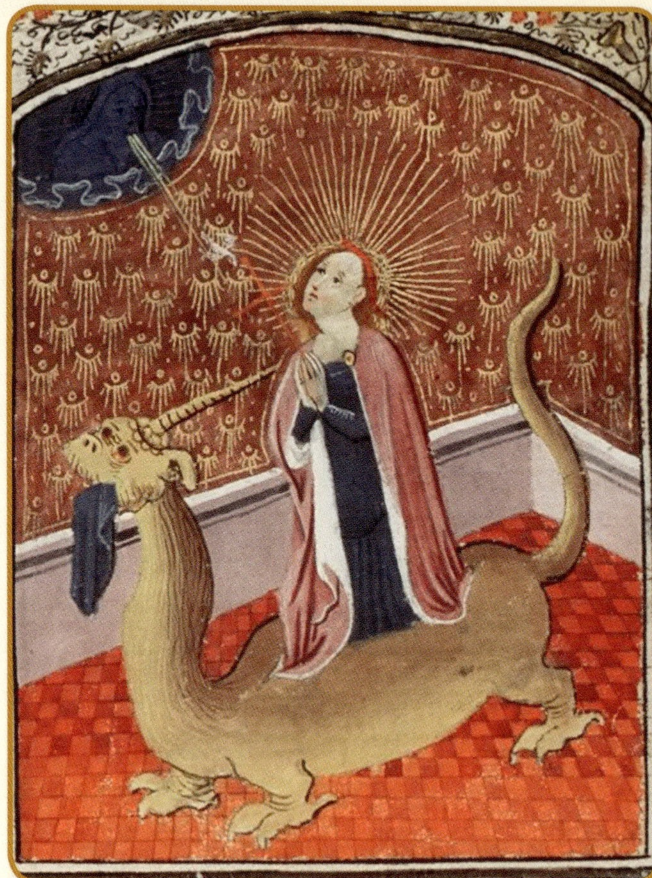

MEMORIAL DAY **July 20, (Eastern Orthodox: July 13)**

PATRONAGE **Sterility, childbirth, pregnancy, kidney diseases, backache, nurses, peasants, people in exile**

LIFE & LEGEND

Margaret, whose name is derived from Greek, meaning "pearl," was fathered by a pagan priest in Antioch, Asia Minor (current Turkey). Because her mother died when she was an infant, Margaret was raised by a Christian woman who adopted her. One day a Roman prefect saw her tending sheep and made sexual advances, which she refused. She was brought to trial as a Christian and, when she refused to sacrifice to the pagan gods, she was first burned and then boiled in a cauldron. She remained unharmed and was ultimately martyred by beheading ca. 304. Legend reports that she was swallowed by the devil in the form of a dragon, but escaped when the cross she was wearing irritated the dragon's intestinal tract. This episode characterizes most of her iconography. She was one of the saints who appeared to Joan of Arc, and she is one of the Fourteen Holy Helpers. Saint Margaret was one of the most popular saints in medieval England, where more than 250 churches were dedicated to her.

REFERENCES 9, 42

315

Margaret Mary Alacoque

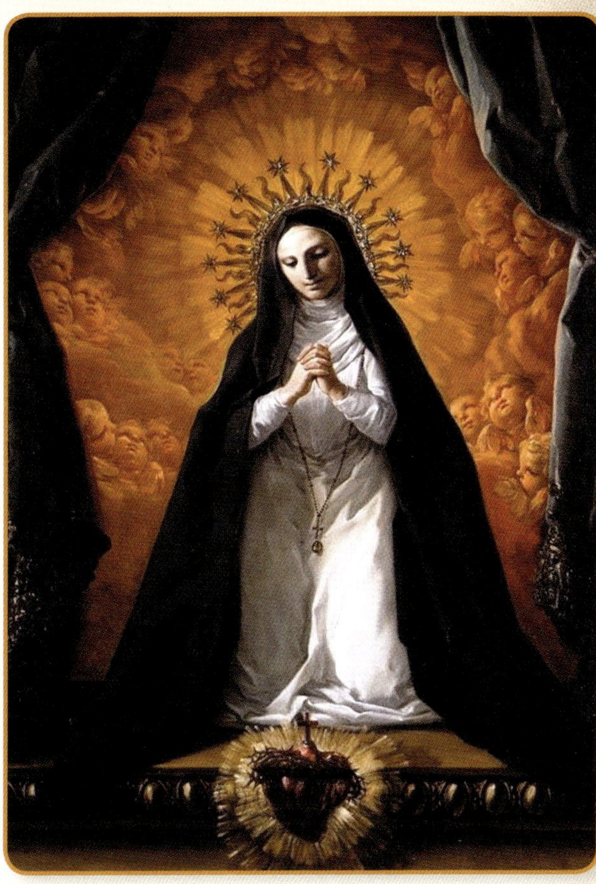

MEMORIAL DAY **October 17**

PATRONAGE **Polio**

LIFE & LEGEND

Margaret Mary was born in 1647 at L'Hautecourt, Burgundy, France. Her father, a prosperous notary, died when she was about 8 years old, leaving the family in financial stress. Margaret was sent to study with the Urbanist Sisters. She enjoyed convent life and decided to become a nun. She practiced corporal mortification until she developed a crippling disorder, either of rheumatic origin or paralysis, that was healed by a vision of the Blessed Virgin. This accounts for her patronage for polio. She joined the Order of the Visitation at Paray-le-Monial in 1671.

She changed her baptismal name to Marguerite-Marie. She received many visions, including one of Christ crucified but alive, claiming His heart was filled with love for her. As a consequence of her visions, she believed that she had been chosen to transmit a new devotion to the Sacred Heart of Jesus, which is the symbol of that boundless love which moved the Word to take flesh, to institute the Holy Eucharist, to take our sins upon Himself, and, dying on the Cross, to offer Himself as a victim and sacrifice to the eternal Father.

Margaret Mary died of natural causes at Paray-le-Monial in 1690, and her body was buried under the altar. When her tomb was opened in the course of her canonization, two miraculous cures immediately occurred. Over the years, her tomb remained the site of many cures. She was eventually canonized in 1920 by Pope Benedict XV.

REFERENCES 6, 9, 42, 45

316 Marguerite d'Youville

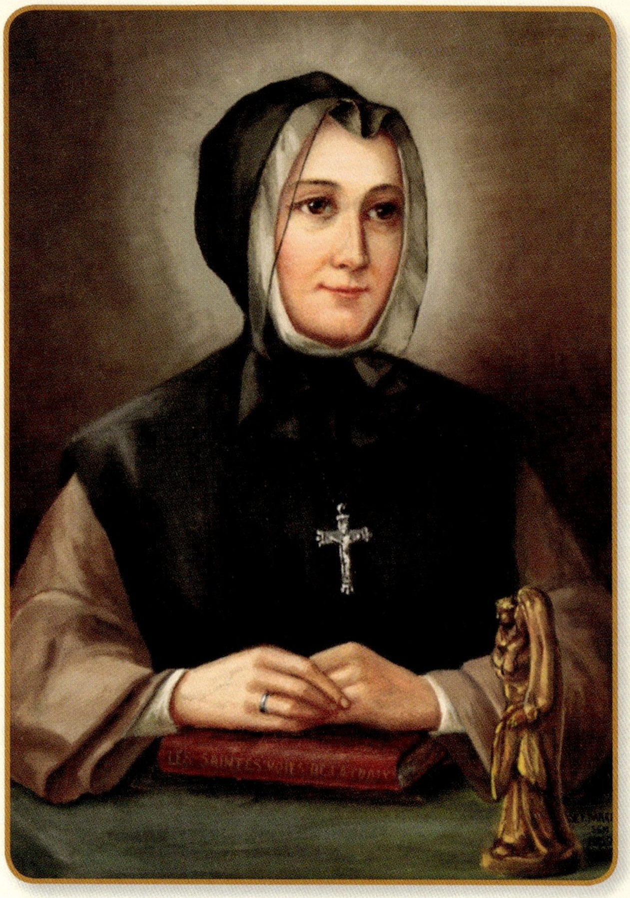

MEMORIAL DAY December 23

PATRONAGE Leukemia, childbirth, difficult marriages, victims of adultery, widows, death of children

LIFE & LEGEND

Marie-Marguerite d'Youville was born October 15, 1701, at Varennes, Quebec, Canada, the eldest of six children of Christophe Dufrost de Lajemmerais and Renee de Varennes, the niece of Laverendrye, who discovered the Rocky Mountains. Marguerite's father died when she was 7 years old, and she was sent to be educated by the Ursulines in Quebec for 2 years. She returned home to help her mother and educate her siblings. Her mother married an Irish physician, and the family moved to Montreal.

At age 21, Marguerite married François d'Youville and bore six children, four of whom died in infancy; the surviving two became priests. Her husband proved to be an adulterer and a provider of liquor to Native Americans. After he died in 1730, she became engaged in charitable works and was joined by three other women who had a deep concern for the poor.

On December 31, 1737, with the help of Father Louis Normant du Faradon, she founded the Sisters of Charity of the General Hospital of Montreal (Grey Nuns). In 1755, the group received diocesan approval. In 1747, she took over as director of the failing Charon Brothers Hospital in Montreal and rejuvenated it. The hospital burned down in 1765, and she directed the reconstruction of the building as a shelter for the poor. She died on December 23, 1771.

Sister communities of the Grey Nuns were established at Saint Hyacinthe, Quebec, Ottawa, and Philadelphia. She was beatified in 1959 by Pope John XXIII and canonized by Pope John Paul II in 1990. The miracle accepted by the Congregation for the Causes of the Saints was the cure of a recurrence of acute leukemia in a young woman who ceased treatment and elected to rely on prayers to Marguerite. With her canonization, Marguerite d'Youville became the first native Canadian saint.

REFERENCES 9, 17

317

Marianus (Marien)

MEMORIAL DAY **August 19**

PATRONAGE **Safe delivery**

LIFE & LEGEND

Marianus was born into a prominent family of Bourges during the sixth century. For reasons unknown, Marianus left his wife and entered the monastery of Pressigny, where he lived 6 years before withdrawing to a forest hermitage near Epineuil in the Bourbonnais. He pursued this solitary life for 44 years, living solely on fruits and honey he found in the wild. Toward the end of his life, Marianus moved to a place near present-day Évaux-les-Bains, where he received those seeking his spiritual guidance. Marianus continues to be venerated at Évaux, where his remains were entombed, and also at Bourges.

REFERENCES 16, 36, 46

318

Martha of Bethany

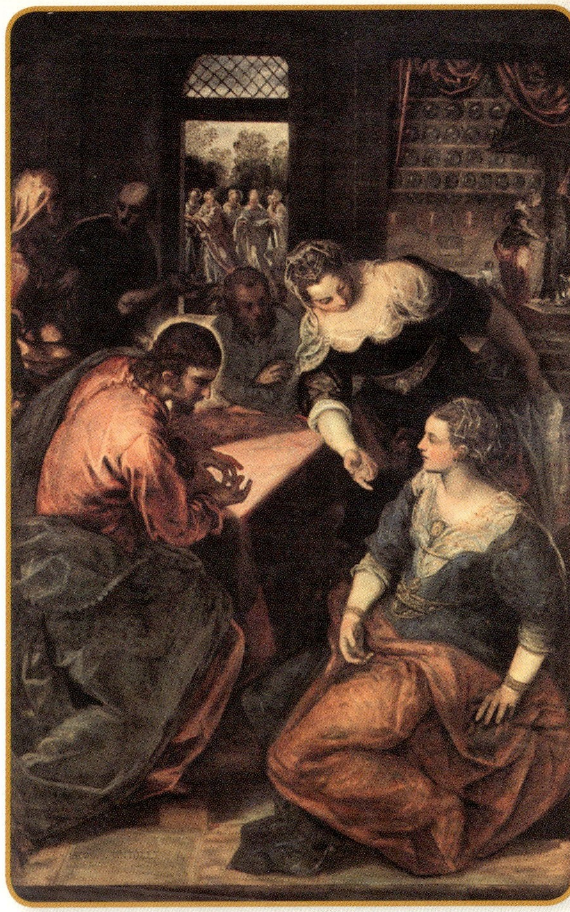

MEMORIAL DAY **July 29**

PATRONAGE **Hemorrhage, plague, hospital administrators, dieticians**

LIFE & LEGEND

Martha, whose name is derived from Aramaic, meaning "lady," was the sister of Mary and Lazarus, with whom she lived two miles from Jerusalem in the village of Bethany. All three were disciples of Jesus, who was a guest in their home when he was preaching in Judea. On one such occasion, Martha's sister, Mary, left Martha alone to manage their guests while Mary "sat at the Lord's feet and listened to his teaching. But Martha was distracted with much serving; and she went to him and said, 'Lord, do you not care that my sister has left me to serve alone? Tell her then to help me.' Jesus responded, 'Martha, Martha, you are anxious and troubled about many things; one thing is needful. Mary has chosen the good portion, which shall not be taken away from her.'" (Luke 10:39-42). Martha is again named in the gospel of John when she went out to meet Jesus, who had come to Bethany after the death of her brother, Lazarus (John 11:1-46).

There are two versions of the subsequent lives of Martha, Mary, and Lazarus. The more reliable sources maintain that Lazarus went to Cyprus, where he became bishop of Kition. Presumably his sisters accompanied him there. In a legend popular in the South of France, Martha, Mary, and Lazarus are said to have been set adrift in an open boat without rudder or oars (by unspecified persons for unspecified reasons), and they came ashore at La Camargue, an island in the delta of the Rhône, in 48 AD. In this legend, Lazarus became the first bishop of Marseilles, in the territory of which his sisters preached the gospel. Martha is said to have proceeded up the Rhône to Tarascon, where she tamed a monster called the Tarasque that had been terrifying the district. As a consequence of Martha's conquest of the beast, the people of Tarascon were converted to the new faith. Martha is said to have died and been buried there in the year 68. Her relics were discovered in 1187 and entombed at Tarascon in the Église Collégiale Sainte Marthe, the construction of which began in 1199.

REFERENCES 6, 36, 46

319

Martial of Limoges

MEMORIAL DAY **June 30**

PATRONAGE **Plague, contagious diseases, epidemic diseases**

LIFE & LEGEND

A ninth-century life of Martial, composed at the monastery of Saint Martial in Limoges, says that the saint was a contemporary of Saint Peter during the first century. Peter dispatched Martial to Gaul as a missionary and as the first bishop of Limoges. From the ninth to the eleventh centuries, the legend of Martial continued to be amplified. The numerous surviving manuscripts of the enhanced legend maintain that Martial was the boy with five barley loaves and two fish from which Jesus fed the five thousand (John 6:9), that he was one of the 70 disciples sent out by Jesus, that he was present at the raising of Lazarus, and that he was seated at the Last Supper. This legend, with all its late medieval accretions, is related faithfully by du Broc de Segange. In reality, Martial was probably a native of Asia Minor and was one of the seven missionaries sent from Rome before the year 250 to evangelize Gaul. Martial was responsible for the evangelization of the Limousin region, where he was bishop of Limoges.

REFERENCES 6, 16, 36, 46

320

Martin of Tours

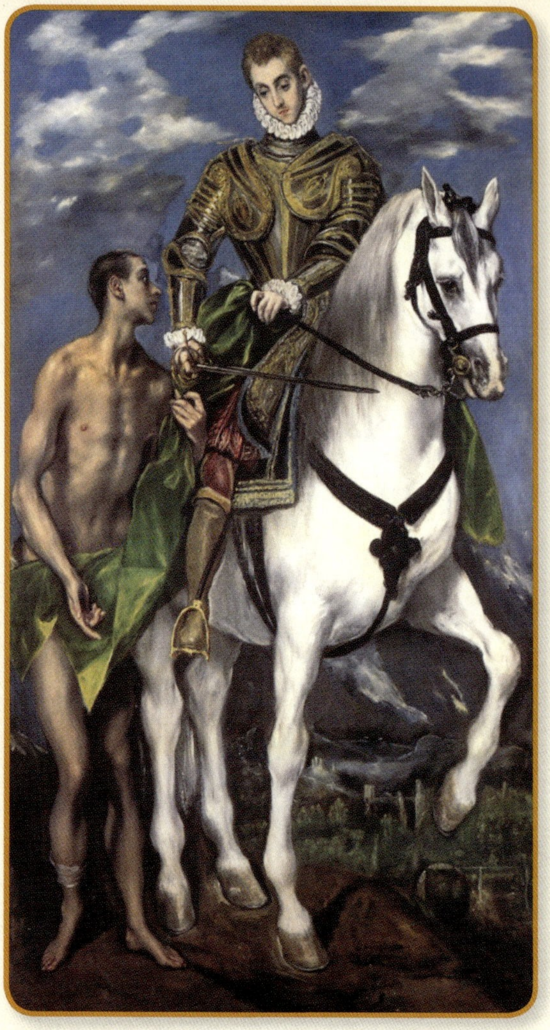

MEMORIAL DAY **November 11**

PATRONAGE **Alcoholism, skin diseases, poverty, horsemen, France, Buenos Aires**

LIFE & LEGEND

Martin, whose name is derived from that of the God of War, Mars, and implies "courage and bravery," was born to pagan parents ca. 316 in what is Hungary today. His father, a military tribune, was transferred to Pavia, Italy, where Martin spent his youth and became attracted to Christianity during his adolescence. He joined the Roman army at age 15 and was assigned to duty in Gaul. It was there that the most celebrated legend associated with him took place.

While on horseback, he encountered an elderly beggar who was sparsely clothed. Martin divided his officer's cloak in two and gave one half to the beggar. That night Martin dreamed that Jesus was wearing the half-cloak that he had given away, and he heard Jesus say to the angels: "Here is Martin, the Roman soldier who is not baptized; he has clad me." In another story, Martin awoke to find his cloak restored, and that cloak is preserved among his relics.

Martin was baptized at age 18, and, on the eve of a battle, he indicated that his faith prohibited him from fighting. He was jailed but released when the battle did not take place. On one occasion he encountered robbers in the mountains of Lombard, and he converted one of the thieves. He also converted his mother to Christianity. Martin became a spiritual student of Saint Hilary at Poitiers. He became a hermit for 10 years in an area now known as Ligugé. He attracted other monks, preached throughout the countryside, and converted many peasants.

He was named bishop of Tours in 371 and moved to a hermit's cell near that city. He built a new monastery at Marmoutier that gained in importance and persists. He died at about age 81 in Candes, France. A chapel was built over his grave, and the building where his cloak was preserved became known as a capella, deriving from "cappa," the Latin word for "cloak," which was converted to the French word, "chapelle." Martin was considered to be one of France's most important saints. His tomb became a national shrine.

In the sixth century, Clovis, the king of the Salian Franks, credited the intervention of Saint Martin with his victory over the Alemanni. He then moved his capital to Paris and is considered the "Founder of France." The cult that was established around Saint Martin is the first to be related to a saint who had not been a martyr. Martin Luther himself was named for Saint Martin, because he was baptized on Saint Martin's memorial day.

REFERENCES 6, 9, 42, 46a

321
Marus

MEMORIAL DAY **January 26**

PATRONAGE **Gout, paralysis, spasms, contractures of limbs**

LIFE & LEGEND

Little is known of Marus other than he was a bishop of Treves in the fifth century. "Nevertheless," writes du Broc de Segange, "tradition informs us that both those who appealed to him while living and those who approached the tomb that held his remains often obtained a cure for the most serious afflictions, particularly gout, paralysis, spasmodic disorders, and contractions in the extremities."

REFERENCES 16, 36

322

Mary of Egypt

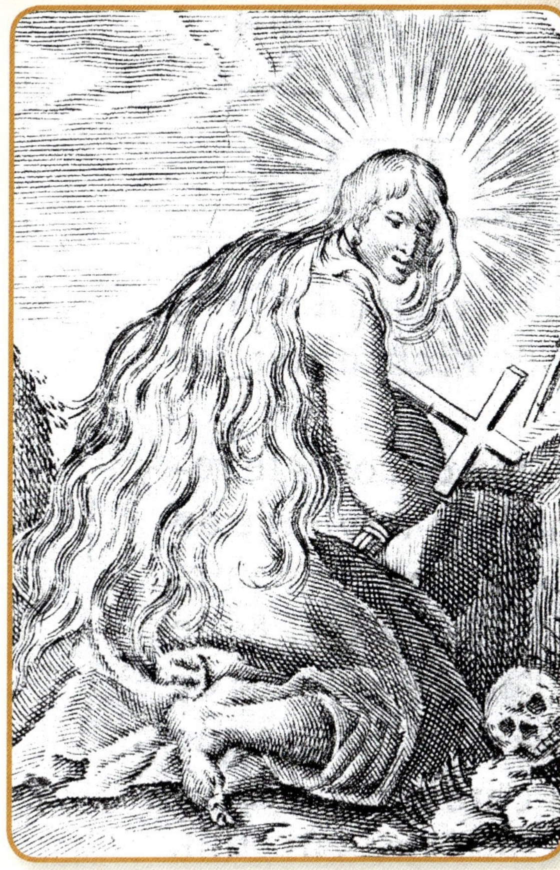

MEMORIAL DAY **April 3 (Greek Orthodox: April 1)**

PATRONAGE **Fever, repentant prostitutes**

LIFE & LEGEND

Mary, who lived during the fifth century, left her parents at age 12 and went to the city of Alexandria, where she supported herself for the next 17 years as a singer, actress, beggar, and prostitute. Out of curiosity, by cajoling the sailors to take her on board, she joined a band of pilgrims traveling from Alexandria to celebrate the feast of the Exaltation of the Holy Cross in Jerusalem. Mary seduced several of her pilgrim companions on the voyage and resumed her dissolute ways in Jerusalem. On the day appointed for the veneration of the Holy Cross, Mary attempted to enter the church of the Holy Sepulchre with the surging crowd, but was repeatedly stopped at the threshold by an invisible force. Withdrawing to the courtyard, she suddenly realized how depraved her past had been, was filled with compunction, and prayed to the Mother of God to help her. The next morning Mary found that she was able to enter the church and venerate the Holy Cross. She immediately left Jerusalem with some loaves of bread and crossed the river Jordan. Mary spent the next 47 years in the wilderness beyond the Jordan, where she lived in solitude and prayer, both repenting of and seeking to forget the pleasures to which she had once been enslaved.

About the year 430, a Palestinian monk named Zosimus was passing through this part of the wilderness when he spied a human form. Assuming it to be a hermit and desiring to obtain the holy man's blessing, Zosimus overtook the fleeing figure. The person he met was the former prostitute Mary, covered only by her white hair, her skin darkened and leathered by the sun. Mary ordered Zosimus to come no closer and told him her story. Zosimus promised to meet her again the following year and to bring her holy communion. The next year he found her waiting for him at the appointed place and gave her communion. When they departed, they agreed to meet the following year. When Zosimus returned 12 months later, he found the lifeless body of Mary wrapped in a mantle he had given her, with a written request, traced on the ground, to bury her body. Having no implement with which to dig her grave, Zosimus was confronted by a lion, which assisted him. On returning to his monastery, Zosimus revealed the story of Mary of Egypt. An English translation of the full text of Mary's life according to Sophronus, bishop of Jerusalem, is provided in Ward's *Harlots of the Desert.* Mary's relics are in Rome, Naples, Cremona, and Antwerp.

REFERENCES 6, 16, 36, 46, 51

323

Mary of Oignies

MEMORIAL DAY **June 23**

PATRONAGE **Fever, childbirth**

LIFE & LEGEND

Born into a wealthy family of Nivelles in Brabant, Belgium, Mary was married at age 14 at the insistence of her parents, in spite of her desire to become a nun. In Butler's words, "Mary, young as she was, acquired a great ascendancy over her husband." She convinced the young man to live with her in celibacy, to distribute their wealth to the poor, and to convert their home into a hospice for lepers. The remarkable austerity and holiness of Mary's life also attracted visitors seeking her spiritual guidance. Late in life, Mary left her home in Williambroux to live as a hermit at Oignies, were she died in 1213.

Mary of Oignies is remembered as a mystic, who received visions and possessed the gift of clairvoyance. Du Broc de Segange relates, "In 1609 her relics were placed under the altar of the church of Notre-Dame d'Oignies. In the time of Molanus, toward the end of the sixteenth century, she was invoked by parturient women who were successfully delivered by touching the saint's woolen shirt. Those suffering from fevers were cured by embracing a fragment of one of her limbs encased in a silver reliquary." In 1817, her relics were transferred to Nivelles.

REFERENCES 6, 14, 16, 36

324

Mathias the Apostle

MEMORIAL DAY **February 24**

PATRONAGE **Infertility, smallpox**

LIFE & LEGEND

Mathias is said to have been one of the 70 disciples who Jesus sent out two by two to preach and work miracles. When, after the Ascension, the disciples gathered to elect a replacement among the twelve for Judas Iscariot, the lot fell to Mathias "and he was enrolled with the eleven apostles" (Acts 1:26). According to tradition, Mathias' apostolic ministry kept him at first in Judea. Some sources maintain that he traveled to Ethiopia. More certainly, he wandered through Cappadocia and as far east as the shores of the Caspian Sea. He is supposed to have been martyred at Colchis. Mathias' remains are said to have been translated from Jerusalem to Rome by Saint Helen, the mother of Constantine.

REFERENCES 6, 16, 36

325

Maturinus (Mathurin)

MEMORIAL DAY **November 1 or November 9**

PATRONAGE **Melancholy, epilepsy**

LIFE & LEGEND

Butler maintains that the life ascribed to Maturinus is entirely legendary. Maturinus is said to have been born to pagan parents in the fourth century in present-day Sens. As a boy, he was irresistibly drawn to the gospels and was baptized at age 12. Maturinus subsequently converted his parents to Christianity and was ordained to the priesthood at age 20. He was so esteemed by his bishop that when the latter had to travel to Rome, he left Maturinus in charge of his diocese. Maturinus was active as a missionary, but he was particularly known for his abilities as an exorcist. He is said to have been sent to Rome expressly to exorcise a demon from a noble maiden, and is said to have died in the Eternal City. His remains were returned to Sens, where they remained until destroyed by the Huguenots. An order of monks in France, known as the Mathurins, maintains a church dedicated to the saint in Paris.

REFERENCES 6, 14, 36, 46

326

Matrona of Capua

MEMORIAL DAY **March 15**

PATRONAGE **Hemorrhage, dysentery**

LIFE & LEGEND

According to du Broc de Segange, Matrona, who lived during the eleventh century, was the daughter of the king of Portugal and "suffered twelve years from a flux of blood. One night in her sleep, she was informed by an angel that if she went to Capua, in Italy, she would find the body of the martyred Saint Priscus in the same place where she would find two heifers that had wandered from their herd. In obedience to this advice from God, the virgin Matrona, accompanied by twelve other maidens and several servants, arrived in Capua, where she did find the body of the saint not far from the city, as indicated by the presence of the heifers. Matrona venerated the remains of the saint and was healed of her illness by her contact with them. In gratitude, Matrona built a church in honor of the saint, as well as a convent in which she and her twelve companions consecrated themselves to the religious life. After having lived a life of great sanctity there, Matrona rendered her soul to God and was placed in a costly tomb. After her death, the sanctity of her life was made evident by many miracles. After all that has been said, it is to be expected that she was invoked in cases of hemorrhage."

REFERENCES 16, 36

327

Maudez (Mawes)

MEMORIAL DAY **November 18**

PATRONAGE **Wounds, ulcers, plaster application to limbs**

LIFE & LEGEND

Maudez was of Irish origin and established a monastery during the sixth century on what is now called the Ile Maudez on the Côtes-d'Armor in Brittany. When the Normans ravaged Brittany in the ninth century, the saint's relics were transferred to Bourges and to Paris. The cult of Saint Maudez is widespread in Brittany (nine churches are named in his honor). There is a village named Saint Maudez in the commune of Guingamp, Côtes-d'Armor; and in England a village near Falmouth is called Saint Mawes. Guyotjeannin relates that, early in the twentieth century, in the village of Landeleau, pieces of earth taken from the site of a long-destroyed chapel to Saint Maudez were used in the preparation of remedies and for plasters applied to wounds and ulcers.

REFERENCES 14, 32

328

Maurice (Moritz)

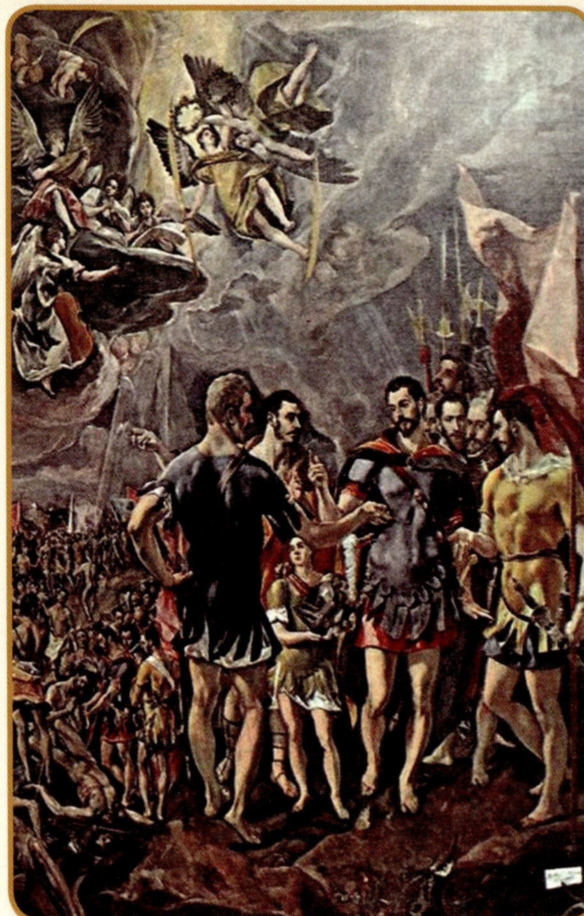

MEMORIAL DAY **September 22**

PATRONAGE **Cramps, gout, children's diseases, alpine troops, infantrymen, swordsmiths, weavers, Austria, Sardinia, Pontifical Swiss Guards**

LIFE & LEGEND

Maurice, whose name is derived from Latin, meaning "moor," was a leader of the Roman Theban Legion in the third century. The legion, which was composed entirely of Christians, was transported from Thebes, Egypt, to Gaul to assist Emperor Maximian Herculius. When the soldiers refused to participate in pagan sacrifices before battle and to act against fellow Christians, every tenth soldier was executed (known as decimation). That did not alter the stance of the remaining 6000 members of the legion who were then massacred en masse. This occurred ca. 287 at Agaunum, now Saint-Maurice-en-Valais, Switzerland, the site of an abbey bearing the name. Saint Maurice became a patron saint of the Holy Roman emperors. The sword of Saint Maurice was used as part of the regalia at coronations of the Austro-Hungarian emperors until 1916.

REFERENCES 6, 42

329

Maurus

MEMORIAL DAY **January 15**

PATRONAGE **Rheumatism, gout (mal de saint Maur), headache, paralysis, scrofula, colds**

LIFE & LEGEND

Maurus was born to a Roman family of the senatorial class, and at age 12 he was placed by his father under the direction of Benedict of Nursia at Subiaco. Maurus remained with Benedict into adulthood. When Benedict retired to Monte Cassino, Maurus succeeded him as abbot of the monastery at Subiaco (ca. 529). An unreliable version of Maurus' life and acts is related in a ninth-century biography composed by Odo, abbot of the monastery at Glanfeuil. In Odo's version, the monk Maurus came to France, where he founded the monastery at Glanfeuil (later called Saint-Maur-sur-Loire) with the support of King Theodebert. Maurus directed this monastery until age 70, when he withdrew into solitude to prepare himself for death in 584. Du Broc de Segange melds both versions, maintaining that Maurus accompanied Benedict from Subiaco to Monte Cassino, and that he was sent to France by Benedict at the request of Bertingran, bishop of Mans, who wished to have a monastery on the Benedictine model in his diocese.

REFERENCES 6, 16, 36

330

Maximilian Kolbe

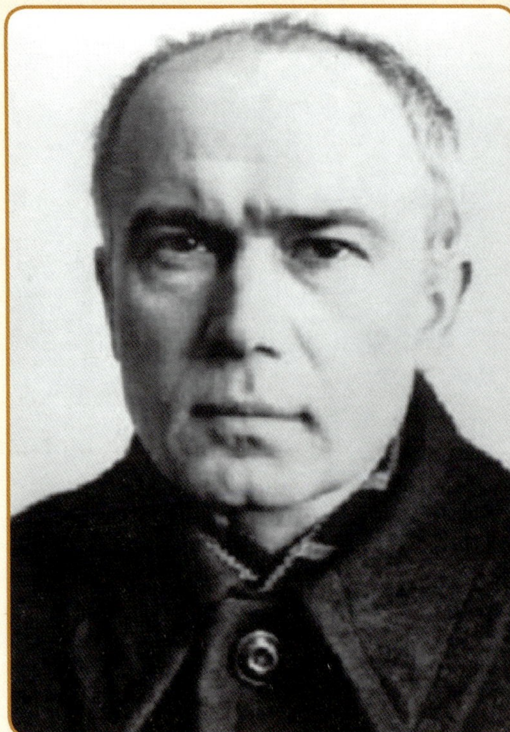

MEMORIAL DAY **August 14**

PATRONAGE **Drug addicts, political prisoners, journalists, pro-life movement, "Our Difficult Century" (declared by Pope John Paul II)**

LIFE & LEGEND

Maximilian was born Rajmund Kolbe in 1894 into a poor but pious family in what was, at the time, Russia-occupied Poland. His father fought for Polish independence and was hanged by the Russians as a traitor in 1914. His mother later became a Benedictine nun. At the time of Rajmund's first communion at age 12, he had a vision of the Virgin Mary. She came to him holding a red crown and a white crown; the white one indicated that he would maintain his purity, and the red one was emblematic of his becoming a martyr. When offered either, he accepted both.

In 1910, he became a novice in the Conventional Franciscan Order and took the name Maximilian, the diminutive of "the greatest." He studied philosophy in the Jesuit Gregorian College from1912 to 1915 and theology at the Franciscan Collegio Serafico in Rome from 1915 to 1919. He was ordained in 1918. While still at the seminary, he and six friends founded the Immaculata Movement devoted to the conversion of sinners. After he was stricken with tuberculosis, he returned to Poland to teach history in 1919. Three years later he received a Doctor of Theology degree.

From August 1920 to April 1921, he was actively treated for tuberculosis. Shortly after he returned from a medical leave, he began the magazine *Knight of the Immaculate* to fight religious apathy. At its peak, the periodical had a monthly press run of 750,000. He had recurrence of active tuberculosis that required another medical leave. In 1927, he founded the City of the Immaculate Monastery near Warsaw. By 1938, that monastery housed almost 800 men, the largest in the world at the time.

Maximilian went to Japan with four brothers in 1930. There he published a version of the magazine *Knight of the Immaculate* in Japanese and founded a monastery at Nagasaki. The magazine grew to a circulation of 65,000, and the monastery, which survived the bombing in World War II, remains the center for Franciscan work in Japan. In 1932, Maximilian went to India, where he built another monastery, but it did not survive.

In 1936, he returned to the monastery near Warsaw. After the Nazi invasion of Poland, he and his brothers housed 3000 Polish refugees, two thirds of whom were Jewish, at the monastery. In February 1941, he was imprisoned in Pawiak and transferred to Auschwitz that May. In July, a prisoner from his barracks disappeared. In retaliation, 10 men from the barracks were picked to starve to death. One of the selected men, Francizek Gajownicezek, bemoaned the potential loss to his family, and Maximilian took his place. After 3 weeks of starvation and dehydration, Maximilian was put to death with an injection of carbolic acid.

He was beatified as a confessor by Pope Paul VI in 1971 and canonized as a martyr by Pope John Paul II in 1982. Maximilian Kolbe is recognized in the Jewish Virtual Library and is one of ten twentieth-century martyrs depicted in statues above the Great West Door of Westminster Abbey, London.

REFERENCES 9, 34

331

Maximinus of Besançon

MEMORIAL DAY **May 29**

PATRONAGE **Gout, foot problems, cripples, wounds and injuries of the lower limbs**

LIFE & LEGEND

Du Broc de Segange relates that Maximinus was consecrated bishop and sent to Besançon by Pope Caius. On the forum of Besançon, Maximinus built a church in honor of Saint John the Baptist, a baptistry, and a religious house for men. After completing these projects, Maximinus pursued his desire to live a hermetic life by withdrawing into the countryside near the city. When he was informed mystically of his impending death, Maximinus consecrated his successor to the see of Besançon and prepared in solitude for death in 291. A chapel was erected in the forest of Foucheraux where he died. As early as the sixth century, this chapel was the site of pilgrimages by those seeking the relief of their illnesses.

Du Broc de Segange also notes: "Since 1754, during the episcopacy of Cardinal Choiseuil-Beaupré, the idea began to circulate that Saint Maximin, bishop of Besançon, never existed, and that the relics that were venerated there were actually those of Saint Maximin, bishop of Treves, who died ca. 347. About 1777, the curé of Foucherans demolished the chapel, but devotion to the saint continued, even during the disorders of the Revolution. After 1801, the pilgrimage to Saint Maximin revived. Each year several healings were confirmed—especially among the crippled and those suffering from diseases or injuries of the legs."

REFERENCES 16, 36

332
Mazerand

MEMORIAL DAY **October 29**

PATRONAGE **Fever**

LIFE & LEGEND

Mazerand's dates and origin are unknown. He is supposed to have been a solitary in the vicinity of Brou in the diocese of Moulins. Mazerand is the patron saint of this place. Near the local church is a fountain that bears his name. According to du Broc de Segange, "Local tradition maintains that for all time people of the region have come seeking its waters and invoking Saint Mazerand for the healing of their different maladies, and especially of fevers."

REFERENCES 16, 36

333
Medard

MEMORIAL DAY **June 8**

PATRONAGE **Sterility, mental illness, toothache, fever, bad weather, prisoners, peasants, vineyards**

LIFE & LEGEND

Medard was born into a pious and noble family in Picardy, France, ca. 456. His brother, and perhaps twin, was Saint Gildard, the archbishop of Rouen. From early childhood, Medard manifested compassion for the poor. As a young man, he prophesied that he would become the bishop of Tournai. He was ordained at age 33. In 530, he became the bishop of Vernand and later transferred the seat to Noyon. He also was named to the post at Tournai, uniting the two dioceses. He died at Noyon, France, in 545, and his relics were maintained at the royal manor at Crouy, where a Benedictine abbey was built over his tomb.

Medard became one of the most revered bishops of his time and is the subject of several legends. He is depicted as laughing with his mouth open, which led to his patronage against toothaches. It is also related that, as a child, Medard was protected from the rain by an eagle that hovered over him, leading to his patronage of good weather.

REFERENCE 42

334
Medicus

MEMORIAL DAY **June 26**

PATRONAGE **Diverse diseases**

LIFE & LEGEND

Medicus is said to have been a native of Ocriculum, an unwalled city on the Via Flaminia below the present Otricoli in Umbria. He supposedly changed his name from Maleficus after his conversion to Christianity, which occurred after he witnessed miracles performed by Saint Victor. Medicus was later denounced for his faith, arrested, tortured, and finally decapitated at Ocriculum in 172. His body was removed during the night of his martyrdom and buried in a grotto near the church of Saint Vittore. This tomb was rediscovered in 1611 and the saint's relics removed.

Medicus is regarded as one of the patron saints of Otricoli and is also invoked for the healing of all manner of disease. There is some debate regarding the saint's curious name—medicus meaning "physician" in Latin. Some maintain that Medicus is actually the saint's name, but does not imply he was a physician; others maintain that the name Medicus refers to the saint's profession, but was not his personal name, which may have been Maleficus or even Benedictus.

REFERENCES 42, 50

335

Méen (Main, Mewan)

MEMORIAL DAY **June 21**

PATRONAGE **Skin diseases, scabies, dandruff, tinea, leprosy, rickets, rheumatism, scrofula, cerebral disorders**

LIFE & LEGEND

Méen was born during the sixth century at Gwent in South Wales. As an adolescent, he was placed under the tutelage of Saint Samson, who was a relation (perhaps his uncle), and who established the monastery at Llanwit, Glamorgan. He accompanied Samson, first to Cornwall, and later across the channel to Brittany, where Méen founded one monastery at Gaël (later named in his honor) and another near Angers. The monastery at Gaël is supposed to have received its water supply from a spring that appeared in the spot where Méen planted his staff. These waters were also famous for the miraculous healing of le mal de saint Méen, or scabies.

REFERENCES 6, 16, 32, 36

336
Mennas

MEMORIAL DAY **November 11**

PATRONAGE **Scabies**

LIFE & LEGEND

Our knowledge of the life of Mennas is limited to his Egyptian birth, his martyrdom, and his burial in his native land. In most versions of his life, it is related that Mennas was an Egyptian serving in the Roman army. When the persecution of Diocletian began, Mennas is said to have deserted his unit at Cotyaeum in Phrygia to live as a recluse in the nearby mountains. Mennas returned to Cotyaeum and publicly declared himself a Christian during games taking place in the amphitheater. He was immediately arrested, tortured, and then beheaded ca. 300. His remains were returned from Phrygia to Egypt, and his place of burial (at present-day Karm Abu-Mina near Alexandria) became a popular place of pilgrimage where many miracles were reported. Between 1905 and 1908, excavations at Karm Abu-Mina revealed a basilica, a monastery, and a complex of other buildings dedicated to the saint. The cult of the warrior saint was popular in Egypt and the East, and phials that once contained water from a well at Mennas' Egyptian shrine have been found elsewhere in north Africa and in Europe.

REFERENCES 6, 14, 36, 46

337

Menoux (Menulphus)

MEMORIAL DAY **July 12**

PATRONAGE **Headache, nervous disorders, mental disorders**

LIFE & LEGEND

Menoux was born in Ireland during the sixth century and emigrated to Armorica (Brittany), where he became bishop of Quimper. After returning from a pilgrimage to Rome, Menoux took ill and died at the village of Mailly (Allier). The cult of Menoux originated and flourished in the Bourbonnais rather than in Brittany. Writing in 1904, Henry Meige relates, "A curious practice of the cult of Saint Menoux has continued to our own day. In the very beautiful church which dominates the village of Saint-Menoux, one sees behind the main altar the saint's sarcophagus. One side of this enormous stone is pierced with an opening large enough to insert one's head. Those who wish to implore saint Menoux for the cure of headache or of a mental disorder introduce their heads into the opening and in this posture make their supplications."

REFERENCES 16, 36, 38

338

Meriadoc (Meriasek)

MEMORIAL DAY **June 7**

PATRONAGE **Headache, deafness**

LIFE & LEGEND

Meriadoc was probably of Welsh origin and was active in Cornwall before crossing over to Brittany. He is said to have been born into a wealthy family and to have given away his inheritance to provide for the poor. He may have been an itinerant missionary bishop among the Bretons during the seventh century. Some sources maintain that Meriadoc was bishop of Vannes, but Butler and others deny that he ever held this see. According to du Broc de Segange, "There are in Brittany several chapels dedicated to Saint Mériadec. The chapel at Stival, near Pontivy, is still an active site of pilgrimage. They preserve there the head of the saintly bishop and display an ancient cone-shaped bell [or hat] of yellow leather that is said to have belonged to Saint Mériadec, that is placed on the heads of those afflicted with deafness. At Plumergat, where the saint is also invoked against deafness and headache, one sees two pieces of quartz with which they rub the head of the afflicted." His legend is the subject of the medieval Cornish miracle play Beunans Meriasek.

REFERENCES 6, 16, 36

339

Michael the Archangel

MEMORIAL DAY **September 29 (Michaelmas)**

PATRONAGE **Ambulance drivers, emergency medical technicians, radiologists, radiation therapists, plague, artists, bakers, bankers, boatmen, coopers, grocers, haberdashers, hatters, sailors, soldiers, Germany, Israel, many cities and regions throughout the world**

LIFE & LEGEND

In the realm of hagiography, the term "saint," when applied to Michael the Archangel, means "holy," and is distinct from that designating canonization, referring to a human soul in heaven. Devotion to Michael is common among Jews, Christians, and Muslims. In the Old Testament of Judaism, Michael is the field commander of the Army of God. In Daniel's vision, he is described as an advocate of Israel. According to the Talmud, his name means "who is like El (God)."

In Christian tradition, in Revelation, there was a great battle in heaven, during which Michael and his angels fought with the dragon representing Satan, who was thrown out of heaven. Early Christians made Saint Michael the patron of the sick who required care. When the Archangel was first venerated, it was related to his prestige as a healer. Legend states that, in the earliest ages, Saint Michael created a medicinal spring near Colossae, and all the sick individuals who bathed in it and invoked the Trinity were cured. When his name was invoked by Saint Gregory I the Great, Saint Michael purportedly caused the plague to cease. In Eastern Orthodoxy, at Constantinople, Saint Michael was regarded as a heavenly physician. In later medieval Christianity, Michael, along with Saint George, became the patrons of chivalry.

REFERENCES 9, 42

340

Millefort (Quinnefort)

MEMORIAL DAY **November 5**

PATRONAGE **Epilepsy, fever, rickets, worms**

LIFE & LEGEND

Millefort entered the ecclesiastic life in his native Scotland during the twelfth century. He eventually was made a bishop, but he was forced to flee Scotland because of difficulties with a powerful lord. He established himself at Bouvaque near Abbeville and became famous for his preaching throughout Picardy and Normandy. When his enemies in Scotland learned of his whereabouts, they hired local peasants to murder him. After his death, the cult of Millefort became widespread throughout Normandy.

REFERENCES 16, 36

341

Molagga (Laicin)

MEMORIAL DAY **January 20**

PATRONAGE **Plague**

LIFE & LEGEND

Molagga was born in Ireland and became a student of Saint David of Wales. He founded the monastery of Fermoy in County Cork, Ireland, and was its first abbot. He died of natural causes ca. 655.

REFERENCES 16, 36

342

Mommolinus

MEMORIAL DAY **October 16**

PATRONAGE **Speech impediments**

LIFE & LEGEND

A native of Coutances, Scotland, Mommolinus became a monk at Luxeuil. He was later sent as a missionary to the region around Saint Omer in the Artois. Mommolinus established and headed a monastery there (later named Saint-Momelin). He became abbot of the monastery at Sithiu before succeeding Eligius as bishop of Noyon in 660.

REFERENCES 14, 36

343
Mucius

MEMORIAL DAY **May 13**

PATRONAGE **Blindness, muteness**

LIFE & LEGEND

Mucius was a Christian priest, and he is supposed to have overturned an altar dedicated to Bacchus during a festival of the god at Amphipolis in Macedonia. He was immediately arrested and condemned to be burned alive. While Mucius remained untouched by the flames, the prefect who had condemned him was consumed by the fire. Mucius was then sent to Heraclea, where he was tortured and exposed to beasts in the arena. When the beasts refused to harm him, Mucius was sent to Constantinople, where he was beheaded ca. 304. The cult of Mucius dates to the fourth century. It is speculated that his patronage of the mute is based on the similarity of his name to the Latin word "mutus."

REFERENCES 6, 14, 16, 36

N

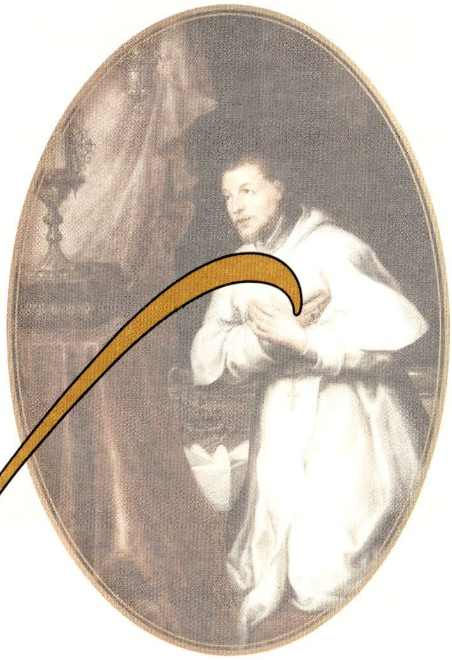

344

Namphanius

MEMORIAL DAY **November 16**

PATRONAGE **Epilepsy**

LIFE & LEGEND

Namphanius, who lived during the eighth century, was of noble birth and a friend of Charlemagne, in whose army he served. Namphanius restored the monasteries of Marcillac and Figeac, and he built another named Lantoy. He then retired to a sanctuary dedicated to Saint Martin near Marcillac, where he led the life of a solitary until his death. Namphanius was buried near a place called Camiac. Numerous miracles occurred at his tomb, especially among those suffering from epilepsy.

REFERENCES 16, 36

345

Nepotianus

MEMORIAL DAY **October 22**

PATRONAGE **Fever**

LIFE & LEGEND

According to Gregory of Tours, Saint Nepotianus counts as the fourth bishop of Clermont-Ferrand (du Broc de Segange maintains he was the fifth). Among a group of envoys sent to Spain from Trier during the fourth century, one of them, a young man called Arthemius, who was remarkable both for his wisdom and his good looks, fell ill of a high fever. The other envoys continued their journey while Arthemius was left behind ill in Clermont. Nepotianus came to see him, anointed him with holy oil, and Arthemius was restored to health. Arthemius forgot both his earthly spouse and his private fortune and became a member of the Holy Church. He was ordained a priest and gained such fame for his saintliness that he succeeded Nepotianus as bishop.

REFERENCES 16, 30, 36

346

Nicasius

MEMORIAL DAY **December 14**

PATRONAGE **Smallpox, plague, cholera, whooping cough**

LIFE & LEGEND

Nicasius was bishop of Rheims in 452, when smallpox was epidemic throughout southern France, and he contracted the disease. He recovered from its attack because, according to his own statement, he had anointed himself with holy oil. Also, while bishop of Reims, Nicasius prophesied the sack of the city by a barbarian army and urged its inhabitants to prepare themselves by prayer and repentance. When the people asked him whether they should yield or fight to the end, he, knowing that the city must fall, replied that they should pray for their enemies. Standing at the door of his church, in endeavoring to save the lives of some, he exposed himself to the infidels, who cut off his head ca. 452. Saint Florentius, his deacon, and Saint Jucundus, his lector, were massacred by his side. His sister, Saint Eutropia, threw herself on her brother's murderer and kicked and scratched him until she, too, was killed.

REFERENCES 6, 36, 47

347

Nicholas of Bari

MEMORIAL DAY **December 6**

PATRONAGE **Rheumatism, infertility, [apothecaries],* thieves, pawnbrokers, sailors, children**

LIFE & LEGEND

Considering the widespread and enduring popularity of Saint Nicholas (apart from his transformation into Santa Claus), it is remarkable how little we actually know of the saint's life. He is thought to have been born into a wealthy family of Patara in Lycia, and to have been elected bishop of the Lycian city of Myra (present-day Kale in the Turkish province of Antalya). When a local poor man was planning to sell his daughters into prostitution, Nicholas went to their home during the night and threw three bags of gold through the window and saved the daughters from their plight. The three bags of gold served as the basis of the three golden balls that identify a pawnbroker's shop.

Nicholas is supposed to have worked numerous miracles during his lifetime, and is said to have been recognized as a saint even while living. He returned three boys to life, who had been murdered and pickled in a barrel of brine to hide the crime. This accounts for his patronage of both children and barrel makers. He also induced thieves to return their loot, which forms the origin of reference to thieves as Saint Nicholas' clerks. Nicholas was imprisoned for his faith during the persecution of Diocletian, but he was held in such esteem by Emperor Constantine that he was released. Nicholas was present at the Council of Nicea (325), where he denounced Arianism. He died of natural causes at Myra ca. 346 and was buried in its cathedral.

*Proposed patronage

Nicholas of Myra became known as Nicholas of Bari when sailors from the Puglian port took advantage of the unsettled state of Asia Minor during the Turkish invasions and stole Nicholas' remains from the church where they were entombed. In May, 1087, Nicholas' remains were landed at Bari, where construction began on a grand new church to house the newly acquired relics. Although the cult of Saint Nicholas was popular in the West even before the removal of his relics to southern Italy, their enshrinement made Bari one of the great pilgrimage sites of medieval Europe. The list of trades and classes of persons for whom Nicholas of Bari is the patron saint is a lengthy one. His patronage of sailors is perhaps the best known, although he is also a patron saint of apothecaries. Whole nations look to Nicholas as their protector, such as Russia and Greece, as do regions such as Puglia, Sicily, and even Lorraine.

REFERENCES 6, 14, 36, 46

348
Nomadia (Néomaie)

MEMORIAL DAY **January 14**

PATRONAGE **Epilepsy, fear, shepherds, domestic animals**

LIFE & LEGEND

Little is known of Nomadia other than her birth into a prominent family of Poitou during the sixth century.

REFERENCES 16, 36

349

Norbert

MEMORIAL DAY **June 6**

PATRONAGE **Safe delivery**

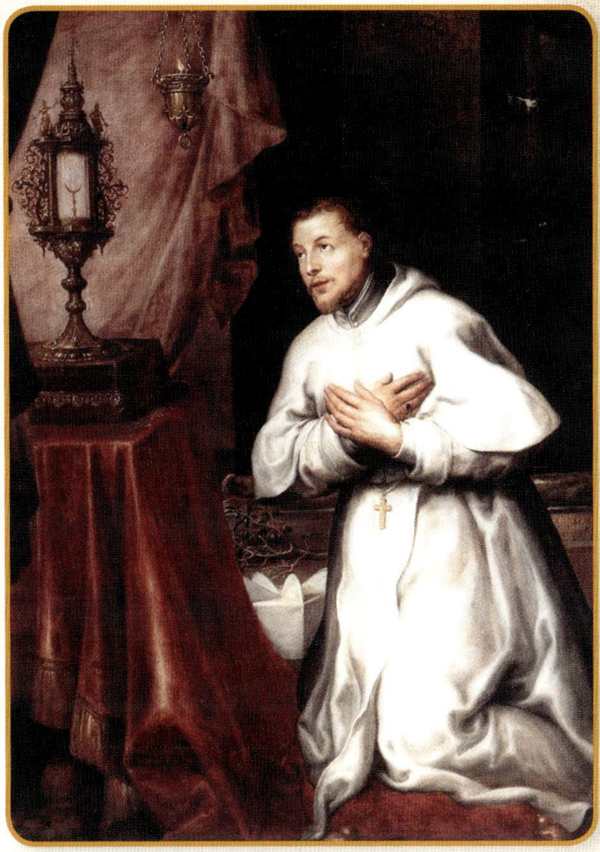

LIFE & LEGEND

Norbert, whose name is derived from Germanic, meaning "bright north," was born at Xanten in the duchy of Cleves, Prussia, the son of Count Heribert of Gennep, a relative of the emperor, and Hedwig of Guise, a member of the house of Lorraine. Although he received minor orders, Norbert chose a life of pleasure and ease, first in the service of the archbishop of Cologne, and later at the court of the emperor, Henry V, who appointed him almoner. Norbert avoided ordination to the priesthood and declined the bishopric of Combrai when it was offered him. In 1115, while on a journey, his horse was panicked by lightning and Norbert was thrown to the ground. On regaining consciousness, he clearly heard the words that had been delivered to Paul on his way to Damascus. Accepting the portent, Norbert immediately altered his way of life. He sought ordination, sold all his worldly belongings, took the monastic habit, and began to wander barefoot preaching repentance to both laity and clergy. His fellow canons at Xanten were not amused by Norbert's new earnestness, and saw to it that he was expelled from the city. Norbert resigned his office and journeyed to Languedoc, where he visited the exiled Pope Gelasius II. With a papal blessing, Norbert journeyed as an itinerant preacher throughout the North of France.

In 1120, he received a gift of land from the bishop of Laon at a place called Prémontré in the forest of Coucy. This was the first house of the Canons Regular of Prémontré, which in time grew to eight men's and two women's monasteries. The new order combined traditional monasticism with an evangelic mission that took its members outside the monastic enclosure to evangelize the secular world. In 1125, Norbert went to Rome to solicit papal approval of the new order. A year later he was appointed archbishop of Magdeburg by Emperor Lothair II. Norbert's insistence on maintaining ecclesiastic rights against the abuses of secular officials and his zeal for reforming a corrupt and indifferent clergy earned him many enemies in Magdeburg. Attempts were made on his life. In the controversy between Innocent II and the antipope Anacletus II, Norbert convinced Lothair to support the former, and, in 1133, he accompanied the imperial army that marched on Rome to restore Innocent to the papal throne. Norbert was then named chancellor of Italy by Lothair, but died in 1134, soon after his return to Magdeburg. His relics were transposed to Prague. He was canonized in 1582 by Pope Gregory III.

REFERENCES 6, 14, 16, 36, 46

350
Notburga

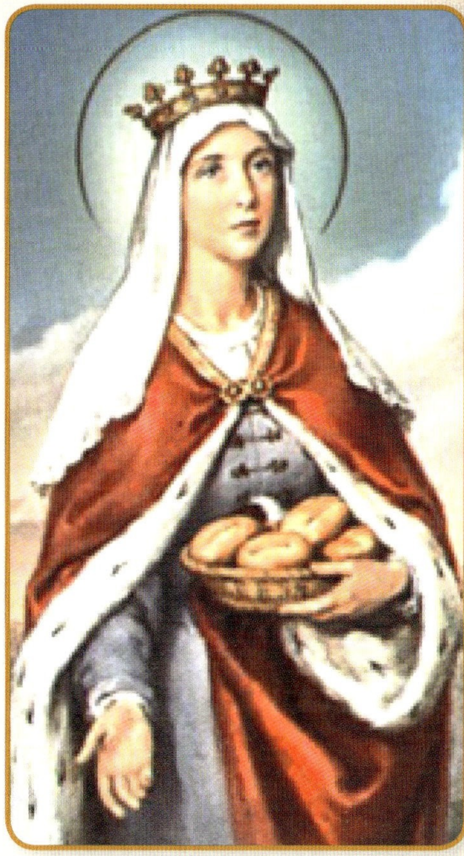

MEMORIAL DAY **September 14**

PATRONAGE **Childbirth, peasants**

LIFE & LEGEND

Notburga was born into a peasant family at Rattenberg in the Austrian Tyrol. As a girl, she entered into service as a kitchen maid in the household of Count Henry of Rattenberg. Some time later, Notburga was dismissed by Henry's wife, Ottilia, for giving leftover food to the poor rather than to the pigs. Notburga then entered the employ of a nearby farmer. When the bells rang for vespers one Saturday, Notburga stopped reaping in the farmer's fields. When he told her to resume work, she refused, pointing out that Saturday vespers mark the beginning of Sunday. When the farmer argued that the fine weather might take a turn for the worse, Notburga threw her sickle into the air where it remained suspended—looking like the first quarter of the harvest moon, which is a sign of good weather. After the death of Ottilia, Henry remarried and hired the saintly Notburga as his housekeeper. She remained in his service the rest of her life. Before her death, Notburga requested that her body be placed on a wagon drawn by oxen and that it be buried wherever the oxen stopped. Her request was respected, and the oxen halted at the church of Saint Rupert in Eben, where Notburga was buried in 1313. She was canonized by Pope Pius IX in 1862.

REFERENCES 6, 14, 16

O

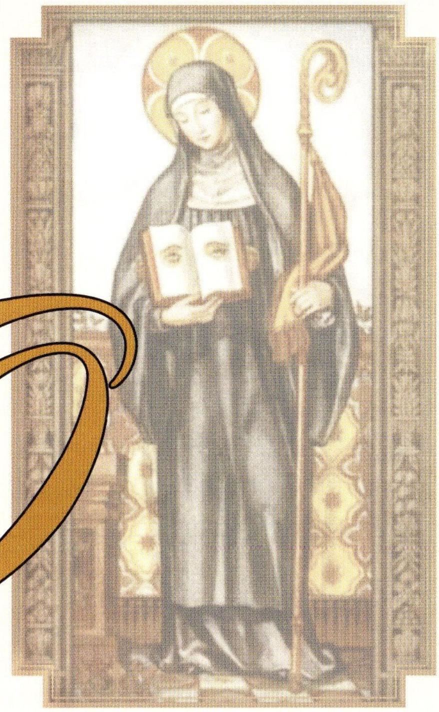

351 Odile

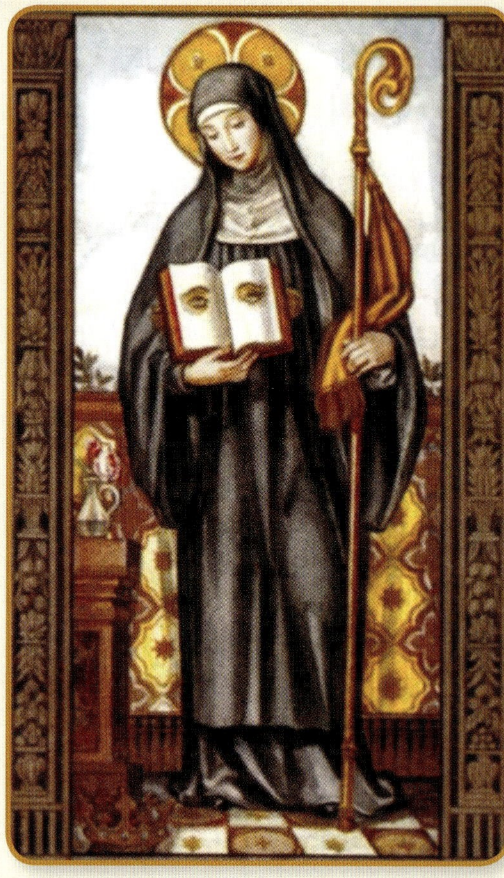

MEMORIAL DAY **December 13**

PATRONAGE **Blindness, eye diseases, headache**

LIFE & LEGEND

Odile, whose name is derived from a Germanic word meaning "wealth," was born blind ca. 662, the daughter of Etichon, the duke of Alsace. Her father was displeased that he had not sired a son, and he discarded her and her mother, who took her to Burgundy where she was raised. When she was 12, an itinerant bishop named Erhard of Regensburg was led by an angel to baptize Odile (an anagram of Sol Dei) at Palma. She immediately recovered her sight.

Her younger brother brought her home, and this enraged her father to the point that he murdered her brother, whom she miraculously revived before leaving home again. She fled to Breisgau, Germany, and hid in a cave. Her father, who tried to capture her, was prevented by falling rocks. Later when her father became ill, Odile nursed him back to health, thereby gaining his acceptance. Her father assisted her in founding the Augustine monastery of Mount Saint Odile in Hochwald, Bas-Rhin, where Odile became abbess. Later, she was led by a vision of Saint John the Baptist to found a second monastery and hospital at Niedermünster, where a local well is still said to cure diseases of the eye. Odile died ca. 720 at Niedermünster and was buried at Saint Odile. She was made Patron saint of Alsace in 1807 by Pope Pius VII. The larkspur plant is connected to Saint Odile and is believed to cure eye diseases.

REFERENCES 6, 9

352

Omer

MEMORIAL DAY **September 9**

PATRONAGE **Blindness, eye diseases**

LIFE & LEGEND

Omer was born near Coutances in Manche. After his mother died, both he and his father became monks at Luxeuil, then under the direction of Saint Eustace. After 20 years at Luxeuil, Omer was chosen bishop of Thérouanne in 637. He was rigorous in restoring discipline to the clergy of his diocese and in evangelizing the region's largely non-Christian population. He also established the monastery of Sithiu, which would become one of the great spiritual centers of France. Late in life, Omer became blind, accounting for his patronage.

REFERENCES 14, 16, 36

353

Onenna

MEMORIAL DAY **April 30**

PATRONAGE **Edema, hydrops**

LIFE & LEGEND

One tradition maintains that Onenna was born ca. 604 in Brittany, the daughter of King Hoël and his wife, Pritel. Another indicates that she was the sister of Judicael, king of Domnonée in northern Brittany. Although she may not have taken the veil, Onenna lived a secluded life tending geese on a farm near present-day Tréhorenteuc. She died ca. 630. There is a wooden statue of Onenna of considerable antiquity that depicts her in a reclining position dying of edema.

REFERENCES 16, 36

354

Orana

MEMORIAL DAY **September 15**

PATRONAGE **Deafness, vertigo**

LIFE & LEGEND

Orana, who lived during the fourteenth and fifteenth centuries, is said to have been deaf and afflicted with chronic vertigo. She is supposed to have received an estate from her father at Eschweiler, near the present German-Belgian-Dutch frontier, where she lived a life devoted to God with a faithful maid, who is honored along with Orana in this region.

REFERENCES 18, 36

355

Ortarius

MEMORIAL DAY **May 21**

PATRONAGE **Paralysis, gout, arthritis, joint diseases**

LIFE & LEGEND

At age 12, Ortarius, who lived during the seventh century, entered the monastery of Landelle in Normandy. He founded a monastery in the forest of Andaine and later retired to a hermitage near Beauménil. After the death of their abbot, the monks of Landelle chose Ortarius as their head, because his reputation for holiness was known to them. A miracle attributed to Ortarius during his lifetime resulted in the cure of a young girl whose hands were paralysed and whose knees too weak to support her, thereby accounting for his patronage.

REFERENCES 16, 36

356
Osmund

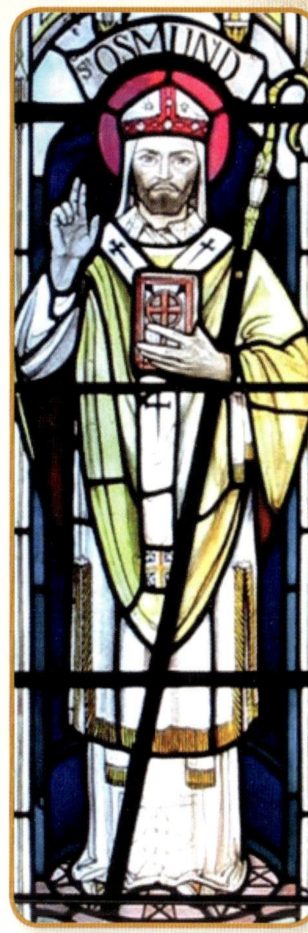

MEMORIAL DAY **December 4**

PATRONAGE **Mental illnesses, paralysis, rupture, toothache**

LIFE & LEGEND

Osmund, whose name is derived from English, meaning "God, protector," was born in Normandy, France, ca. 1050. He was the son of Count Henry of Seez and Lady Isabella of Normandy, one of King William the Conqueror's siblings. He accompanied King William as part of the invasion force in 1066. After the Battle of Hastings, he was made royal chaplain and Earl of Dorset or Somerset. He was promoted to chancellor in 1072.

After that, he embraced an ecclesiastic life and became bishop of Sarum (Salisbury) in 1078. As bishop, he compiled a constitution for the administration of his cathedral that was used as a model for cathedrals throughout England. He took part in preparing the Domesday Book commissioned by William. The first draft was completed in 1086 and included a list of the holdings in 13,418 settlements in the English counties south of the Ribble and Tees Rivers (the border with Scotland at the time.)

Bishop Osmund died of natural causes in 1099 and was buried in the cathedral at Old Sarum. His relics were translated to the new cathedral at Salisbury in 1457, and that shrine was destroyed during the reign of Henry VIII. In the twelfth century, Osmund's reputation for miracles became widespread. Diseased persons with mental illness, paralysis, rupture, and toothache reported cures after they exposed themselves to so-called healholes in his shrine. As a consequence, Gregory IX initiated the process of canonization in 1228, which was not completed until 1456 by Pope Callistus III.

REFERENCES 6, 9, 42, 45

357 Oswald of Northumbria

MEMORIAL DAY **August 5 or August 9**

PATRONAGE **Plague**

LIFE & LEGEND

Oswald was the son of the pagan king, Aethelfrith, and Princess Acha of Deira. After his uncle, King Edwin, died in battle in 633, Oswald mustered what forces he could and marched south to meet King Cadwalla in battle near Hexham (Heavenfield). Although most of his soldiers were pagan, Oswald, a convert, erected a large wooden cross in his camp on the eve of battle and requested his army to kneel before it and pray for victory. His soldiers complied, and during the night a vision of Saint Columba of Iona promised Oswald victory. On the day of battle the superior forces of Cadwalla were defeated, and the British king himself was killed. A church was later erected at Hexham, where the cross was long venerated. In the days of the Venerable Bede, pieces of this cross were steeped in water that was either drunk by or sprinkled on the sick.

After the defeat of King Cadwalla, which Oswald attributed to his faith, Oswald took the throne of Northumbria. Because he was converted to Christianity in Iona, he brought Saint Aidan to Northumbria as bishop to evangelize the region.

Oswald's kingdom eventually stretched as far north as the Firth of Forth and included Britons, Picts, Scots, and English. He was recognized by other monarchs as first among the kings of Britain.

Oswald was killed in his thirty-eighth year in a battle against King Penda of Mercia and his Welsh allies. Recognized as a just and even saintly man in his lifetime, Oswald's relics were widely distributed in the decades that followed. In 1828, his head was found in the coffin of Saint Cuthbert at Durham, where it had been placed in 875. The cult of Oswald was popular not only in England, Scotland, and Ireland, but as far away as Portugal, northeastern Italy, Switzerland, southern Germany, and Bohemia.

During Oswald's reign the plague struck all of England. The king came to the aid of his people with every means at his disposal, until finally he himself was struck down by the malady. He offered himself as a sacrifice for the salvation of the lives of his subjects. A band of angels descended to comfort him and to inform him that his prayers had been granted by the Lord and his people would be spared. The absence of plague at Sauris in Carnia (Friuli) in 1348 was attributed to the intervention of Saint Oswald.

REFERENCES 6, 8, 44, 46

358

Otto of Bamberg

MEMORIAL DAY **July 2**

PATRONAGE **Fever, rabies**

LIFE & LEGEND

Born into a noble Swabian family, Otto was ordained a priest as a young man. He entered into the service of the emperor Henry IV, who made Otto his chancellor in 1101. In spite of his position at the imperial court, Otto sided with the Holy See when Henry broke with Rome over the investiture of a priest, a controversy that culminated with Henry's establishment of an antipope. Otto's loyalty to Rome did not cost him the emperor's respect or trust, and he was nominated bishop of Bamberg. Otto refused to assume the episcopal throne, however, until he was consecrated in Rome by Pope Paschal II in 1106. Otto continued to work toward reconciliation between the papacy and the emperor after Henry V assumed the imperial throne. At the invitation of Boleslaus II of Poland, Otto headed a party of missionaries sent to eastern Pomerania in 1124, a territory recently conquered by the Polish king. Some 20,000 persons were converted as a result. Otto returned to Pomerania in 1128 to reconvert cities that had lapsed back into paganism. He died in Bamberg in 1139, and was canonized in 1189 by Pope Clement III.

REFERENCES 6, 14, 36

359

Ouen of Rouen (Owen, Aldwin)

MEMORIAL DAY **August 24**

PATRONAGE **Deafness**

LIFE & LEGEND

Ouen was born at the beginning of the seventh century at Sancy, France, the son of Saint Authaire. The name Owen is derived from Gaelic, meaning "well-born." Aldwin comes from Old English and means "old friend." Ouen was educated at Saint Medard Abbey, and served in the courts of King Clotair I, King Dagobert I, and King Clovis II. Before he was ordained, he founded a monastery at Rebais in the forest of Brie in 634. In 641, he was appointed bishop of Rouen and later convened a synod to fight simony. He brokered a peace between Neustria and Austrasia for King Thierry III. During his tenure as bishop, he founded several monasteries in his see. He died at Clichy-la-Garenne near Paris in 683. Ouen's relics were brought to Rouen and interred in the abbey of Saint Pierre, which took his name. They are maintained at Saint Ouen's cathedral in Rouen and have been reported to cure deafness on many occasions.

The abbey in Rouen was a Benedictine monastery of great antiquity, dating to the Merovingian period (500 to 752). It is now a glorious church that surpasses the Cathedral of Rouen in size and beauty and is characterized by one of the finest interiors in the world. Saint Ouen is the name of a commune that was incorporated into the city of Paris and is noted for containing the famous Paris flea market.

REFERENCES 9, 42

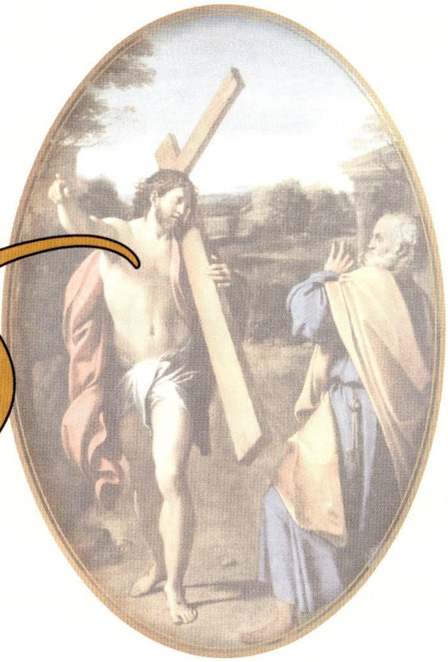

360

Pacificus

MEMORIAL DAY July 10

PATRONAGE Fever

LIFE & LEGEND

Pacificus was one of the favorite companions of Francis of Assisi, from whom he received the name by which he is known. In all likelihood a native of the Marche, Pacificus joined Francis after hearing him preach at San Severino Marche ca. 1212. Five years later Pacificus introduced the Franciscan Order into the region that is presently the Franco-Belgian frontier. He later returned to Italy and, in 1227, was appointed spiritual director of the Franciscan houses in Siena. In 1230, he was invited by Brother Elias to once again cross the Alps and direct the Franciscan province in northern France.

REFERENCES 36, 46

361
Pancras of Rome

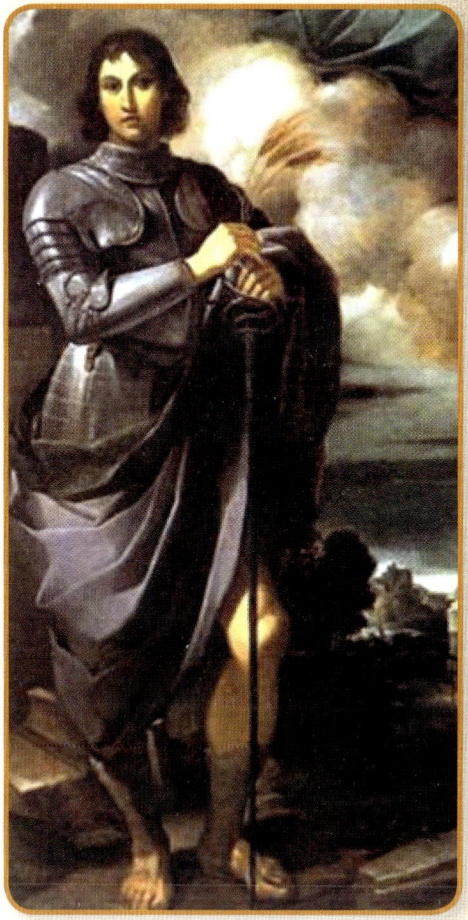

MEMORIAL DAY **May 12**

PATRONAGE **Cramps, headache, perjury, oaths, treaties**

LIFE & LEGEND

Pancras, whose name literally means "the one that holds everything" in Greek, is to be distinguished from Saint Pancras of Taormina. Pancras of Rome was born in Phyrgia ca. 289 to parents of Roman citizenship, and he was brought to Rome as a 14-year-old orphan by his uncle, Saint Dionysius. He was converted to Christianity and zealously followed the faith. He was martyred ca. 304, during Diocletian's persecution, when he refused to sacrifice to the Roman gods and was beheaded on the Via Aurelia in Rome for championing his faith in public.

His relics were initially interred in the Saint Pancras church in Rome that was destroyed in 1798. His head is still in the basilica of San Pancrazio in Rome. At the end of the sixth century, Pope Vitalian sent his relics to England to be installed in a new church as part of the evangelization, Saint Augustine of Canterbury dedicated the first church in England to Saint Pancras, and other churches also bore his name. The district in London that houses the British Library is named Saint Pancras.

REFERENCES 9, 42, 45

362
Pantaleon

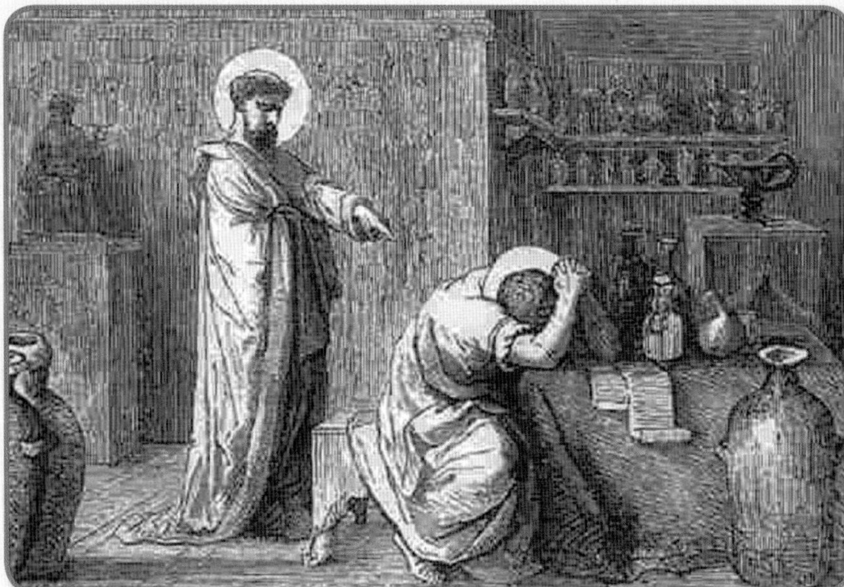

MEMORIAL DAY **July 27**

PATRONAGE **Physicians, midwives, consumption (tuberculosis), bachelors**

LIFE & LEGEND

Pantaleon, whose name translates from Greek, meaning "all compassionate," is one of the Fourteen Holy Helpers. He was born in Nicomedia ca. 275, the son of a wealthy pagan father and Christian mother, Saint Eubula. When his mother died, Pantaleon left the church and studied medicine under Euphrosinos. Pantaleon became physician to Emperor Maximian, but returned to Christianity when he was convinced by Saint Hermolaus that Christ was the better physician.

Pantaleon, who is depicted carrying a medicine box, was used as an example for the thesis of the church that faith was to be trusted over medical advice and treatment, a dictum that persisted until the sixteenth century.

Pantaleon miraculously returned sight to a blind man and, consequently, convinced his own father to convert to Christianity. When his father died and left Pantaleon a fortune, he distributed the wealth among the poor and freed slaves. During the Diocletian persecution, Pantaleon refused to declare apostasy, and as evidence of his faith he cured a paralytic. Condemned to death, he underwent a series of tortures accompanied by miraculous interventions. When his flesh was burned, Christ appeared in the image of Hermolaus and healed Pantaleon. When Pantaleon entered a cauldron of molten lead, Christ accompanied him and the lead became cold. When he was thrown in the sea laden with a heavy stone, the stone floated. When he was thrown to beasts, the beasts fawned over him. When he was bound on a wheel, the ropes broke and the wheel shattered. An attempt was made to behead him, but the sword bent, and the executioners were converted to Christianity. Pantaleon implored that those who tortured him be forgiven, thereby accounting for his name. Eventually, when he was ready to die, he was beheaded at Nicomedia in 303.

His relics were initially venerated at Nicomedia and then transferred to Constantinople. Relics are maintained at Saint Denis in Paris, and his head is venerated in Lyon, France.

REFERENCES 9, 42

363

Patroclus

MEMORIAL DAY **November 19**

PATRONAGE **Madness, fever, skin diseases**

LIFE & LEGEND

Born during the sixth century at Bourges (ancient Avaricum), Patroclus was ordained archdeacon at age 25 and served at the court of Clodomir as tutor to the king's sons. In his desire for a life of greater holiness, Patroclus left the court and set out into the wilderness to live as a hermit. He did not long enjoy the solitary life, because his reputation attracted many disciples to his rustic cell at Colombier. There Patroclus established a monastery, where he died after a life of great austerity. There still exists at Colombier a fountain that was discovered by Patroclus, the water from which is reputed to be effective in the healing of skin diseases.

REFERENCES 36, 46

364

Paul of Narbonne

MEMORIAL DAY **March 22**

PATRONAGE **Blindness, paralysis**

LIFE & LEGEND

Paul of Narbonne was among the party of missionaries sent from Rome in the middle of the third century to evangelize the Roman province of Gaul. His fellow missionaries included the martyred Saturninus of Toulouse and Dionysius (or Denis) of Paris. The name of Paul is associated with the city of Narbonne, of which he was probably bishop. Du Broc de Segange is among those who equate Paul of Narbonne with Sergius Paulus, the proconsul of Cyprus who was converted to Christianity when Paul blinded the magician Elymas at Paphos (Acts 13:6-12). According to this legend, Paul miraculously restored sight to the son of a widow near Rome—another source, perhaps, of Paul's patronage of those who are blind.

REFERENCES 6, 16, 36

365

Paulina do Coração Agonizante de Jesus (Pauline of the Agonizing Heart of Jesus)

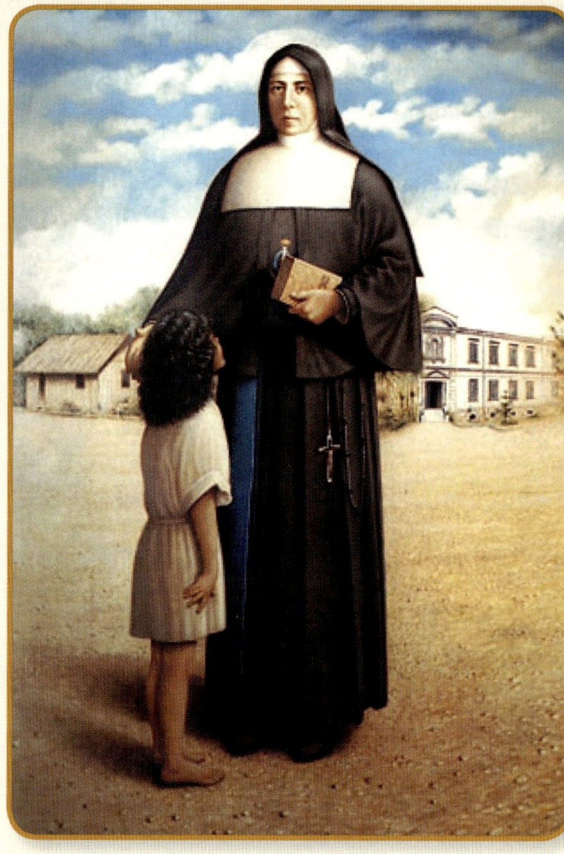

MEMORIAL DAY **July 9**

PATRONAGE **Diabetes**

LIFE & LEGEND

Paulina was born Amabile Lucia Visintainer in a poor but pious family at Vigolo Vattaro, Italy, on December 16, 1865. Ten years later, her family and about 100 neighbors emigrated from Italy to the state of Saint Catherine in Brazil. In her early teens she began teaching the catechism to children, tended the sick, and cleaned the church. While caring for a cancer patient, she and a friend began the Congregation of the Little Sisters of the Immaculate Conception, which was approved by the bishop. In 1890, she took her vows and her new name. The congregation grew rapidly, and, in 1903, Sister Paulina was elected superior general for life.

Shortly thereafter, she left to work with orphans and aged slaves in Saõ Paulo. In 1909, she was sent to work with the sick at the Hospice of Saint Vincent de Paul at Bragança Paulista. In 1918, she was recalled to the Congregation's mother house at Ipiranga where she lived for 20 years, caring for sick sisters.

Paulina had a long history of diabetes mellitus, which became increasingly apparent after 1938. Her right arm was amputated because of vascular complications, but she continued to sew and clean the convent. She died of complications of diabetes on July 9, 1942. She was beatified in 1991 by Pope John Paul II, and, in 2002, she became the first Brazilian to be canonized.

366
Peregrine Laziosi

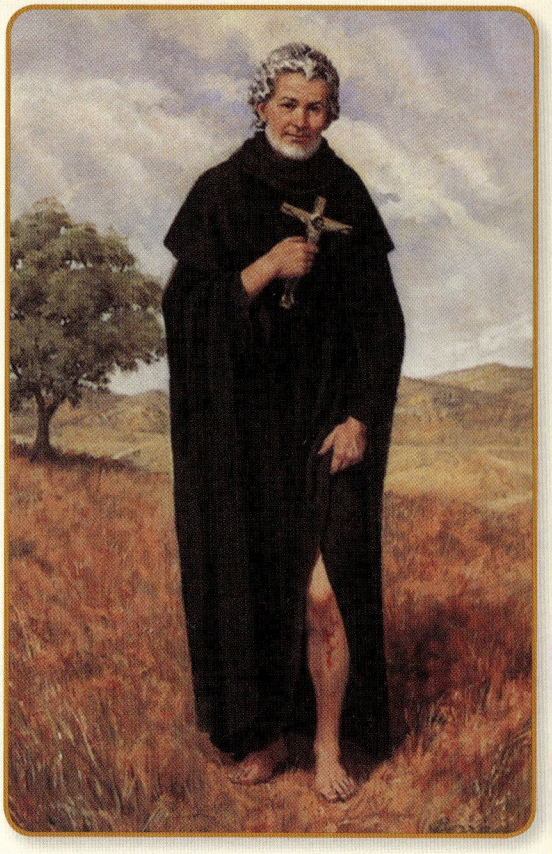

MEMORIAL DAY **May 1**

PATRONAGE **Cancer, breast cancer, skin diseases, open sores, AIDS patients, childbirth, pregnancy, leg injuries**

LIFE & LEGEND

Peregrine, whose name is derived from Latin, meaning "foreigner," was born at Forli, Italy, in 1260 into a wealthy family. He was involved in politics during his early life and took a strong antipapal stance. At the time of an uprising by the antipapal party, Peregrine struck the pope's mediator, Saint Philip Benizi, in the face. When, in response, Saint Philip turned the other cheek and prayed for his assailant, Peregrine, then about 30 years of age, converted and turned his energies to the church and the performance of good deeds. He received instructions from the Virgin Mary in a vision to go to Siena and join the Servites, and he was ordained there. He returned to his hometown of Forli, and lived in complete silence without sitting down for 30 years as penance.

He then became a preacher and orator and founded a Servite house at Forli. At the age of 60, he developed an aggressive cancer in his lower leg and foot. On the eve of a proposed amputation, Peregrine's prayers resulted in a vision of Christ leaving the cross and touching the diseased leg. He awoke to find the tumors gone, and the cure was sustained throughout his life. He died at age 85 in Forli and was canonized in 1726 by Pope Benedict XIII. Peregrine is generally referred to as "the Cancer Saint," and a specific novena is addressed to him.

REFERENCES 6, 9

367

Peter of Alcántara

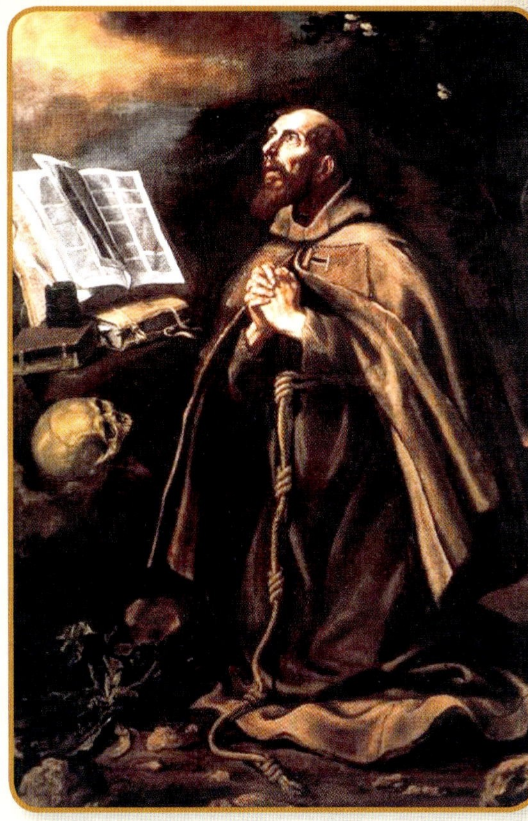

MEMORIAL DAY **October 19**

PATRONAGE **Fever**

LIFE & LEGEND

Peter Garavita was born in 1499 at Alcántara in the province of Estremadura, Spain, where his father was a lawyer and local governor. He was sent by an uncle to study at the university in Salamanca, and, at age 16, he joined the Observant Franciscans. Peter progressed rapidly in his spiritual life and, at age 22, was sent to found a monastery at Badajoz. In 1524, he was ordained to the priesthood, and later he served as director of several monasteries before being sent to Lapa, a remote place where he was made abbot, but better able to pursue his desire for solitude. Peter served as court chaplain to King John III of Portugal, who was unable to retain the ascetic Peter in his court. In 1538, Peter was elected minister provincial of the Observant Franciscans of Saint Gabriel and Estremadura, but he resigned this office in 1540 when he was unable to impose a stricter rule on the members of his province. He subsequently went to live in a remote hermitage near Lisbon and was named superior of the community at Palhares. Still seeking to form a community of greater strictness, Peter traveled to Rome barefoot to obtain the approval of the pope. He succeeded in obtaining the blessing of Julius III and returned to Spain to found a monastery near Pedrosa. The foundation of this establishment marked the beginning of the Franciscan branch later known as the Alcantarines. In 1560, Peter met Teresa of Ávila and became her confessor and spiritual adviser. Peter was a mystic writer whose works were used by Saint Francis de Sales. He died in Estremadura in 1562.

REFERENCES 6, 9, 16, 36, 42, 45

368 Peter the Apostle

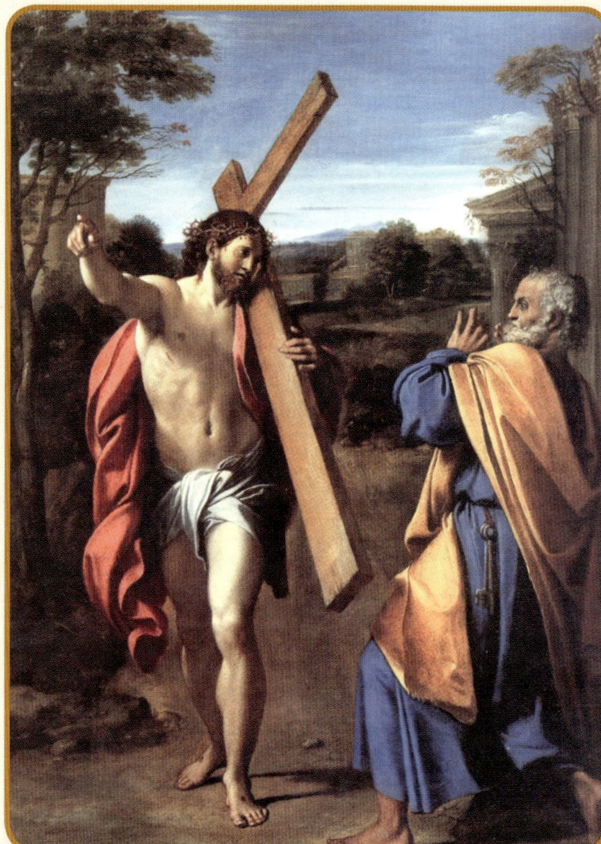

MEMORIAL DAY **June 29 (feast of Peter and Paul)**

PATRONAGE **Fever, foot problems, [podiatry],* bakers, bridge workers, butchers, clock makers, cobblers, locksmiths, masons**

LIFE & LEGEND

Peter was born as Simon in Bethsaida on Lake Genesareth. He settled in Capharnaum and worked as a fisherman on the lake. He was married and had children. As was the case of many of his contemporary Jews, Simon was attracted by the preaching of John the Baptist. Jesus changed Simon's name to Peter (actually Cephas, which translates into Latin as Petrus, meaning "rock"). Christ

*Proposed patronage

accorded Peter the prime position among the Twelve Apostles. Peter's were the first feet Christ washed before the Last Supper, accounting for Peter's patronage of foot ailments.

Peter's earliest apostolic activities took place in Jerusalem, Judea, and north to Syria. He proceeded in his missionary activities to the coastal regions of Lydda, Joppe, and Caesarea. It was there that he cured the palsied Eneas, raised Tabitha from the dead, and received the first non-Jewish Christians into the Church.

Peter founded a church in Antioch and pursued his recruitment of Church members throughout Asia Minor. During the last years of his life, he labored in Rome where he was martyred. There are varied reports of his death and martyrdom. It is purported that he was executed as part of Emperor Nero's persecution in 67 and 68. He was crucified with his head down at his own request, because he believed he was not worthy to die in the same manner as Christ. It is believed that the execution took place in the Neronian Gardens at the foot of the Vatican Hills. For a time, his remains shared a place with those of Paul on the Appian Way, where the church of Saint Sebastian now stands. They were restored to their initial resting place, and a basilica was erected over the grave. The basilica was replaced by Saint Peter's cathedral in the sixteenth century.

REFERENCES 6, 9, 33, 42, 45

369

Peter Chrysologus

MEMORIAL DAY **July 30**

PATRONAGE **Fever, rabies**

LIFE & LEGEND

Peter Chrysologus was born at Imola, in Emilia, Italy, where he was educated and also ordained. In 1433, he was consecrated bishop of Ravenna, a city that served as capital to Emperor Honorius and as the major point of contact between the Greek east (Constantinople) and an Italy that was under constant pressure from Gothic invaders. As bishop, Peter sought to reform the laxity of both clergy and laity in his diocese and to convert the remaining pagan population. His preaching toward those ends was so effective that he was given the Greek title "Chrysologus" or golden-worded. Many of his sermons survive. Peter so impressed Honorius' sister, Galla Placidia, that she generously supported him in the ambitious building projects that still grace the historic center of Ravenna. Peter Chrysologus also officiated at the funeral of Germanus of Auxerre, who died at Ravenna 2 years before Peter's own death in 1450 in his native Imola.

REFERENCES 36, 46

370
Peter Damian

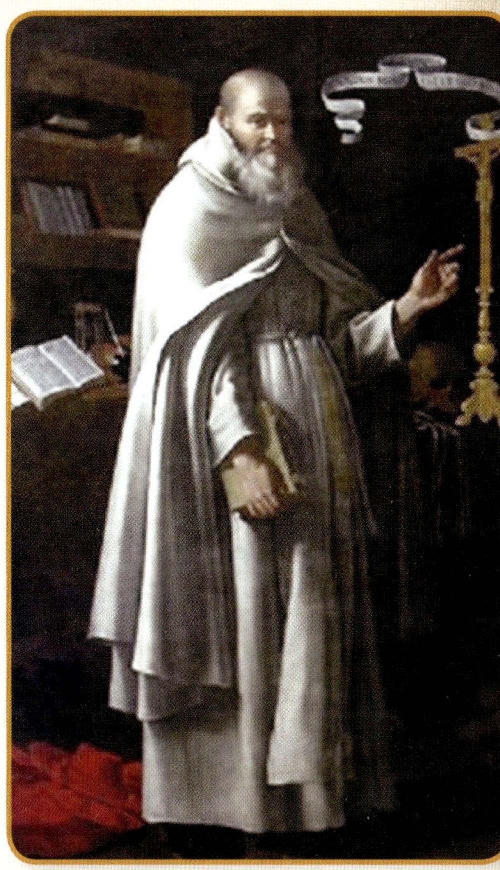

MEMORIAL DAY **February 21**

PATRONAGE **Headache, sore throat**

LIFE & LEGEND

Peter was born at Ravenna ca. 1077, the youngest child of an impoverished family. When he was orphaned early in life, he was sent to live with a brother who mistreated him. He then moved to live with another brother, Damian, an archpriest at Ravenna, whose name Peter took. Peter was an impressive student of theology and canon law at Ravenna, Faenza, and Parma, and became a professor at age 25. In 1035, he gave up his teaching and became a Benedictine monk. His extremes of self-mortification affected his health, and he was assigned teaching roles during his recovery. In 1043, he became Enonomus of Fonte-Avellana, a position he held for the rest of his life. He founded sister hermitages in San Servino, Gamungo, Murciana, Acreta, San Salvatore, Sitria, and Ocri.

Peter was in Rome when Clement II crowned Henry II and attended a synod in which decrees were passed against simony. In 1050, he published *Liber Gomorrhianus,* a treatise of the vices of priests. He condemned the study of philosophy and indicated that it was not necessary for salvation. Peter was consecrated cardinal-bishop of Ostia in 1057. He supported Pope Alexander II and opposed the antipope, Benedict X. Peter died in 1072 of fever at Ravenna and was buried at the monastery church. He was declared a Doctor of the Church in 1828. His relics were removed several times and have been in the chapel of Saint Peter Damian in the cathedral of Faenza, Italy, since 1898.

REFERENCES 6, 9, 42

371

Peter Thomas

MEMORIAL DAY **January 6**

PATRONAGE **Plague, contagious diseases**

LIFE & LEGEND

Peter Thomas was born in 1305 in the diocese of Sarlat in the southwest of France. In spite of his humble origins, Peter's intellectual abilities attracted notice, and he was admitted to the Carmelite Order at Condom. In 1342, he was appointed procurator general of the order, headquartered at Avignon, which at the time was also residence of the pope. His proximity to the papal hierarchy wrought considerable changes in his life.

In the confined environment of Avignon, Peter's many abilities became obvious to the papacy, which engaged him in a variety of diplomatic and military initiatives for the remainder of his career. He was sent as papal legate to negotiate a solution to the troubles among Genoa, Milan, and Venice. In 1354, he was consecrated the bishop of Patti and Lipari, and he represented the pope at the coronation of Emperor Charles IV as king of Italy. Peter also served as papal intermediary between Venice and the kingdom of Hungary over their conflicting interests in Dalmatia, and he was sent to Constantinople to try to resolve the schism between the western and eastern churches.

In 1359, Peter returned to Constantinople with an army. He came as Universal Legate to the Eastern Church and imposed himself on the Byzantines as patriarch of Constantinople in place of the legitimate Greek hierarchy. In 1363, he was appointed archbishop of Crete and Candia. In 1365, he commanded an attack on Muslim-held Alexandria. Three months after the failure of this expedition, in 1366, he died on Cyprus of wounds sustained during the siege.

In spite of the worldly nature of much of his career, Peter's biographers emphasize the monastic ideals to which he adhered, his many austerities, his concern for the poor, and his missionary zeal. Venerated by the Roman church as a bishop martyr, he has not yet been canonized. After describing the bishop's death, du Broc de Segange relates: "After his death the aura of sanctity shone upon his grace-filled face and body which, still fresh and rosy, was covered with an abundant and fragrant exudation. They wiped this up with cotton which was used to effect astonishing and numerous healings. This is certainly the reason why he is invoked against the plague and contagious diseases."

REFERENCES 6, 9, 14, 16, 36

372

Peter of Verona (Peter Martyr)

MEMORIAL DAY **April 29**

PATRONAGE **Headache, women in labor**

LIFE & LEGEND

Born in 1205 at Verona to parents who belonged to the neo-Manichean sect of the Cathari, Peter was nonetheless sent to Catholic schools and was educated at the University of Bologna. He entered the Dominican Order and became famous in Milan and throughout Lombardy for his preaching and miraculous healings. About 1234, he was appointed inquisitor general for the Milanese territories, which then embraced most of northern Italy, apart from Venetia. In this role he earned such enmity among the Catharists that they plotted his assassination. On April 6, 1252, on the road from Como to Milan, Peter and his companions were attacked by a party of Catharists. Peter was mortally wounded in the head by a man named Carino, who later repented his crime, abjured Catharism, and became a Dominican lay brother at Forlì.

REFERENCES 6, 16, 36, 46

373

Petronilla

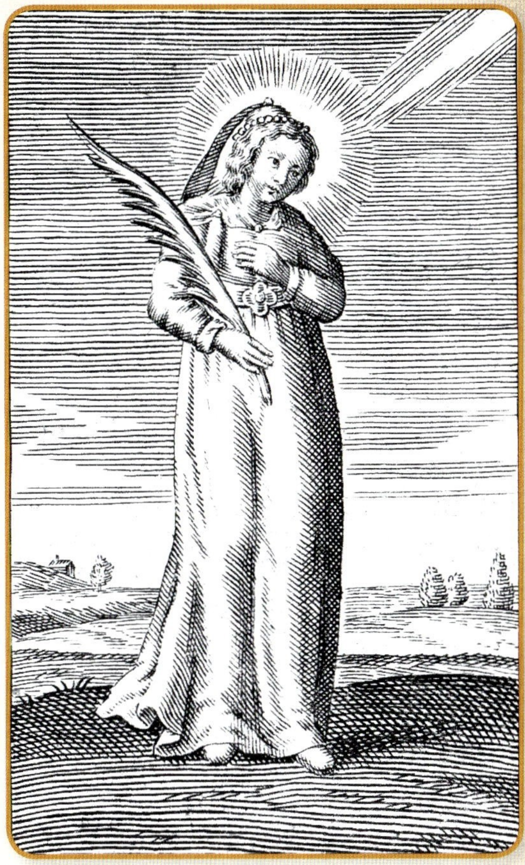

MEMORIAL DAY **May 31**

PATRONAGE **Fever**

LIFE & LEGEND

The belief that Petronilla was the daughter of Saint Peter was prevalent in the sixth century and possibly earlier. Du Broc de Segange and others were of the opinion that she was the spiritual daughter of Peter rather than his real daughter. According to legend, the Christian virgin, Petronilla, expired on the last of 3 days given her to consider a marriage proposal from a pagan Roman patrician named Flaccus. In some versions of this legend, she had suffered years before from a fever that Saint Peter declined to heal, because he thought she would benefit spiritually from her malady. God eventually did heal Petronilla, however, and the beautiful young virgin became an object of desire for the noble Flaccus.

The actual Petronilla may have lived two centuries later than the legendary daughter of Peter. A fresco dating from the late fourth century in the cemetery in Domitilla on the Via Ardeatina in Rome identifies Petronilla as a martyr.

REFERENCES 6, 9, 16, 36, 42, 45, 46

374

Phaletrus

MEMORIAL DAY **November 23 or November 25**

PATRONAGE **Infertility, splenic diseases**

LIFE & LEGEND

Born near present-day Limoges in the latter half of the fifth century, Phaletrus made pilgrimages to the holy sites of Rome and Jerusalem as a priest before entering the monastery at Fleury-sur-Loire on his return to Gaul. Phaletrus later withdrew into the wilderness near Chabris, where he directed a small community of like-minded contemplatives. Phaletrus was recognized for his holiness and miraculous healing of the sick. He died ca. 525.

REFERENCES 16, 27, 36

375
Pharaildis (Varelde)

MEMORIAL DAY **January 4**

PATRONAGE **Sick children**

LIFE & LEGEND

The cult of Pharaildis, who was the sister of Saint Gudule and the niece of Saint Gertrude of Nivelles, was once widespread in Flanders, where she was known as Varelde, Veerle, or Verylde. Pharaildis was born in Ghent ca. 650 and had made a vow of virginity, but her parents betrothed her against her will to a noble suitor. Her husband treated her badly, and Pharaildis maintained her vow and refused him conjugal rights.

Pharaildis was freed from this unhappiness only by the death of her spouse. She is supposed to have lived to her ninetieth year, a long life during which she devoted herself to prayer, abundant acts of charity, and the working of miracles. She is said to have caused a fountain to rise from the ground at Brouay, the waters from which, according to du Broc de Segange, "have the power to heal children afflicted with wasting diseases. Every Friday, in the chapel of the saint in the church at Brouay, one sees pilgrims imploring the saint for the healing of their children."

REFERENCES 6, 9, 14, 16, 36, 45

376

Philip (Filippo) Benizi

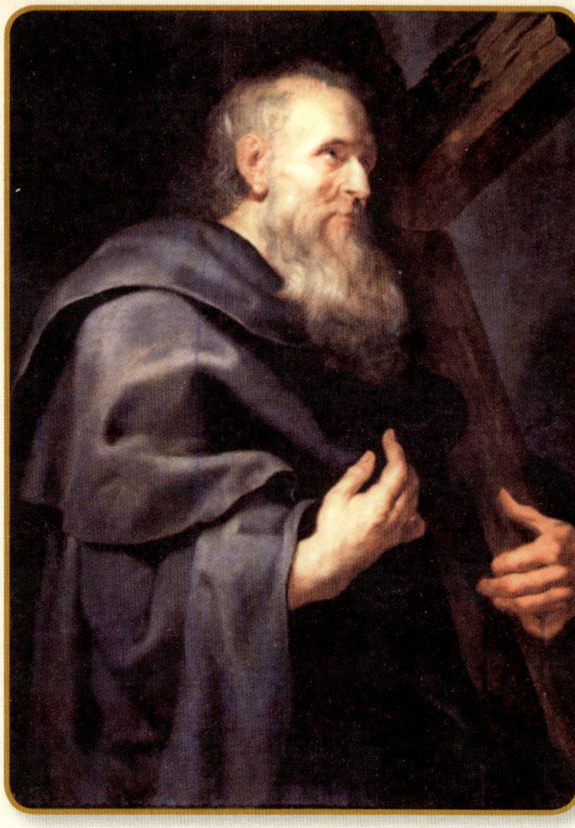

MEMORIAL DAY **August 23**

PATRONAGE **Leprosy, epilepsy (particularly in children)**

LIFE & LEGEND

Philip, which is a name derived from Greek, meaning "lover of horses," was born into a noble Florentine family in 1233. At age 13 he was sent to Paris to study medicine. He continued these studies in Padua, where he received a degree of doctor of medicine and philosophy at age 19. He then returned to Florence, were he practiced medicine. In 1254, he joined the recently formed Servites (Servi di Santa Maria). In spite of his desire to remain a simple monk, Philip was ordained to the priesthood in 1258, served as superior in several friaries, and was eventually elected prior general of the order. He was sent to Forli, Italy, to resolve a conflict between the pope and the emperor. He declined the archbishopric of Florence when it was offered to him, and, after learning that he was seriously being considered as a candidate for the papacy, he went into hiding on Mount Tuniato until the accession of Gregory X. Philip resigned the generalship of his order in 1285 and retired to a Servite house in Todi, where he died that same year. Numerous miraculous healings were attributed to Philip, even during his lifetime. He once met a leper on the road, to whom he gave his cloak, resulting in an immediate cure. Philip Benizi was canonized 1671 by Pope Clement X.

REFERENCES 6, 9, 14, 36, 42, 45, 50

377

Philip Neri

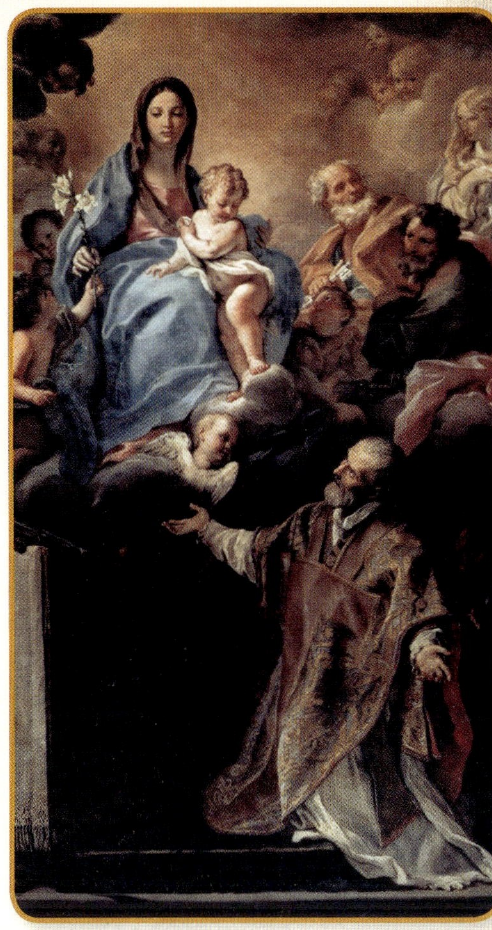

MEMORIAL DAY **May 25**

PATRONAGE **Limb problems, heart diseases, infertility, joint diseases, [cardiology],* Rome, U.S. Special Forces**

LIFE & LEGEND

Philip Neri was born on May 25, 1515, in Florence, Italy. He was the son of a poor notary and received his early education from the Dominican friars of San Marco in Florence. When his father's property was destroyed, Philip was sent to his uncle at San Germano near Monte Cassino, where he had a conversion. He moved to Rome in 1533.

During his first 17 years in Rome, Philip was a layman who traveled throughout the city, directing disreputable and irreligious people to the parishes. He continued this activity throughout his life, earning him the title, "Apostle of Rome." According to Bacci, his biographer, while Philip was in prayer in 1544, a ball of fire entered his mouth and lodged in his chest. This caused a pulsating swelling in the region of his heart. After Philip died years later and his body was studied by physicians, two broken ribs were noted, and the curvature formed an arch that allowed for a markedly dilated but otherwise normal heart.

*Proposed patronage

In 1548, along with his confessor, Father Persiano Rossa, he founded the Confraternity of the Most Holy Trinity, which focused on the care of pilgrims and those convalescing from illness. Philip was ordained a priest in 1551 and settled at the hospital of San Girolamo della Carità, where he initiated meetings in the Oratory consisting of prayers, readings, lectures, and musical selections. Participants conducted mission work throughout Rome, preached sermons in different churches in the city, and heard confession. This was the genesis of the Congregation of the Oratory, a community of secular priests that was formally recognized by Pope Gregory XIII in 1575 and was given the church of Saint Maria in Vallicella. Cardinal John Henry Newman, the most influential Catholic thinker and writer in the nineteenth century, joined an English chapter of the Congregation of the Oratory in 1847.

In his later years, Philip had a series of ailments that were cured by prayer. He died of natural causes in 1595, and his body was interred in Chieza Nuova in Rome. He was beatified by Pope Paul V in 1615 and canonized by Pope Gregory XV in 1622.

REFERENCES 6, 9, 42, 45

378 Philomena

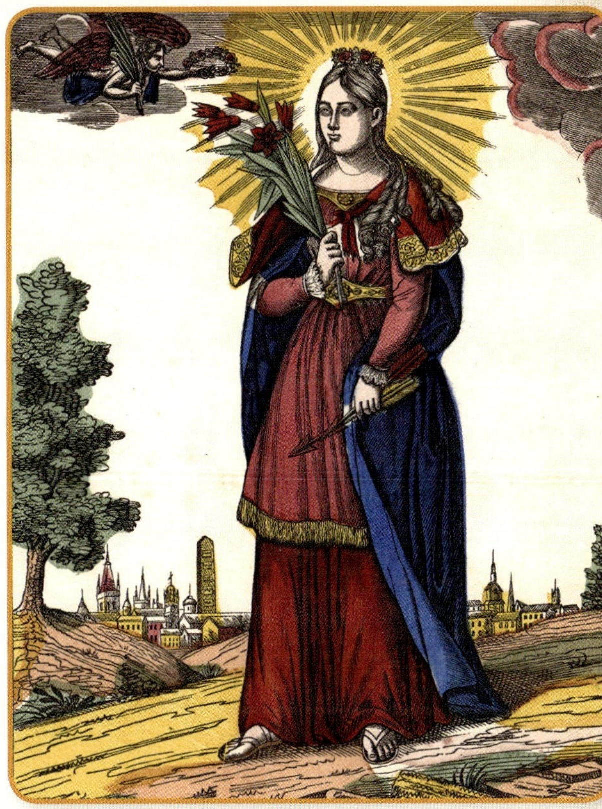

MEMORIAL DAY **August 11 (removed in 1961 by Pope John XXIII)**

PATRONAGE **Infertility, cancer, heart ailments, children, desperate causes, orphans, the poor**

LIFE & LEGEND

The Legend of Saint Philomena, whose name literally means "love of strength" in Greek, and who is referred to as the "Wonder Worker of the Nineteenth Century," is unique in the annals of hagiography. She is the only individual who was beatified based on miraculous intercessions. Nothing is known about her life, with the exception of what she revealed in a private revelation to a nun, which indicated that she was martyred as a teenager in the early days of the Church.

In 1802, the remains of a young girl, about 13 years of age, were found in the catacombs of Saint Priscilla on the Via Salaria in Rome. The body, along with drawings of two anchors, three arrows, and a palm, was covered with stones, and a small glass phial containing the remains of blood. A set of tiles that accompanied the remains spelled out the words "LUMENA PAXTE CUMFI," which are meaningless. But, they were rearranged to read "PAX TECUM FILUMENA" (Peace with you, Filumena). Three years later, Canon Francis de Lucia of Mugnano, Italy, was standing over her relics, which at the time resided in the Treasury of the Rare Collection of Christian Antiquity in the Vatican, when he had a spiritual experience that led to his request to install the relics in a chapel in Mugnano.

Once the relics were enshrined, miracles began to occur there. Cancer patients were cured, wounds were immediately healed, and the Venerable Pauline Jaricot was cured of her debilitating heart ailment overnight. Pope Leo XII had altars and churches erected in honor of Philomena, and she was canonized by Pope Gregory XVI in 1837. In 1961, Saint Philomena's feast day was removed from the liturgical calendar, but that did not affect her canonization.

REFERENCES 6, 9

379

Piat

MEMORIAL DAY **October 1**

PATRONAGE **Fever, heart palpitations**

LIFE & LEGEND

A native of Benevento, Piat left Italy, perhaps in the company of Saint Denis, to evangelize Tournai, in Belgium, and Chartres, in Gaul. Piat converted thousands of people in the vicinity of Tournai. He was tortured and martyred in the persecutions of Emperor Maximian Herculeus ca. 286 by having large nails driven through his body at Seclin, a village between Lille and Tournai. His body was discovered in the seventh century by Saint Eligius who built a reliquary for them. Piat is interred at Chartres where miracles were reported to have occurred at the tomb.

REFERENCES 6, 16, 27, 36, 45

380
Pirminus

MEMORIAL DAY **November 3**

PATRONAGE **Pregnancy, labor, plague, poisoning, snakebite**

LIFE & LEGEND

The monk Pirminus, a native of southern Aragon or Gaul, fled the Moors and migrated to the Grisons (Graubünden), where he rebuilt the Swiss Dissentis abbey that had been destroyed by the Avars. He later founded the monastery of Reichenau on an island in Lake Constance; and then, having been exiled for political reasons, went to Alsace, where he founded the Murbach monastery. Pirminus' final monastic foundation was the abbey at Amorbach in lower Franconia. He was consecrated a regionary bishop and was the author of a catechism titled the Dicta Pirmini. He was one of the great Apostles to German lands. Pirminus died in 753 and was buried at Hornbach.

REFERENCES 14, 36

381

Placido of Recanati

MEMORIAL DAY **June 5**

PATRONAGE **Fever, epidemics**

LIFE & LEGEND

Placido was born in 1328 in the small city of Recanati in the Italian Marches, was orphaned young, and was raised by an uncle who took great care in his nephew's education. While pursuing his studies, Placido made the decision to enter the religious life, knowing that in doing so he would disappoint his uncle. To this end, he traveled to Rome and joined an order commonly known as the Apostolini. When his uncle died, Placido was left a considerable sum, with instructions that it be used for the construction of a religious house and church for the order to which he belonged in Recanati. Placido was sent back to Recanati by his superiors, and, in 1370, was made prior of the religious house he founded. He died in 1398, and his remains were interred in the church of San Giovanni Evangelista, where numerous miracles were recorded at his tomb.

REFERENCES 16, 36

382

Polycarp

MEMORIAL DAY **February 23**

PATRONAGE **Earache, dysentery**

LIFE & LEGEND

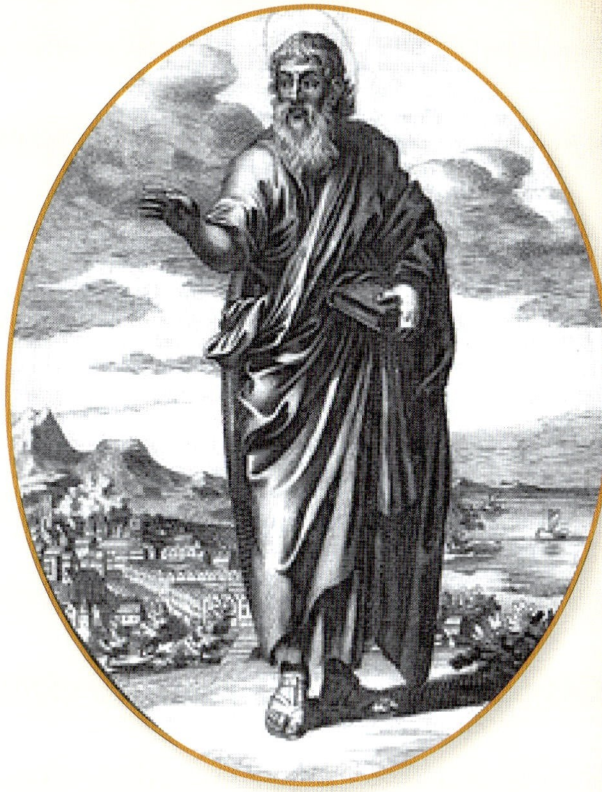

Polycarp was born ca. 69 and is thought to have been a disciple of John, the author of the Fourth Gospel. He served as the bishop of Smyrna (currently Izmir, Turkey). A letter that he wrote to the Philippians is one of the earliest Christian documents to survive. The Martyrdom of Polycarp, which is a circular letter from the church of Smyrna, represents one of the earliest authentic accounts of a specific Christian martyrdom, reporting the fatal stabbing of the 86-year-old Polycarp after an attempt to burn him at the stake failed to do any harm.

REFERENCES 6, 9, 33

383

Porcarius

MEMORIAL DAY **August 12**

PATRONAGE **Blindness, eye injuries**

LIFE & LEGEND

Porcarius was the abbot of 500 monks at the monastery founded in the fifth century by Saint Honoratus of Arles on the island of Lérins in Provence, opposite Cannes. After a dream presaging an attack on the monastery by Moorish raiders, Porcarius sent away as many of the novices and monks as the only ship available could accommodate. He then prepared the remainder of his community to meet death. All the monks were killed ca. 739 by the Moors except four, who were taken into slavery. According to Kerler, Porcarius was blinded by his captors, accounting for his patronage.

REFERENCES 6, 14, 36, 46

384

Portianus

MEMORIAL DAY **November 24**

PATRONAGE **Blindness, eye diseases**

LIFE & LEGEND

Portianus was born a slave on an estate near the village that today bears his name in the department of Allier, France. A pious young man, Portianus commonly used to visit the nearby monastery of Mirande for spiritual consolation. His difficult master noted Portianus' frequent absences, had him followed to the monastery, and accused the abbot of trying to steal his servant. When the abbot and Portianus' master became involved in an increasingly bitter dispute over the pious slave, the layman was suddenly struck blind.

Repenting of his conduct, the man begged the abbot's forgiveness and asked him to pray for the restoration of his sight. The abbot ordered Portianus to make the sign of the cross on his master's eyes, and, when he did so, the man's sight was restored. Portianus was freed and immediately entered the abbey of Mirande. He was ordained a priest there and was later made abbot. He demanded that the Merovingian king, Thierry of Austrasia, release his Auvergnate prisoners, and the king complied. Portianus died of natural causes in 533.

REFERENCES 16, 36

385

Praejectus (Prix, Priel, Priest) of Clermont

MEMORIAL DAY **January 25**

PATRONAGE **Fever, incurable diseases**

LIFE & LEGEND

A native of Clermont, France, Praejectus was reputed to be a man of exceptional learning, eloquence, and piety. In 666, he was made bishop of Auvergne with the approbation of Childeric II, king of Austrasia. Praejectus was zealous in founding churches, monasteries, and hospitals in his diocese. He is invoked against fever because of his miraculous healing of the future Saint Amarin, abbot of a monastery at Voussac in the Bourbonnais, of a dangerous fever. Praejectus was murdered at Volvic on January 25, 676, while returning from court to Clermont. The reason for his death was revenge for his supposed involvement in the arrest and execution of Hector, count of Marseilles, by Childeric. After Praejectus' death, numerous miracles were recorded at his tomb.

REFERENCES 6, 16, 36

386

Priscus (Brix)

MEMORIAL DAY **May 26**

PATRONAGE **Sick children**

LIFE & LEGEND

During the third century, Priscus, his friend Cottus, and other Christians of Besançon fled that city during the persecutions of the emperor Aurelian and sought refuge in the forests surrounding Auxerre. They were hunted down, however, and martyred. Priscus himself was beheaded ca. 272. In the fifth century, the martyrs' place of burial was discovered by Saint Germanus, who rebuilt the tombs and effectively established their cult. Du Broc de Segange quotes a magazine article published in 1850 that describes the celebration of the feast day of Saint Priscus and his companions in the village of Saint-Brix, including the practice of women who "bring their sick children—the ones who have been pronounced incurable and have been abandoned by the physicians—in a final act of desperate hope. It is not uncommon to encounter on this day wagons filled with women and their children and to see mules whose panniers have been loaded with two or three of these poor creatures, their faces pale and suffering."

REFERENCES 6, 16, 36

387

Psalmodius

MEMORIAL DAY **June 15**

PATRONAGE **Blindness, labor, childhood diseases, colic, herpes, worms**

LIFE & LEGEND

Psalmodius was born into a noble British family and received a thorough education in the Christian tradition. He had performed miraculous cures even before he resolved to leave Britain for France. Psalmodius' reputation for holiness and working miracles preceded him. After landing at Saintes in the Saintonge, Psalmodius was received by the bishop, Leontius, who saved water in which Psalmodius had washed his hands to restore sight to a blind woman by washing her eyes with this liquid. Psalmodius withdrew deep into the forest around Limoges. It was there, apparently, that the recluse received his name because of his unceasing recitation of the psalter. Psalmodius' reputation for holiness and miracle working followed him even in the depths of the forest. His successful intercession for a woman who lay dying after a long and painful labor marked the beginning of his invocation for women in parturition. He died in 589. Psalmodius is also called on for those who are dying, so that they may have adequate time to prepare their souls, and for various diseases of childhood, including colic, stomach disorders, and worms.

REFERENCES 16, 36

2

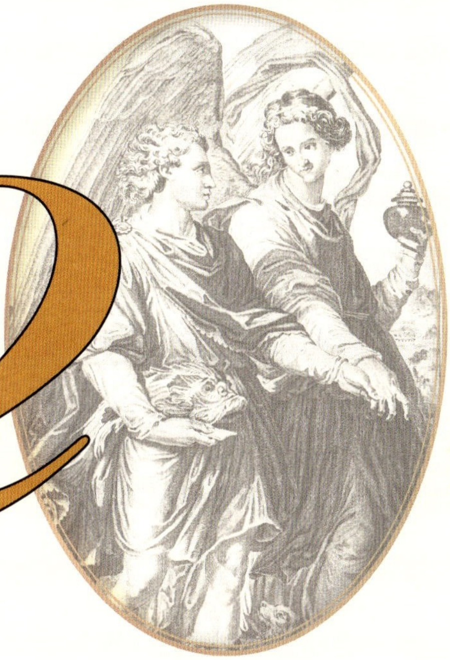

388
Quintianus

MEMORIAL DAY **November 13**

PATRONAGE **Fever**

LIFE & LEGEND

A North African, Quintianus sought refuge in Gaul from the Arian persecution of orthodox Christians. Settling at Rodez (Aveyron), he was almost immediately chosen to occupy the episcopal throne of this city, which happened to be vacant. As the new bishop, he erected a church in memory of his predecessor, Saint Aman, and transferred the holy man's relics there. When the city of Rodez was threatened by Visigoths, an Arian tribe, Quintianus was forced to seek exile in Clermont. He returned to Rodez after the defeat of the Visigoth army by Clovis, but when Rodez fell into the hands of the Arians after Clovis' death, Quintianus found himself back in Clermont, this time as its bishop (ca. 515). His episcopate was a difficult one, because he had enemies within and outside his diocese, but he met these difficulties with gentleness and charity. He died in 527.

REFERENCES 16, 36

389

Quintinus (Quentin)

MEMORIAL DAY **October 31**

PATRONAGE **Dropsy, cough, surgeons**

LIFE & LEGEND

Quintinus, the son of a Roman senator, converted to Christianity and went as a missionary to Gaul with Saint Lucian of Beauvais. Quintinus was active in the area of Ambianus (Amiens), where he was arrested and tortured for his missionary work by the military prefect Rictiovarus. With the assistance of an angel, Quintinus escaped from prison, but was again arrested while preaching in the marketplace of Amiens. He was conducted to Augusta Veromanduorum (present-day Saint-Quentin), where he was beheaded and his body thrown into the Somme in 286. According to Butler, Quintinus' body was immediately recovered and buried by the faithful. Other sources maintain that the body of the saint lay at the bottom of the Somme for 55 years before being recovered, identified, and buried. This may be the origin of Quintinus' patronage of those suffering from dropsy. His tomb was known as a site for miracles, and his relics were later discovered by Saint Eligius.

REFERENCES 6, 16, 36, 46

390

Quirinus

MEMORIAL DAY **March 30 or April 30**

PATRONAGE **Scrofula, diseases of the leg, paralysis, gout, epilepsy, plague, ear diseases, throat disorders, ulcers**

LIFE & LEGEND

Quirinus was a military tribune entrusted with the execution of Pope Alexander and other Christians during the reign of Emperor Trajan. He was converted to Christianity after witnessing miracles performed by Alexander, and was baptized with his daughter, Balbina. As a consequence, Quirinus was arrested, tortured, and martyred by decapitation in the third century. He was buried in the catacombs of Pretestatus on the Via Appia. In the tenth century, Quirinus' remains were given by Pope Leo IX to an abbess named Gepa (perhaps Leo's sister), who deposited them in the city of Neuss on the Rhine, where they are still venerated in the church named in his honor.

From Neuss, Quirinus' cult spread along the Rhine to Cologne and westward into France and Belgium. Du Broc de Segange relates that one of the miracles witnessed by Quirinus was Alexander's miraculous cure of his daughter, Balbina, of the scrofula from which she suffered. He also describes the tortures that Quirinus endured before his decapitation, including the removal of his tongue and the amputation of his hands and feet. He continues, "In memory of the cure from scrofula of his daughter by Pope Alexander, Quirinus himself was invoked against this and related disorders: purulent abscess, fistula, and affections of the ears caused by an internal abscess . . . In France, at a time when the saints were still held in honor, scrofula (les humeurs froides) and fistula were always designated with the name Saint Quirinus' disease (le mal de saint Quirin), and in Belgium, those ulcers which one sees on the neck were called ulcus Quirini or ulcer of Saint Quirinus, which sufficiently demonstrates that Saint Quirinus was the specially designated physician of all such disorders . . . As for the invocation of the saint against diseases of the legs, the gout and paralysis—this stems from having all his limbs broken and not being able to move so that he had to be transported by oxen to his place of execution. The invocation of Quirinus in cases of epilepsy is a little more difficult to explain." Kerler adds that Quirinus was also invoked in time of plague.

REFERENCES 16, 36, 46

391

Quiteria

MEMORIAL DAY **May 22**

PATRONAGE **Rabies, madness, palpitations, plague, leprosy, wounds**

LIFE & LEGEND

Quiteria was the daughter of a Galician nobleman. Unbeknownst to her parents, Quiteria was baptized a Christian and vowed to remain a virgin. When her father attempted to marry his daughter to a suitor, he learned of her conversion and her vow and demanded that she renounce her faith. Quiteria refused and fled home. She was tracked down by her father's men at Aire (Landes) in the southwest of France, and executed there on his orders. Fay maintains that after being decapitated, Quiteria picked up her head and carried it into the city of Aire, where her remains were preserved.

The cult of Saint Quiteria was popular in the South of France, Spain, and Portugal. According to Fay, "between Lannemaignan and Tachousin (Gers), a fountain rises on the side of a hill with miraculous powers that is dedicated to Saint Quiteria. There is a pool about 200 meters from the church where the sick—especially those afflicted with leprosy—come to bathe." Fay dates Quiteria to the third or fourth century, Butler dates her to the fifth century, and du Broc de Segange places her in the seventh century.

REFERENCES 6, 16, 23, 36

R

392

Radegunde

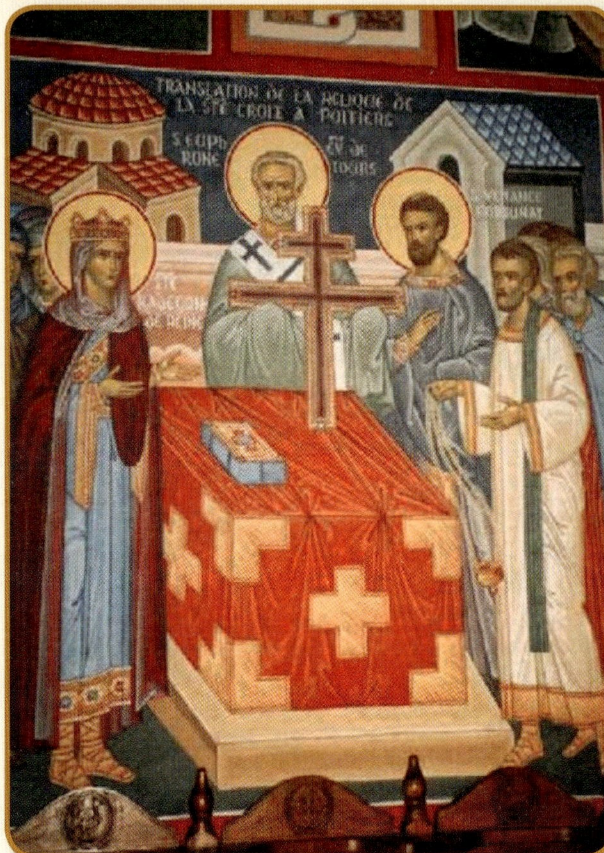

MEMORIAL DAY **August 13**

PATRONAGE **Fever, leprosy, scabies, ulcers**

LIFE & LEGEND

Radegunde was born in Saxony in 518, the daughter of Berthaire, one of three Thuringian pagan kings. Her father was murdered by her uncle, who brought her up until the Frankish king, Clotaire I, defeated the Thuringians. Radegunde was abducted by Clotaire and taken to his castle to become his queen. Although she married the king ca. 540, she converted to Christianity and maintained a devout life. She used the money she received at the wedding to found several hospices, one of which still exists at Athies.

After 10 years in an abusive marriage, she fled the court and took the veil from Saint Medard, the bishop of Noyon. She escaped the territory over which Clotaire ruled and settled in Poitiers, where she founded a convent. To sanctify the convent, the patriarch of Jerusalem sent a fragment of the True Cross on which Christ was crucified. Radegunde never left the convent and devoted her life to prayer and meditation, although Clotaire eventually asked for her pardon.

Radegunde died in 587. She is the patron saint of Jesus College, Cambridge, that was founded in 1496. A stained glass window at the college represents scenes from her life, and a statue of her looks down to one of the college's gates.

REFERENCES 29, 45

393

Raphael

MEMORIAL DAY **September 29**

PATRONAGE **Blindness, eye diseases, physicians, nurses, mental illness, travelers**

LIFE & LEGEND

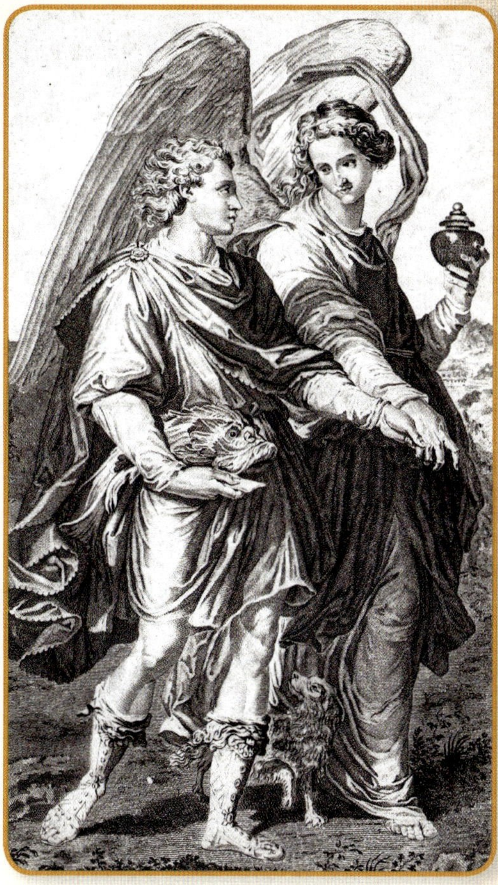

Raphael, whose name in Hebrew means "God has healed," is one of the seven archangels. The Hebrew word for "doctor of medicine" has the same root as Raphael. Of the seven archangels, only three, Michael, Gabriel, and Raphael, are mentioned by name in the scriptures. Raphael, who is venerated in Judaism, Christianity, and Islam, is the central figure in the Deuterocanonical Book of Tobit. In that writing, Raphael appears in human form, calling himself "Azarias the son of the great Ananias," as the traveling companion of the younger Tobias. During travel through the desert of upper Egypt, Raphael delivered Sarah, the daughter-in-law of the elder Tobias, from the demon that had killed seven of her husbands. After returning from the desert travels, Raphael healed the blindness of the elder Tobias and then revealed himself as "the angel Raphael." The Gospel of John reports the legend of a pool called Probatica with healing power associated with Raphael.

Raphael was added to the Roman Catholic calendar for saints in 1921 with a feast day of October 24. This was changed in 1969 when September 29 became the joint celebration for the three archangels, Michael, Gabriel, and Raphael.

REFERENCES 6, 9

394

Ratho

MEMORIAL DAY **May 17 or June 19**

PATRONAGE **Calculi, hernia**

LIFE & LEGEND

Ratho Graf von Andechs was known in Bavaria as Saint Grafrath. He was famed as a young knight for his stature and his military virtues. He distinguished himself in fighting against the Hungarians, but, after peace was restored, he laid down his arms and made pilgrimages to Rome and to the Holy Land. Ratho acquired numerous relics in Rome, Constantinople, and Jerusalem, which remain at Andechs. On his return from the East, Ratho built a Benedictine monastery on an island that he named Wörth in the river Amper. Both the monastery and the church were destroyed by the Hungarians not long after Ratho's death in 953, although his tomb survived.

REFERENCES 6, 14, 16, 36

395

Raymond Nonnatus

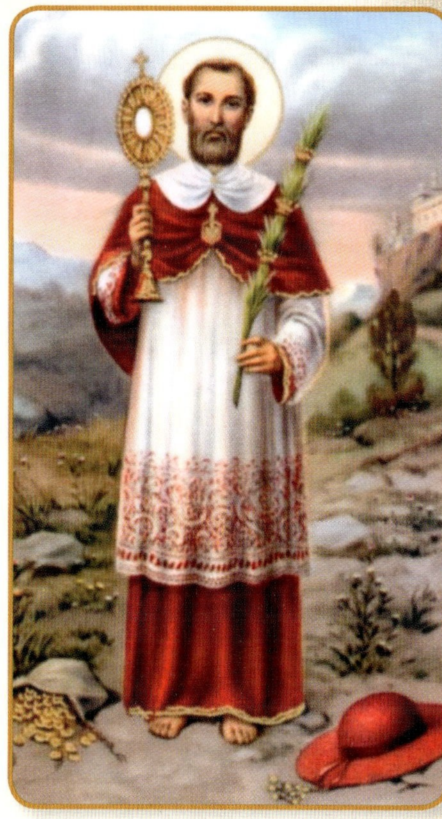

MEMORIAL DAY **August 31**

PATRONAGE **Pregnancy, newborns, fever, midwives, [obstetrics]***

LIFE & LEGEND

Nonnatus in Latin means "not born" and refers to the fact that the saint was delivered by caesarian section after his mother died in childbirth. He was born in 1204 at Portello in Catalonia, Spain, into a relatively poor but noble family. He was well educated at the court in Aragon and, from an early age, felt drawn to a religious life. He joined the Mercedarian Order, which was founded to ransom Christian captives of the Moors in Africa.

He went to Algiers, where he spent his own estate to retrieve many hostages. When his money ran out, he surrendered himself to free another hostage. He was imprisoned and tortured, but converted some of the guards. To prevent him from preaching, a hole was bored through his lips and a padlock was passed through them. He was eventually ransomed and returned to Barcelona. He served as master-general of the Mercedarian Order.

In 1239, he was made a cardinal by Gregory IX. On his way to Rome the following year he took ill and died. His body was interred at a chapel near his family farm. He was canonized in 1657 by Pope Alexander VII. His liturgical celebration is no longer included among those that are necessarily commemorated.

*Proposed patronage

REFERENCES 6, 9, 11

396

Raymond of Toulouse

MEMORIAL DAY **July 3**

PATRONAGE **Plague**

LIFE & LEGEND

Raymond Gayard, whose surname is derived from Germanic, meaning "advice, decision," was born at Toulouse, where, at an early age, his parents placed him in the service of the church of Saint-Sernin, named in honor of the first bishop of Toulouse. Raymond became a chanter at Saint-Sernin, although he remained a layman and happily married. After the death of his wife, Raymond placed all his goods at the service of the poor. He founded an almshouse for 12 poor men and paid for the construction of two stone bridges over the river Hers. Eventually, Raymond became a canon of the church of Saint-Sernin, and he assumed responsibility for completing construction of the church that had begun early in the eleventh century. The church became a popular pilgrimage site. Raymond died in 1118 and was buried in the almshouse that he founded; numerous miracles were said to have been worked at his tomb.

REFERENCES 6, 14, 16, 36, 46

397

Regina of Alise

MEMORIAL DAY **September 7**

PATRONAGE **Skin lesions, scabies**

LIFE & LEGEND

Regina was the daughter of Clement, a pagan residing in present-day Alise in Burgundy. When Regina's mother died giving birth to her, the infant was placed in the care of a Christian woman, who raised the child in her faith. Clement subsequently refused to have anything to do with his daughter, who continued to live with her nurse, earning her keep as a shepherdess. When Regina's beauty attracted the attention of the prefect Olibrius, Clement resumed interest in his daughter's affairs and tried to persuade her to renounce her faith and to marry the distinguished prefect. Regina refused both her father and her suitor. She was imprisoned, but remained obdurate. An enraged Olibrius then ordered her to be tortured and beheaded ca. 286.

REFERENCES 6, 14, 16, 36, 45

398

Reginald

MEMORIAL DAY **September 17**

PATRONAGE **Fever, infertility**

LIFE & LEGEND

A native of Picardy, Reginald, whose name is derived from Germanic, meaning "ruler with counsel," was a member of the Canons Regular of Saint-Jean-des-Vignes in Soissons when he heard of hermits living in the forest of Craon under the direction of Robert d'Abrissel. In spite of the efforts of Saint Ivo of Chartres to convince him to remain in a cenobitic monastery, Reginald left Soissons for the wilderness of Craon. When Robert d'Abrissel later departed to found the monastery at Fontevrault, Reginald continued the hermetic life with several disciples in the forest of Mélinais near La Flèche in the diocese of Angers. In 1104, many decades after his death, Henry II, king of England, constructed an abbey of the Canons Regular of Saint Augustine on the site of Reginald's tomb.

REFERENCES 16, 36, 46

399

Regulus

MEMORIAL DAY **March 30**

PATRONAGE **Fever, Senlis (France)**

LIFE & LEGEND

Ostensibly of Greek origin, Regulus was a companion of Saint Denys in the evangelization of Gaul and became the first bishop of Senlis during the third century.

REFERENCES 6, 16, 36

400
Reineldis

MEMORIAL DAY **July 16**

PATRONAGE **Eye diseases, skin diseases, ulcers, wounds**

LIFE & LEGEND

Reineldis was the daughter of Saint Amalburga and the sister of Saint Gudula and Saint Emebert. When her parents embraced the monastic life, Reineldis followed her father, Witger, to the abbey at Lobbes, hoping to remain there with him. When this proved impossible, she made a pilgrimage to the Holy Land, from which she returned after 7 years to settle in Saintes, where she devoted herself to a life of prayer and charity. Reineldis, along with her servant, Gundulf, and the subdeacon, Grimoald, was killed at Saintes in 784 by raiding barbarians. Kerler relates that those suffering from wounds, ulcers, and sores would often be healed by bathing in a spring associated with Reineldis near the church at Saintes.

REFERENCES 6, 14, 36, 46

401

Remaclus

MEMORIAL DAY **September 3**

PATRONAGE **Infertility**

LIFE & LEGEND

A native of Aquitaine, France, Remaclus grew up around the royal court. He trained under Saint Sulpicius of Bourges before his ordination to the priesthood as a Benedictine monk in 625. Remaclus was appointed by Saint Eligius to be the first abbot of the monastery he had founded at Solginac. Remaclus next undertook direction of the monastery at Cugnon in Luxembourg before being summoned to the court of Sigisbert III, with whose support he founded the double monasteries of Stavelot and Malmédy in the Ardennes. Remaclus was the missionary bishop of Maastricht in the Netherlands (meaning he did not have a fixed see). From Stavelot and Malmédy he was active in evangelizing a still largely pagan population. Remaclus life of prayer and asceticism served as an inspiration to the monks under his charge and to laymen who sought his spiritual direction. Remaclus constantly worked to spread monasticism and was the spiritual teacher of Saint Trond, Saint Babolen, Saint Theodard, and Saint Lambert. He died ca. 673 and was buried at Stavelot in current Belgium.

REFERENCES 6, 36, 45

402

Remigius (Rémy)

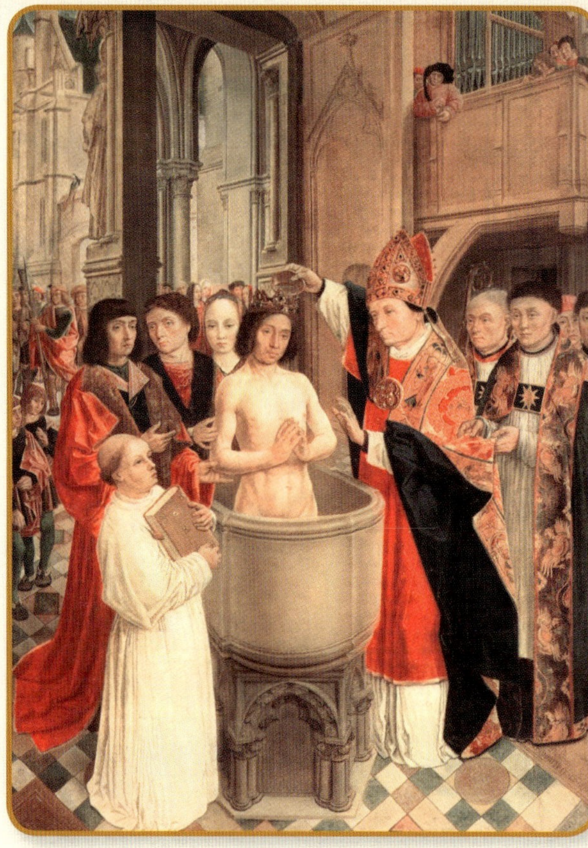

MEMORIAL DAY **October 1 (January 13 in Rheims)**

PATRONAGE **Fever, throat ailments, plague, epidemics**

LIFE & LEGEND

Remigius was born ca. 438, the son of Count Emilius of Laon and Saint Celina. When still in his twenties, Remigius was made bishop of Rheims, where he served for 74 years. He was noted for his oration and devoted himself to evangelizing the Frankish tribes that, late in the fifth century, were wresting Gaul from Roman dominion. Remigius' efforts were facilitated by the conversion of the Merovingian king, Clovis, who, during the deciding battle against the Alemanni, had invoked Christ and was later instructed in the Christian faith by Remigius. Later known as the "Apostle of the Franks," Remigius baptized Clovis, members of his family (his wife Clotilda was already Christian), his chieftains, and three thousand of his followers in 496. This constituted the beginning of the conversion of all Franks and the establishment of the Church in France.

Remigius was also a zealous opponent of the Arian heresy that was rife among the invading German tribes. He was blind at the time of his death on January 13, 533. In 1049, his relics were transferred to the Basilica Saint-Rémy when he was canonized by Pope Leo IX.

REFERENCES 9, 14, 33, 36

403

Rene Goupil

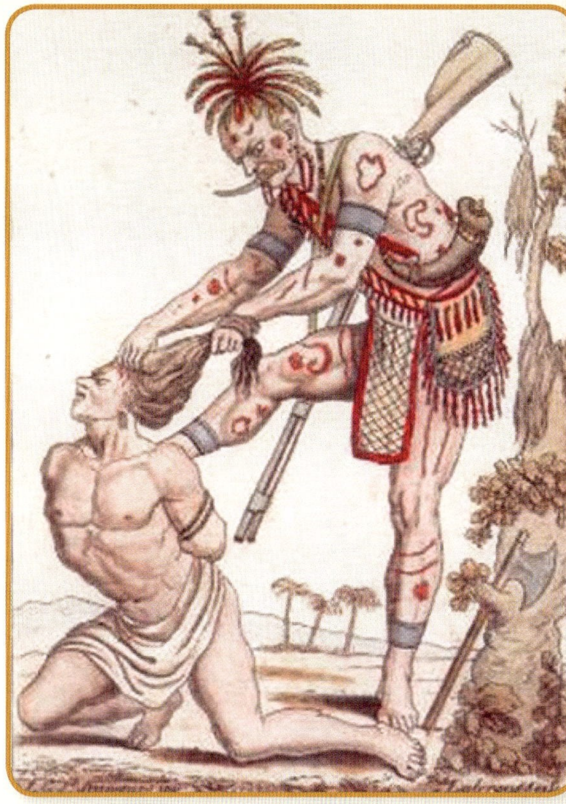

MEMORIAL DAY **October 19 (United States); September 26 (Canada)**

PATRONAGE **Anesthesia, anesthesiologists**

LIFE & LEGEND

Rene Goupil was born in 1606 in the village of Saint Martin in Angers, France. He became a novitiate in the Jesuit Order in Paris, but he could not be ordained because of his deafness and ill health.

He studied medicine and, in 1639, arrived in North America to work without pay as a layman with the Jesuits. He performed menial chores around the Jesuits' house and cared for the sick and wounded in the hospital in Quebec for 2 years before embarking on a mission with Saint Isaac Jogues in August, 1642. Jogues' narrative, which was sent to Jemme Lalemant, the Jesuit superior at Quebec, in early May, 1646, provides a detailed eyewitness account of the suffering and death of Rene, the first North American martyr.

After they set out in canoes from Three Rivers, Canada, accompanied by Hurons, the missionaries were ambushed by the Iroquois near Lake Saint Peter. Rene and Isaac Jogues were tortured throughout the 13-day trek to the Iroquois country. Torture included beatings, tearing nails out, and amputating fingers at their joints. Although he was badly wounded, Rene cared for others who were wounded, among both the prisoners and the enemy. On Lake Champlain they were again tortured by a group of Iroquois. It was at this point that Rene's thumb was amputated, his chest was burned with hot coals and ashes, and he was placed, half-dead, on a scaffold in the middle of the village. Rene recovered, and the prisoners were moved to the Indian village of Andagaron, near Auriesville, New York, where Rene was caught making the sign of a cross over a child's head while instructing the children in Christianity. This stimulated an old Iroquois to order a young warrior to deliver a fatal hatchet blow to Rene's head. As Rene was dying, Isaac Jogues received him into the Jesuit Order and later referred to him in the letter to his superior as "a martyr of Jesus Christ." Rene was beatified in 1925 and canonized by Pope Pius XI in 1930.

The National Shrine of North American Martyrs in Auriesville, New York, depicts a group of eight who were martyred during their religious duties.

REFERENCES 9, 35, 45

404

Richarius

MEMORIAL DAY **April 26**

PATRONAGE **Fever**

LIFE & LEGEND

Richarius was born into a wealthy family of Ponthieu. A landowner and person of some substance in the vicinity of Abbeville, Richarius provided shelter and protection to two Irish missionaries, Cadoc and Frichor, who had landed on the coast and were in danger from the largely pagan population. Inspired by the words of his guests, Richarius was converted to Christianity and decided to enter the priesthood. After a period of study and spiritual preparation, Richarius was ordained and then lived for a time in England. He returned to France, preaching and evangelizing in the northern reaches of the country. His reputation for holiness and rhetorical skill brought him into the presence of King Dagobert, who supported Richarius in his work, including the establishment of a monastery at Celles. Worn out by his labors, Richarius later withdrew into a hermitage on land provided him by Dagobert in the forest of Crécy. The place where he lived and died in seclusion in 645 later became the site of the Forêt-Moutier monastery.

REFERENCES 6, 16, 36, 46

405

Rigobert (Robert)

MEMORIAL DAY **January 4**

PATRONAGE **Fever, toothache**

LIFE & LEGEND

Rigobert was of an ancient family of Porçain. He entered the monastic life as a Benedictine monk in the abbey of Orbais, of which he may have been abbot when called to the episcopal throne of Rheims ca. 695 to 699. He was zealous in the reform of his diocese, and he was highly regarded by Pepin d'Hérstival, who entrusted Rigobert with the education of his son, Charles Martel. Charles later banished Rigobert to Gascony for failure to support him politically. It is not clear whether the saintly Rigobert was eventually recalled to his see or whether he was simply allowed to return to his house at Gernicourt near Rheims, where he died ca. 750. Throughout his life he was noted for his patience and as a miracle worker.

REFERENCES 6, 16, 27, 36, 46

406

Rita of Cascia

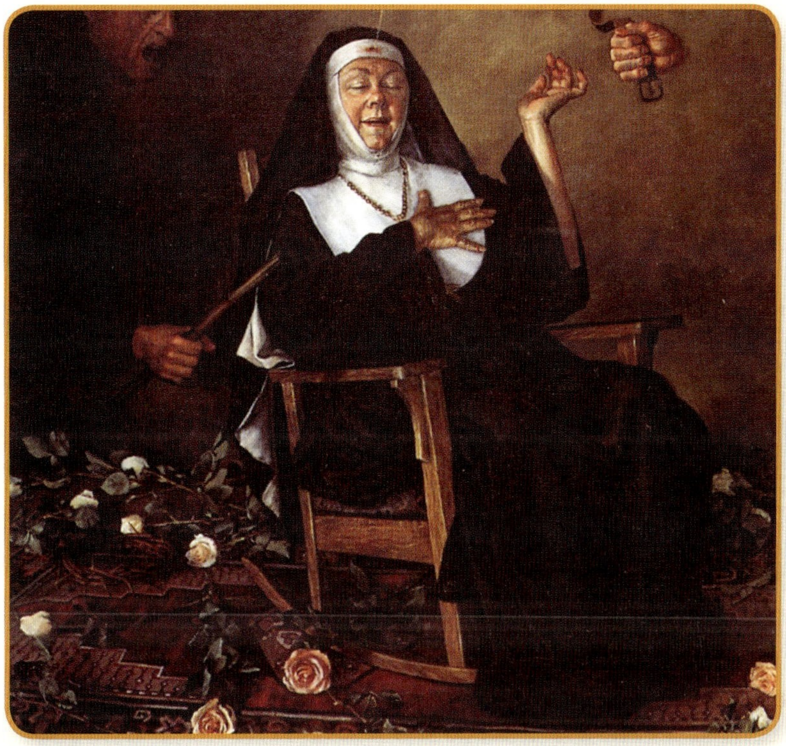

MEMORIAL DAY **May 22**

PATRONAGE **Smallpox, wounds, childbirth, abused women, desperate causes**

LIFE & LEGEND

Rita, whose name is a contraction of Margherita, was born in 1381 at Roccaporena in Umbria, Italy. Although she wished to enter a convent as a young girl, she acquiesced to her parents' desire and married at age 12. She bore her husband, who was abusive and immoral, twin sons. After enduring about two decades of abuse from him, her husband died of a stab wound. Her sons sought revenge, and when Rita could not dissuade them, she prayed to God to take them rather than allow them to commit a sin. The sons then died of natural causes.

Rita wanted to enter the Augustine convent at Cascia, but initially she was refused because she was not a virgin. At age 36 she was finally accepted. Her entrance into the convent is related as a miracle. Although the doors were locked and all the sisters were asleep, Rita was transported within by her patron saints, Saint John the Baptist, Saint Augustine, and Saint Nicholas of Tolentino. One day in the convent, she prayed to be allowed to suffer like Christ. Suddenly, a thorn from the figure of the crucifixion of Jesus Christ fell and wounded her forehead. She remained in the convent until she died in 1457.

Rita was beatified by Pope Urban VIII in 1627 and canonized by Pope Leo XIII in 1900. She is often depicted with a wound of her forehead. She is also represented with the symbol of a rose. Legend states that when she was secretly delivering bread to the poor, her husband demanded that she uncover what she was carrying. The bread became roses. Also, when she was bedridden late in life and a friend asked whether she desired anything from her old home, Rita replied that she would like a rose. When her friend went to Rita's home on a winter day, she found a single rose in bloom and brought it to the convent.

REFERENCES 6, 9, 42, 45

407

Roch (Rocco, Roque)

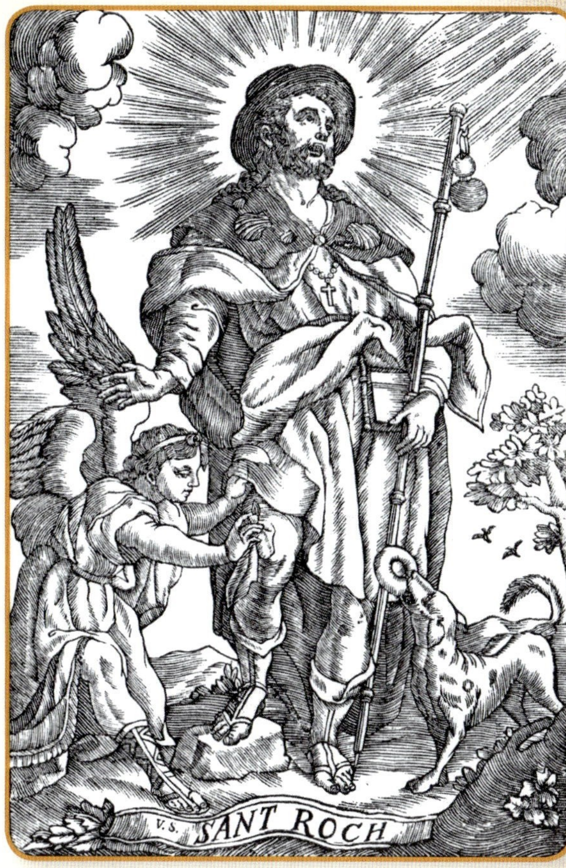

MEMORIAL DAY **August 16**

PATRONAGE **Cholera, invalids, knee problems, plague, skin diseases, rashes, contagious diseases, dysentery, epidemic diseases, pharmacists, physicians, surgeons, grave diggers, diseased cattle, dogs, tile makers**

LIFE & LEGEND

Roch, whose name is derived from Germanic, meaning "battle cry," was born into nobility at Montpellier, France, in 1295. At birth he was noted to have an image of a red cross on the front of his chest, which grew as he did. His parents died when he was 20, at which point he dispensed of his inheritance and became a mendicant pilgrim. He traveled to Italy, where, while tending to victims of the plague in public hospitals at Acquapendente, Cesena, Rome, Mantua, Modena, and Parma, he was credited with performing many miraculous cures. At Rome, Roch cured the cardinal of Angeleria by marking his forehead with a cross that remained.

At Piacenza, Roch was stricken with the plague and withdrew to the forest, where he was supplied with water from a spring that arose miraculously where he built his hut. His food was supplied by a nobleman who was led to him by the nobleman's dog. As a sign of his asceticism, Roch castrated himself and threw his testicles to the dog. When Roch's health improved, he returned to Montpellier, where he was arrested as a spy and thrown into prison. He died in 1327 after 5 years of imprisonment, having never revealed his name to avoid worldly glory.

According to the Golden Legend, after Roch died, an angel placed a tablet with letters of gold under his head. The words indicated that whoever invoked Saint Roch would not be hurt or afflicted by pestilence. Roch was recognized by his birthmark after he died, and, shortly thereafter, he was canonized and a church was erected in his name. In 1414, when the Council of Constance was affected by the plague, a procession invoking Saint Roch's intercession took place, and it was deemed responsible for stopping the outbreak. His relics are maintained in Venice.

Saint Roch is represented as a pilgrim with a lesion on his exposed leg, accompanied by a dog bearing a loaf of bread in its mouth. The skin lesion accounts for his patronage of the plague or of skin disease, and the location accounts for his patronage of knee problems. It has been suggested that the apparent lesion depicts blood from the castration on his leg and that the dog is shown devouring the testicles.

REFERENCES 6, 9, 33, 42

408
Roland of Chèzery

MEMORIAL DAY **January 16**

PATRONAGE **Eye diseases, headache, stomach ailments**

LIFE & LEGEND

Roland, whose name has a Germanic derivation, meaning "famous country," was born into a notable British family and emigrated to France to flee worldly honor and humble himself in a religious life. He entered the monastery at Chèzery in the diocese of Geneva, where he became abbot in 1170. Roland was zealous in fulfilling his duties, and, according to du Broc de Segange, "at last, having filled the entire country with the fragrance of his virtues, rendered his soul to God circa 1200." Du Broc de Segange makes mention of "a fountain located half-an-hour from the church [where Roland is buried] called the 'holy fountain' or 'Fountain of Saint Roland,'" where the sick bathed in the hope of being healed.

REFERENCES 16, 36

409

Roland de'Medici

MEMORIAL DAY **September 15**

PATRONAGE **Headache**

LIFE & LEGEND

Roland was born into the Medici family of Milan. He wanted to lead the life of a recluse, so withdrew alone into the woods between Tabiano and Salsomaggiore. For 26 years he lived in silence, living on what the forest provided, clothed in goatskin, and devoting himself to constant prayer. Worn out by his labors, Roland's body was discovered in 1386 near the castle of Bargone. He was buried at the church of Saint Trinità in Busseto.

REFERENCES 36, 46

410
Rolande

MEMORIAL DAY **May 13**

PATRONAGE **Urinary retention, calculi, intestinal disorders, hernia, blindness**

LIFE & LEGEND

The virgin Rolande is said to have been born into the royal family of France during the eighth century, and to have fled to Cologne to escape the attentions of a Scottish king who wished to marry her. She died young. Du Broc de Segange transcribes the epitaph on her tomb, which expands the list of maladies she is credited with healing: "Here lies the noble Rolande, daughter of the great Didier, king of France. Here my mortal remains repose. I have cured, by the grace of God, urinary retention, hernia, blindness, and other infirmities. Call upon me, you who have need of my help."

REFERENCES 36, 46

411

Romanus of Rouen

MEMORIAL DAY **October 23**

PATRONAGE **Mental illnesses**

LIFE & LEGEND

Romanus's father, Benoist, a counselor of King Clotaire II, was converted to Christianity by Saint Remigius. Benoist placed his son in the court of Clotaire at an early age. Romanus followed a religious vocation and was chosen bishop of Rouen ca. 630. He was zealous in the conversion of his fellow Franks, and personally destroyed the temple of Venus in Rouen. He is said to have worked many miracles during his lifetime. He died in 639.

REFERENCES 6, 16, 36, 45

412

Rosalia

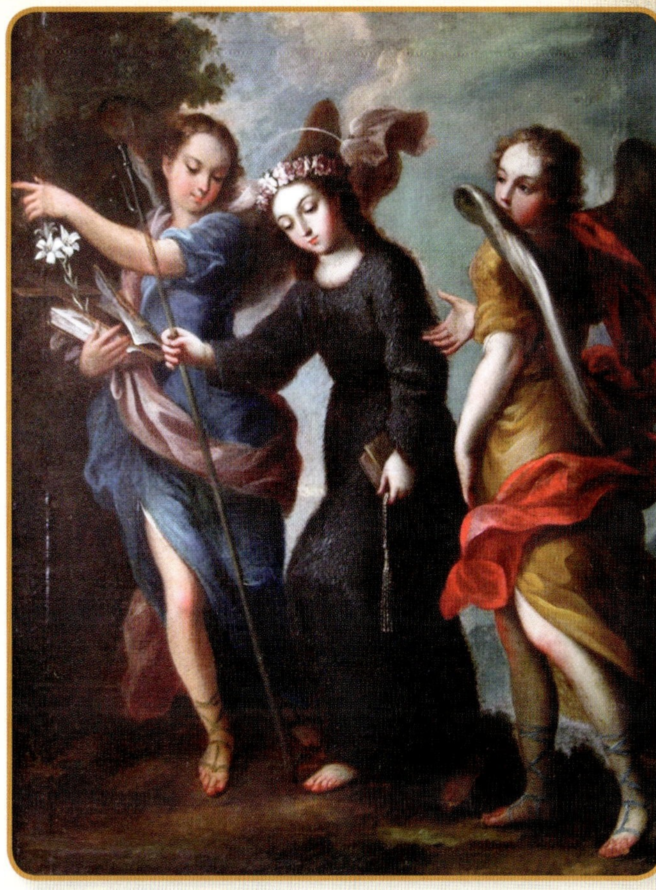

MEMORIAL DAY **September 4**

PATRONAGE **Plague, Palermo**

LIFE & LEGEND

Rosalia, who was born ca. 1130, was a daughter of Sinibaldo, the feudal lord of Quisquinia, in Sicily, and of Maria Guiscarda, a cousin of the Norman king, Roger II. Rosalia's beauty at court attracted the attention of many noble suitors, including no less a figure than Baldwin, the crusader and future king of Jerusalem. Rosalia's interests lay elsewhere, however. She withdrew to a cave on Monte Coschina near Bivona. She later moved to a cave on Monte Pellegrino outside Palermo, where she continued a life of solitude and prayer.

According to one version of her life, Rosalia's body remained in the cave where she died ca. 1160, and in time it was entirely covered with stalactitic deposits. The saint's remains were discovered centuries later, when, during the epidemic of plague that struck Palermo in 1640, one of the plague's victims was visited by Rosalia in a vision, revealing to him the location of her remains. These were subsequently found, placed in a reliquary, and processed throughout the city, lifting the plague. She was declared patron of the city, and her feast day was made a holy day by Pope Pius XI in 1927.

REFERENCES 6, 36, 45, 46

413

Rose of Lima

MEMORIAL DAY **August 24**

PATRONAGE **Wounds, smallpox, parturition, Latin America, Peru, Lima, the Philippines**

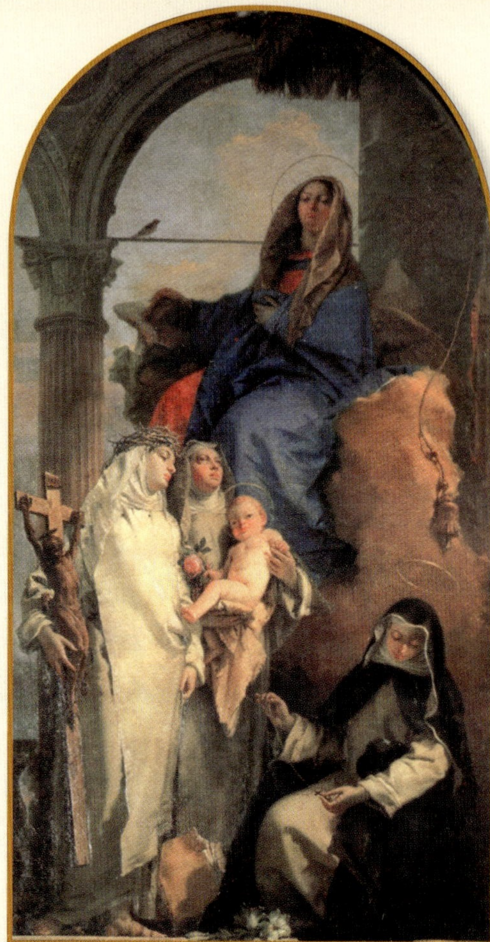

LIFE & LEGEND

Rose was born into a large family in Lima, Peru, on April 20, 1586, and given the baptismal name of Isabel Flores de Oliva. A servant claimed that she saw the baby's face become a rose, accounting for Isabel's adoption of the name of the flower. As a young child, she revered God and began a life of prayer and mortification. She purposefully patterned herself after Saint Catherine of Siena with fasting and penances. She cut off her hair and scarred her face with pepper and astringents. This disfigurement might serve as the basis for her patronage of wounds.

She related many visions and revelations and took a vow of virginity. She fasted frequently and abstained from meat. She cared for the poor and sick while she produced embroidery, which she sold to support her family. She spent time as a recluse living in a grotto, but, when she was 20 years old, she entered a Dominican convent. She spent the next 11 years in continuous self-martyrdom until she died on August 24, 1617, at age 31. Throughout her time at the convent she wore a metal spiked crown covered with roses and an iron chain around her waist. Her funeral was attended by a large crowd of dignitaries, and the eulogy was given in the cathedral by the archbishop. Many miracles occurred when her name was invoked. She was beatified by Pope Clement IX in 1667, and her canonization by Pope Clement X in 1671 made her the first saint to come from the western hemisphere. Initially her feast day was August 30 so that it would not interfere with the August 24 feast of Saint Bartholomew the Apostle, but when the Roman Calendar of Saints was reformed in 1969, the date was made August 23. In Peru and other Latin American countries, her feast continues to be celebrated on August 30.

REFERENCES 6, 9, 42, 45

S

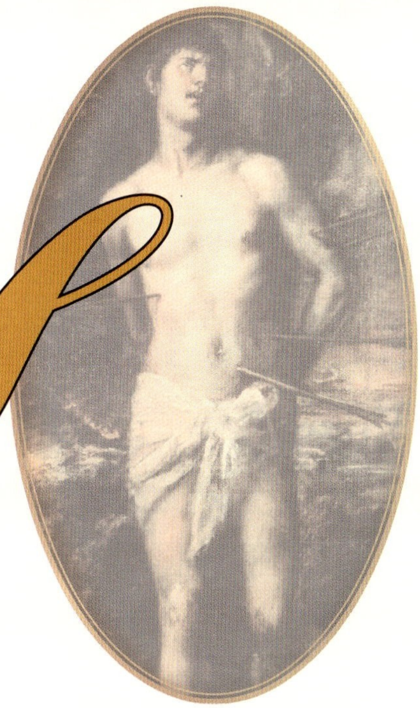

414

Sabina

MEMORIAL DAY **August 29**

PATRONAGE **Hemorrhage**

LIFE & LEGEND

The very beautiful fifth-century Basilica of Santa Sabina on the Aventine in Rome provides an interesting insight into the kind of biographic knowledge we have of many saints. The church is a titulus, or one of the early churches of Rome that are ascribed to a founding patron. In the case of Santa Sabina, the church was constructed over a large private house that had been used for liturgical and other purposes by Christians since the second century—a house that may have originally belonged to a patrician woman named Sabina. Often the title "saint" was prefixed to the name in later centuries.

The earliest account of Sabina's life and martyrdom was written in the sixth century and is regarded as unreliable. The barest relation of her life maintains that Sabina, whose name is derived from the Latin, meaning "of the Sabine tribe," was a member of a patrician Roman family who was converted to Christianity in the second century by her Syrian servant Serapia. Both women were arrested and martyred within a month of one another.

REFERENCES 6, 36, 46

415
Salvator of Horta

MEMORIAL DAY **March 18**

PATRONAGE **Fever**

LIFE & LEGEND

Born at Santa Columba in the diocese of Gerona in Catalonia, Salvator, whose name is derived from Latin, meaning "saving one," was orphaned as a child. He was working as a shoemaker in Barcelona when, at age 20, he joined the observant branch of the Franciscans. Salvator lived in several monasteries—much of the time at the Franciscan house in Horta. He eventually returned to Barcelona, but died at Cagliari in Sardinia in 1506.

Salvator's reputation for holiness was notable, in part because of the numerous healing miracles attributed to him. His cell was a destination for pilgrims, and he is said to have cured as many as 2000 in one day. Du Broc de Segange maintains that Salvator was passed from one Franciscan house to another, and finally to Sardinia, because of the unruly crowds he attracted and the desire of his superiors to be rid of him. He notes also that the number of the sick whom Salvator healed was "incroyable" and that he raised three persons from the dead. Salvator was beatified by Pope Paul V in 1606 and canonized by Pope Pius XI in 1938.

REFERENCES 6, 9, 16, 36, 42, 45

416

Saturninus (Sernin) of Toulouse

MEMORIAL DAY **November 29**

PATRONAGE **Smallpox, headache, plague, vertigo, bullfighting**

LIFE & LEGEND

Saturninus was born in the third century to Roman nobility. He was sent as a missionary from Rome to evangelize on both sides of the Pyrenees. He is believed to have been the first bishop of Toulouse, where he performed many miracles, along with Saint Martial. Butler relates that Saturninus founded a small church in Toulouse and that the "chief [pagan] temple in the city stood between that church and the saint's house. In this temple oracles were given, but they had been long silent, which was attributed to the presence of the Christian bishop. Accordingly the priests seized him one day going by and dragged him into the temple, declaring that he should either appease the offended deities by offering sacrifice to them or propitiate them with his blood." Saturninus refused to sacrifice and was tied by his feet to a bull that had been brought to the temple for sacrifice. The animal was goaded to run downhill, and Saturninus was dragged along behind it to his death ca. 257. His remains were much later enshrined in the church named in his honor (Saint-Sernin-du-Taur).

REFERENCES 6, 9, 36, 42, 45, 46

417

Scholastica

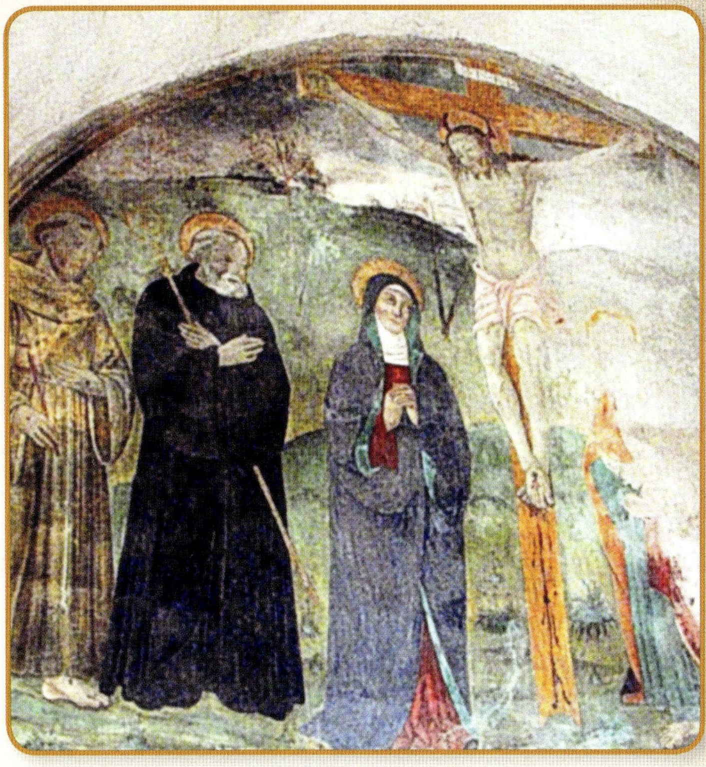

MEMORIAL DAY **February 10**

PATRONAGE **Convulsive children, nuns, rain, storms**

LIFE & LEGEND

Scholastica, whose name means "she who has the leisure to study," was the twin sister of Saint Benedict. The twins were born to a noble family in 480. Their mother died in childbirth, and Scholastica became a nun at an early age. She was a leader of a community for women that was located a short distance from Saint Benedict's abbey at Monte Cassino. Some chroniclers indicate that she preceded Benedict to a life dedicated to Christ. Legend, as related by Pope Saint Gregory the Great, tells that she was accustomed to meet with her brother on an annual basis. The day was spent worshiping together and discussing religious issues.

On one occasion she wished to extend the visit. When Benedict adamantly refused, Scholastica was able, by prayer, to cause a heavy rain fall, as well as thunder and lightning, which precluded Benedict from returning to his cell. As related by Saint Gregory the Great, the sky was clear and cloudless when Scholastica began to cry profusely, but, as she lifted her head, the torrential storm began. She indicated that this was evidence that God acted to grant her desire, and the discussion between the twins continued through the night. Three days later, Benedict saw his 63-year-old sister's soul leave her body in the form of a dove. This accounts for Saint Scholastica's representation as a nun with a crozier and crucifix with a dove flying from her mouth. He removed her body to his monastery and buried her in the grave that had been prepared for him so their bodies would rest next to one another forever.

REFERENCES 6, 9

418 Sebastian

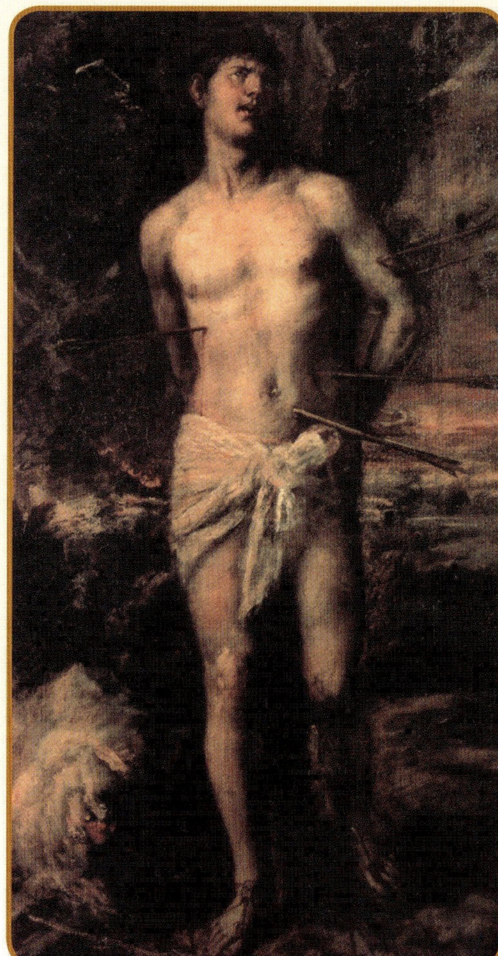

MEMORIAL DAY **January 20**

PATRONAGE **Plague, epidemic diseases, [trauma],* athletes, soldiers, gay men**

LIFE & LEGEND

Nothing is known about Sebastian's birth. His name is derived from the place name, Sebaste. According to Ambrose, Bishop of Milan, who wrote in the fifth century, Sebastian was from Gallia Narbornensis and was a captain in the Praetorian Guard under Diocletian and Maximian, who did not know that he was a Christian. During the persecution of Christians,

*Proposed patronage

Sebastian brought supplies to the prisoners. Sebastian purportedly cured a woman of her muteness with the consequent conversion of 78 gentiles. When Diocletian learned of Sebastian's faith, he had him bound to a stake and shot at by archers. When the widow of Saint Castulus went to retrieve his body, she found that he was still alive and nursed him back to good health. He subsequently returned hearing and sight to a deaf and blind girl. He proceeded to taunt Diocletian, who had him beaten to death ca. 287 and had his body thrown in a latrine.

His relics are housed in the Basilica Apostolorum on the site of what was the provisional tomb of Saint Peter and Saint Paul. A church currently on that site bears the name of San Sebastiano. Paul the Deacon writes that Rome was freed of the plague in 680 by Saint Sebastian's patronage. The same situation occurred in Milan in 1575 and in Lisbon in 1599. Sebastian is one of the most frequently depicted saints, and he is often used to introduce lectures on trauma.

REFERENCES 6, 9, 33, 42, 45

419
Senan of Saint-Pol-de-Léon

MEMORIAL DAY **March 6**

PATRONAGE **Plague**

LIFE & LEGEND

There are more than 20 Irish saints named Senan. The details of the lives of some of these men have doubtless become mixed. The events in the life of the fifth-century Senan of Saint-Pol-de-Léon venerated in Brittany are similar to those of Senan, the sixth-century Irish bishop whose feast day occurs on March 8. Senan of Saint-Pol-de-Léon was a native of Ireland. He was ordained by Saint Patrick, with whom he worked closely in eradicating paganism from Ireland. Having accomplished all he could there, Senan left Ireland with a small band of monks and crossed the sea to the Breton coast near Saint-Pol-de-Léon. At present-day Guic-Sané, he established a small monastery where he lived for many years. Sensing the approach of death, Senan returned to Ireland. According to du Broc de Segange, his remains were buried at Inishcarra, which may mark another point of confusion with the life of the sixth-century Bishop Senan.

REFERENCES 16, 36

420

Serenicus and Serenus

MEMORIAL DAY **May 7**

PATRONAGE **Fever, infantile colic (Serenicus), plague (Serenus)**

LIFE & LEGEND

Serenicus and his brother, Serenus, were born into a patrician family of Spoleto. In spite of their privileged background, the brothers went to Rome, where they joined the Benedictine Order. For a time they lived in a monastic community at Rome, but they later crossed across the Alps into Gaul, where they sought solitude in the vast forest of Charnie near the present-day village of Saulges (Mayenne). The brothers made this decision either under angelic guidance or to escape honors and offices that the pope wished to bestow on them. In spite of their hermetic life, the brothers attracted numerous visitors. In quest of greater solitude, Serenicus left his brother at Saulges and withdrew into the territory of Hyesmes on the banks of the Sarthe. Even there Serenicus' holiness attracted disciples. He eventually formed a monastic community that he directed until his death ca. 669. Serenicus' name is invoked by those suffering from fever and for infants afflicted with colic. Du Broc de Segange relates that to the left of the altar of the church of Saint-Cenery-le-Géré, near Alençon, "one notices a block of granite which was supposed to have been the saint's bed. This stone is scratched by pilgrims, who make their colicky infants swallow the dust."

After Serenicus' departure, Serenus remained at Saulges, where he was known for his mystical life and miracle working. He died ca. 680. When the region was stricken by plague, Berarius, bishop of Le Mans, sought the Serenus' intercession. According to Butler, "The cleansing rain which cleared away the infection and refreshed the earth was attributed by the grateful people to the prayers of Saint Serenus."

REFERENCES 6, 16, 36

421

Servatius (Servatus)

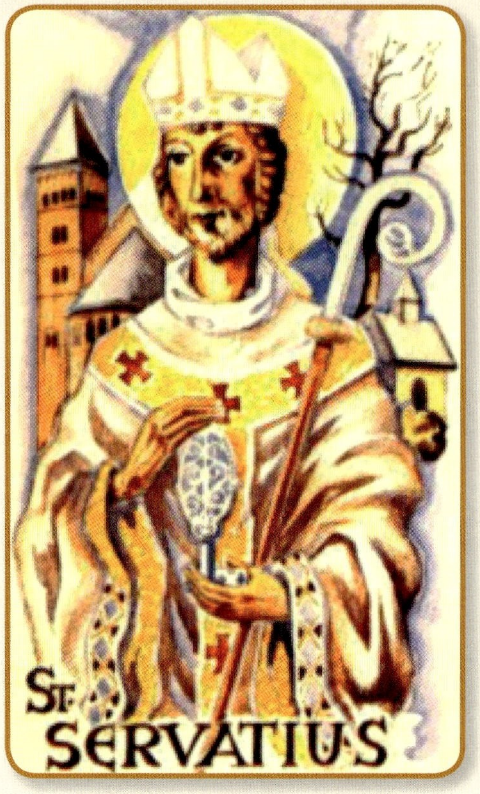

MEMORIAL DAY **May 13**

PATRONAGE **Foot and leg problems, rheumatism, rats and mice, Maastricht (the Netherlands)**

LIFE & LEGEND

The life of Servatius, whose name is derived from Latin, meaning "rescued," is difficult to define, because it was first written about in the sixth century *History of the Franks* by Gregory of Tours. Servatius was born as an Armenian in the early part of the fourth century, and served as bishop of Tongres, Belgium (now part of the Netherlands), for 37 years before he moved to Maastricht. He built basilicas in both cities, and the church at Maastricht remains an important religious site.

Servatius spread Christianity throughout the Low Countries. Legend indicates that he was a distant relative of John the Baptist and Jesus and that, before going to Tongres, he was a guardian priest of the Holy Sepulchre in Jerusalem. He campaigned against the Arians (named for Arius, a presbyter in Alexandria in the fourth century) who denied that Christ was consubstantial, meaning of the same essence and substance with God. Servatius died of fever in Maastricht in 384, and his relics reside at the Saint Servaas Basilica in that city. He was canonized pre-Congregation. Many miracles have been ascribed to him at his tomb, particularly related to lameness. He is often represented with three wooden shoes, perhaps related to three churches in the Netherlands that bear his name.

REFERENCES 6, 9, 45

422

Severinus of Noricum

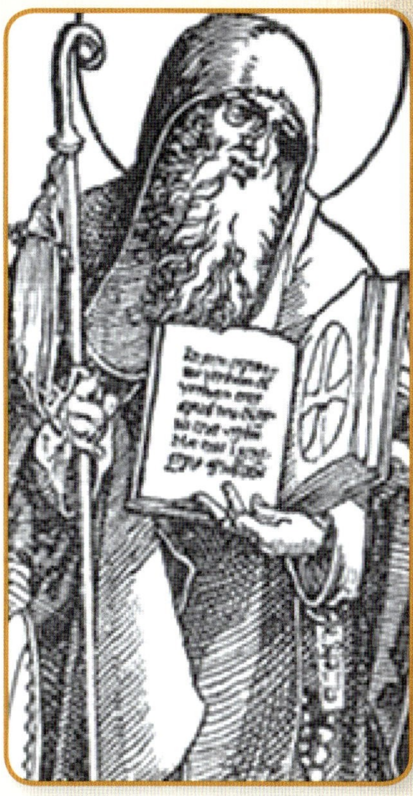

MEMORIAL DAY **January 8**

PATRONAGE **Headache**

LIFE & LEGEND

Severinus, who belonged to a prominent Roman or Italian family, made a sojourn in the eastern parts of the empire, where he lived as a hermit in the Egyptian desert. Ca. 454, he journeyed as a missionary to the frontier of Noricum and Pannonia (in present-day Austria), a region at the time overrun by invading Germanic tribes. In addition to the success of his preaching among the barbarians, Severinus was noted for having established several monasteries in Noricum, and for his gifts of prophecy and working miracles. One winter, in the city of Faviana on the Danube, the populus was starving. Severinus offered a sermon on penance, after which the ice on the river cracked and allowed food to be delivered. He enjoyed the confidence of several barbarian kings, and may have thereby mitigated the ferocity of the invaders on local populations. Although he died in Noricum ca. 482 after he foretold the date of his own death, Severinus' remains were later transferred to Umbria and later still to Naples, where they remain in the monastery of San Severino.

REFERENCES 6, 14, 16, 36, 46

423

Servulus

MEMORIAL DAY **December 23**

PATRONAGE **Paralysis, lameness**

LIFE & LEGEND

Our knowledge of Servulus is derived from the account of him in the fourth dialogue of his contemporary, Pope Gregory the Great. Palsied from birth, Servulus was unable to stand, sit upright, or move himself from one place or even from one side to another. He was carried daily by his mother and brother to the portico of the street leading to the church of San Clemente in Rome, where, chanting prayers and hymns, he lay begging from those entering or leaving the church precinct. Much of what he collected he gave to those needier than himself. With some of his alms he purchased the books of Holy Scripture, which, because he was illiterate, he had others read to him. Like Lazarus at the gate of the rich man (Luke 16:20-25), Servulus lived on what others more fortunate deigned to spare; and, like Lazarus, he lived and died ca. 590 in humble acceptance of his condition and faith in God's ultimate mercy. Gregory the Great relates Servulus' life as an example of those who have become so holy that heavenly music is heard at the moment of their death. Servulus' body was supposed to have been buried within the church of San Clemente, though the site of his grave has never been identified. In the Middle Ages, a chapel in his memory was erected along the street leading to the church, and his remains may have been placed there.

REFERENCES 6, 10, 36, 46

424

Severus of Agde

MEMORIAL DAY **August 21**

PATRONAGE **Fever, headache**

LIFE & LEGEND

Born into a wealthy Syrian family during the fifth century, Severus came into his inheritance at an early age. Dissatisfied with his life, Severus set out on a journey that took him across the Aegean and through the straits of Messina to the coast of Provence, where he landed at Agde. There he handed his wealth over to the bishop, Beticus, whom he asked to reserve half for the poor and half for the ransom of captives. Severus became a solitary and eventually founded a monastery at Agde, of which he was abbot and where he passed the remainder of his life. Severus is invoked by those suffering from fever and from headache, especially migraines.

REFERENCES 16, 36

425
Sigismund of Burgundy

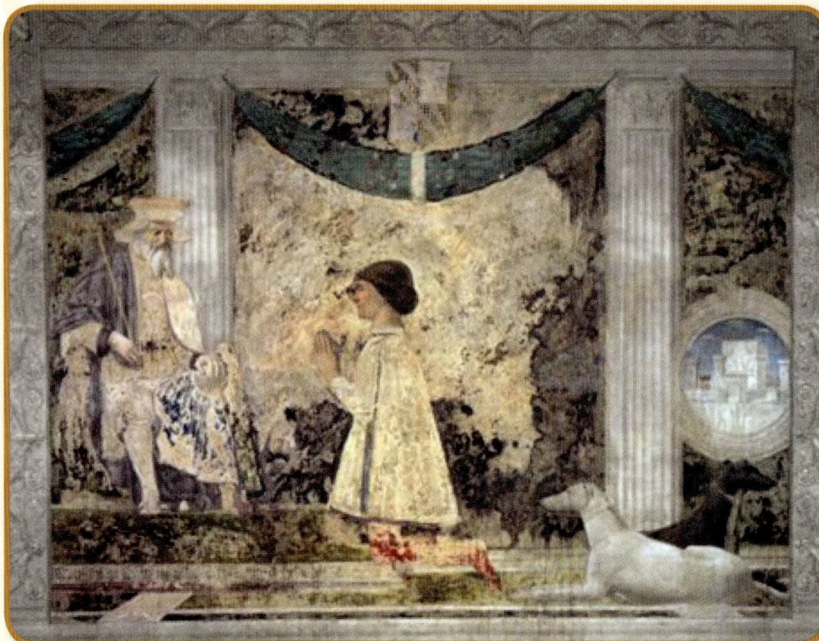

MEMORIAL DAY **May 1**

PATRONAGE **Fever, fractures**

LIFE & LEGEND

Sigismund was the son of Gundebald, the Vandal ruler of Burgundy and an Arian. The young prince was converted to orthodox Christianity in 516 by Saint Avitus of Vienne, a year before his father's death. Based on the accusations of his second wife, Sigismund impulsively ordered that Sigeric, his son by his first wife, be strangled for having designs on his throne. Soon after, Sigismund was stricken with remorse, prayed for forgiveness, and made recompense in generosity to the Church, most notably by restoring and aggrandizing the monastery of Saint-Maurice at Agaunum. Some time later Sigismund was defeated in battle by the three sons of Clovis. He escaped the battlefield and lived for a time as a hermit in the vicinity of Saint-Maurice before being captured and executed in 523 at Orleans by King Clodomir. His body was thrown down a well, but his relics were recovered and placed in a shrine near the abbey of Agaunum. The relics were later translated to the cathedral of Prague.

REFERENCES 6, 16, 36

426

Simplicianus

MEMORIAL DAY **May 31**

PATRONAGE **Headache**

LIFE & LEGEND

Simplicianus, who lived in the second century, was the son of Justinus, a former consul, who had been sent to Aquitania as provincial governor (in the region that is presently Poitou). When Justinus learned that his son had converted to Christianity, he used all his persuasive powers to convince Simplicianus to apostatize. When the young convert remained obdurate, his father had him beheaded. According to legend, when Simplicianus' head hit the ground it made a hollow that became the site of pilgrimages. The pilgrims would place their heads in the hollow to relieve their headaches.

REFERENCES 16, 36

427

Stanislaus Kostka

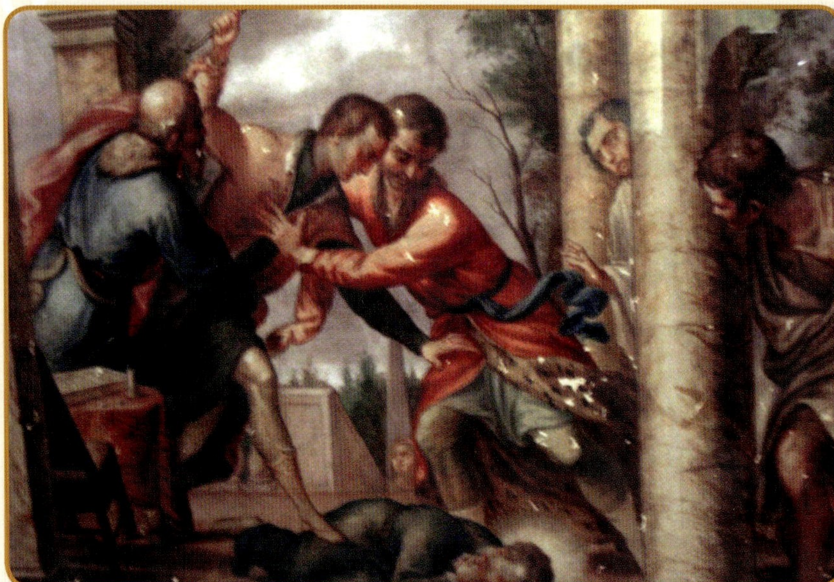

MEMORIAL DAY **August 15**

PATRONAGE **Heart palpitations, broken bones, eye diseases, fever**

LIFE & LEGEND

Stanislaus, whose name is derived from Slavic, meaning "strength" was born into a noble Polish family in 1550. His father was a senator of the kingdom and lord of Zakroczym, and his mother was the aunt of the chancellor of Poland. At the age of 14, he was sent with his older brother, Paul, to Vienna to attend a Jesuit college. During a serious illness, Stanislaus stated that Saint Barbara brought two angels to him to give him the Eucharist and he immediately improved. His brother was annoyed by Stanislaus' extreme piety and consequently harshly thrashed him.

This is depicted in an oil painting and might serve as the basis for his patronage of broken bones.

Stanislaus decided to join the Society of Jesus and, without the knowledge of his brother or tutor, walked to Rome dressed as a mendicant. On the way, he spent a month with Peter Canisius, who later became a saint. Stanislaus arrived in Rome in October, 1567, and became a novitiate in the Society of Jesus. Shortly thereafter, he became seriously ill with a burning fever in his chest that he ameliorated with cold compresses. This accounts for depictions of him at a fountain with a cloth on his chest, and it is also the genesis of his patronage for heart palpitations.

When he felt that death was imminent, he wrote a letter to the Blessed Virgin asking her to call for him, and he died that night in Rome at age 18. The city immediately proclaimed him to be a saint and venerated his remains. His older brother witnessed his official beatification in 1605. Saint Stanislaus was canonized by Pope Paul V in 1726. He remains a popular saint in Poland.

REFERENCES 9, 45

428

Stapinus (Estève, Étienne, Stephanus)

MEMORIAL DAY **August 6**

PATRONAGE **Gout, rheumatism, leg disorders**

LIFE & LEGEND

Stapinus, who lived during the seventh century, was a native of Dourgne (Tarn). Before his selection as the fifth bishop of Carcassonne (Aude), Stapinus lived as a monk in the solitude of the nearby mountains. Although little is known of this saint, his cult began during the Middle Ages and spread throughout several regions of France and to northern Italy, Germany, and Belgium.

REFERENCES 16, 36

429

Sulpicius Pius

MEMORIAL DAY **January 17**

PATRONAGE **Gout, lumbago, kidney diseases**

LIFE & LEGEND

Born into a wealthy family, Sulpicius Pius renounced his inheritance as a young man to devote himself to a life of prayer and devotion to the poor. He was elected bishop of Bourges ca. 624-626, the second Sulpicius to hold that office. He was known for his austere manner of living, his charity, and his intense life of prayer. He is said to have recited the entire psalter each day. He was additionally loved by the people for his defense of them from the oppression of King Dagobert's minister, Lullo. He attended the Council of Clichy in 627. The saintly bishop worked miracles during his lifetime, including the extinction of a dangerous conflagration by making the sign of the cross over the flames. Near the end of his life, Sulpicius asked the king to replace him as bishop so that he might devote his remaining time to the poor. He died in 647.

REFERENCES 6, 16, 36, 46

430

Sulpicius Severus

MEMORIAL DAY **January 29**

PATRONAGE **Infertility, labor**

LIFE & LEGEND

Little is known of Sulpicius Severus other than he was made bishop of Bourges in 584, he attended the Council of Mâcon in 585, and he invoked a provincial Church council at Auvergne. He wrote a popular biography of Saint Martin of Tours that enhanced the reputation of that saint. Sulpicius died in 591.

REFERENCES 6, 16, 36

431
Swithbert

MEMORIAL DAY **March 1**

PATRONAGE **Angina, throat diseases, heart diseases, Drevenack, Germany**

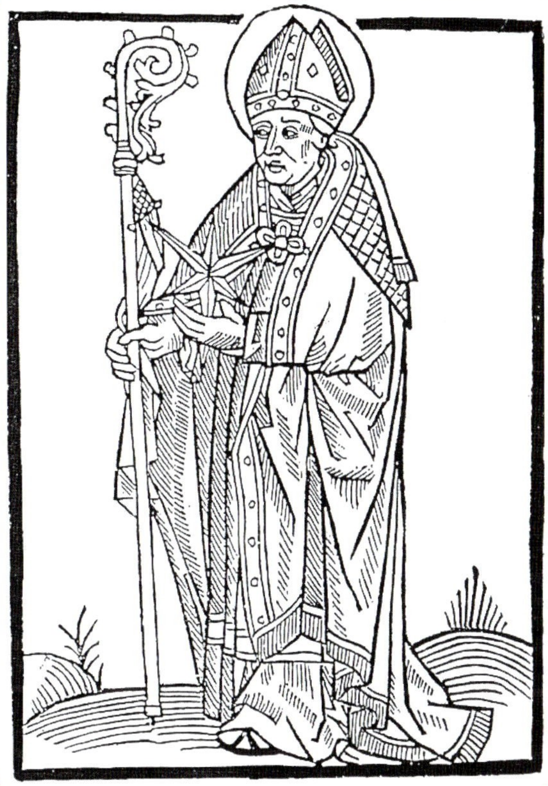

LIFE & LEGEND

Known as the Apostle of the Frisians, Swithbert was born in England in the middle of the seventh century. He studied in Ireland with Saint Egbert and became a Benedictine monk. Swithbert was one of 12 monks sent to evangelize the Frisians. The group headquartered at Utrecht and was extremely successful in its mission.

Swithbert worked mainly in North Brabant and Cleves. He returned to England, and he was consecrated as a missionary bishop in 693. He returned to Frisia where he continued to evangelize. Eventually he withdrew to a small island in the Rhine, 6 miles from Düsseldorf, where he built a monastery and ended his days in 713. His relics were discovered in 1626 in Kaiserwerth, where they are still venerated.

REFERENCES 6, 9, 45

432

Symphorian

MEMORIAL DAY **August 22**

PATRONAGE **Eye diseases, fractures, syphilis**

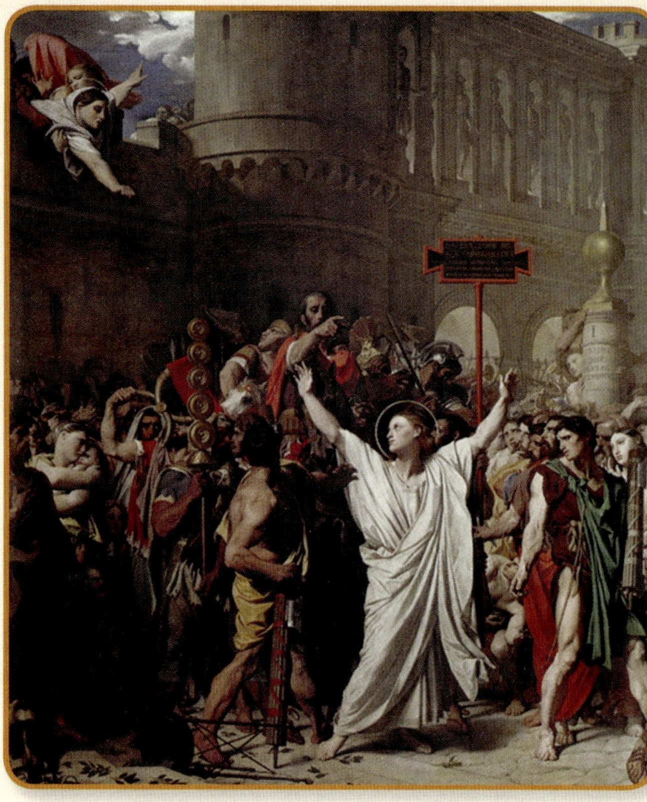

LIFE & LEGEND

Symphorian was the son of Senator Faustus and Blessed Augusta. One day, in the city of Autun in Gaul, Symphorian was heard making derisive remarks while watching a procession pass by honoring the goddess Cybele. He was seized by the crowd and brought before the provincial governor, Heraclius, for having calumniated the deity. After refusing to deny his Christian faith and honor the goddess, Symphorian was taken outside the city to be executed in 178. From high above on the city's walls, his mother shouted encouragement to her son. In 454, a basilica was erected at Autun on the site of Symphorian's execution. His cult subsequently spread throughout Gaul, the Low Countries, and Germany.

REFERENCES 6, 9, 14, 16, 45, 46

433

Syre

MEMORIAL DAY **June 8**

PATRONAGE **Urinary calculi, hernia, fractures, stuttering**

LIFE & LEGEND

Syre was born in the environs of Arcis-sur-Aube toward the end of the third century. She married at age 18, but was soon widowed. Shortly after the loss of her husband, she lost her sight. A convert to Christianity, Syre had been blind 40 years when she heard of the miracles worked by the intercession of Saint Savinian, who had been martyred at Rilly in 275. The location of Savinian's tomb, however, had been forgotten subsequent to the persecution of Christians under Aurelian and Diocletian. With a child as her only guide and companion, Syre set off for Rilly, confident of finding Savinian's burial place. On her way, Syre paused in a grassy field where she suddenly recovered her sight. Syre immediately began digging in the earth beneath her feet and discovered the grave and uncorrupted body of Saint Savinian. A church was built on the site, and Syre, who had taken vows, was made custodian of the saint's tomb. Strangely, she is not customarily invoked for blindness or diseases of the eye.

REFERENCES 16, 36

Z

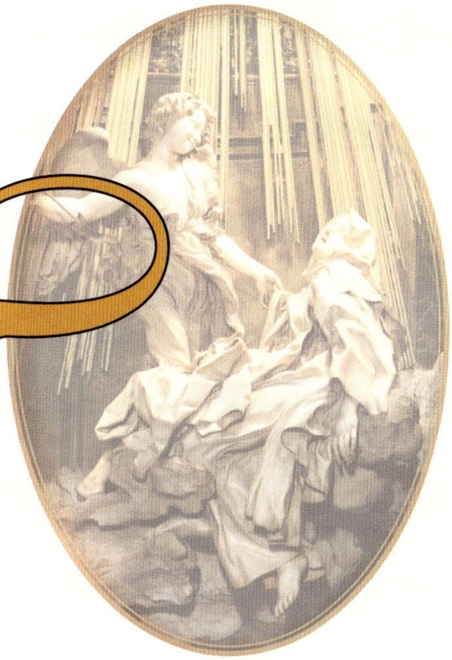

434
Tanche

MEMORIAL DAY **October 10**

PATRONAGE **Hemorrhage**

LIFE & LEGEND

Tanche was a native of Saint-Ouen in the diocese of Troyes. From her childhood she was singularly dedicated to God. According to du Broc de Segange, Tanche's mother and father went to visit the child's godfather, who was upset that the girl had not come with them, and he sent a servant to bring the girl back. The servant had gone only a short distance with her when he began to make improper advances toward her. Tanche resisted the servant, who proceeded to beat her about her face with the pommel of his sword, and she began to bleed copiously from her mouth and nostrils. At this moment, the son of Satan severed her head with his blade. Tanche picked up her bleeding head and carried it to the valley of Lhuître, where angels arrived and buried her corpse ca. 637. After a long period of time, the location of Tanche's grave was divinely revealed, and her remains were transferred to the church at Lhuître, where numerous miracles have been worked at her tomb.

REFERENCES 16, 36

435

Taracus

MEMORIAL DAY **October 11**

PATRONAGE **Headache**

LIFE & LEGEND

Taracus, Probus, and Andronicus were the most celebrated martyrs of Cilicia. Their cult was widespread throughout the East, their relics were diffused from Jerusalem to the Bosphorus, and churches were dedicated in their honor at Mopsuestia and Constantinople. Taracus, a native of Claudiopolis in Isauria, was a career soldier until released from the army at his own request because of his Christian faith. Taracus and two companions, Probus and Andronicus, were arrested at Pompeiopolis in Cilicia during the persecution of Diocletian and Maximian. They were interrogated and beaten by the governor Maximus at Tarsus and later at Mopsuestia before being dispatched by gladiators at Anazarbus ca. 304 after wild animals sent into the arena to kill them refused to do so. The bodies of the three men were recovered by the Christians of Anazarbus, who relayed an account of their martyrdom throughout the region.

REFERENCES 6, 36, 46

436

Teresa and Sanchia of Portugal

MEMORIAL DAY **June 17**

PATRONAGE **Fever**

LIFE & LEGEND

Teresa and Sanchia were two daughters of Sancho I, king of Portugal. Teresa, the oldest of three daughters, married her cousin, Alfonso IX, king of Léon, by whom she had three children. When it was learned that Teresa and Alfonso were cousins, the marriage was annulled. Teresa returned to Portugal and her estate at Lorvao, where she closed a laxly run Benedictine abbey and founded in its place a community of 300 women who lived according to the Cistercian rule. Teresa did not take the veil, however, until after the death of her sister Sanchia in 1229.

Unlike her sister, Sanchia never married, but lived after her father's death on her estate at Alenquer, where she founded a convent for women under the Augustinian rule (Cellas). Sanchia was so impressed after visiting the convent founded by her sister at Lorvao that, on her return to Alenquer, she converted Cellas into a Cistercian community. After Sanchia's death, Teresa surreptitiously removed her sister's body from its grave and reburied her at Lorvao. In 1231, Teresa settled a dispute between her children over the succession to the throne of Léon. Teresa died in 1250, and her remains were laid in a grave beside Sanchia's. Teresa was canonized by Pope Clement XI in 1705.

Citing a memoir of the seventeenth-century Franciscan, Francisco de Macedo, du Broc de Segange relates the following about the two sisters: "just as physicians have remedies that are proven efficacious for curing light fevers and ordinary maladies, so the nuns at Lorvao have a prescription for those suffering from tertian or quartan fevers that cures infallibly. The patient must recite for thirty days consecutively the psalms of penitence. He must then drink a vial of honeyed water with powers derived from the tomb of the two sisters. After making a novena, the patient is then cured."

REFERENCES 6, 16, 36, 46

437

Teresa of Ávila

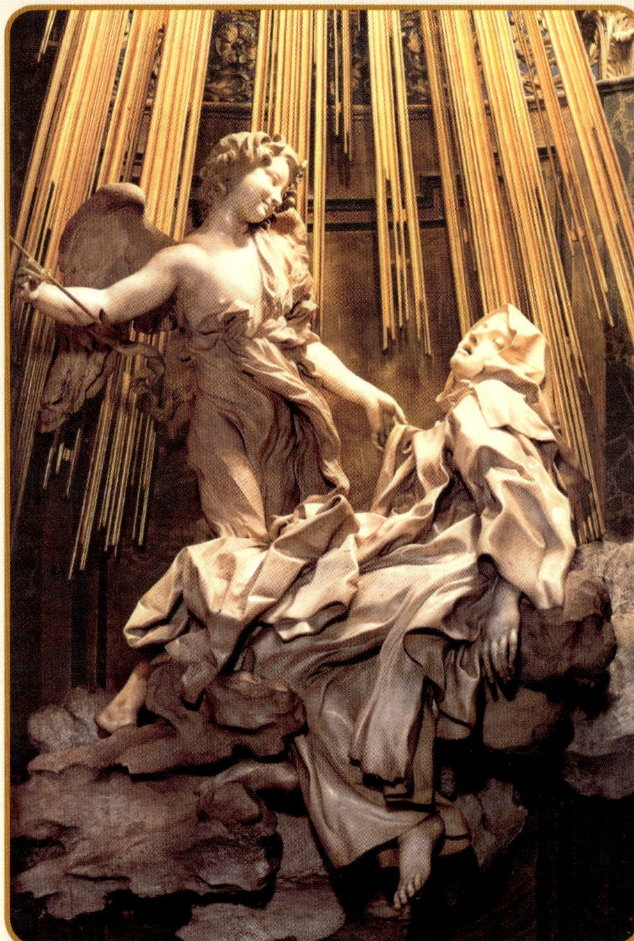

MEMORIAL DAY **October 4**

PATRONAGE **Bodily ills, headache, heart diseases, lace makers, Spain**

LIFE & LEGEND

Teresa was born in Ávila in the old kingdom of Castile in Spain on March 28, 1515. Her paternal grandfather was a Jewish convert to Christianity during the Spanish Inquisition. Her father, Alonso Sánchez de Cepeda, had purchased a knighthood and was very pious, as was her mother, who died when Teresa was 14. Teresa was initially educated by Augustine nuns in her hometown and entered the Carmelite Convent of the Incarnation at Ávila in 1535. Early in her life at the convent she suffered a serious illness that left her impaired for the remainder of her life. At the same time, she experienced spiritual visions and ecstasies. She is purported to have said: "Lord, either let me suffer or let me die," which inspired Bernini's *Ecstasy of Saint Teresa* at Santa Maria della Vittoria in Rome. Her account of her religious experiences are described in her autobiography completed in 1565, which is compared to the "Confessions of Saint Augustine."

In 1562, Teresa founded the convent of the Discalced Carmelite Nuns of the Primitive Rule of Saint Joseph of Ávila. Over the ensuing 15 years she founded eight convents of the same order throughout Spain. In 1576, older Carmelites condemned her work and persecuted her, but King Philip II of Spain came to her defense. She proceeded to found more convents, bringing the total to 16.

Shortly after her death in 1582, Philip II had her manuscripts brought to his palace, where they were edited and published in 1587. Her memorial day was set as October 15 when she was canonized in 1662. In 1970, she, along with Saint Catherine of Siena, were made Doctors of the Church by Pope Paul VI, and these were the first two women to be so honored.

REFERENCES 6, 9, 49

438

Thaumast

MEMORIAL DAY **January 1**

PATRONAGE **Fever, toothache, colic**

LIFE & LEGEND

Nothing is known of Thaumast's origins. He was a regional bishop active in Poitiers, where he died and was buried during the fifth century. Beginning in the sixth century, people afflicted with fevers or with toothaches sought relief from the stone that sealed his tomb. In later times, mothers would bring their colic-afflicted children to the tomb for cure. The stone was used so frequently that it was worn out at several places.

REFERENCES 16, 36

439

Theobald of Provence

MEMORIAL DAY **June 30**

PATRONAGE **Fever**

LIFE & LEGEND

Theobald was born in Brie in 1017, the son of Count Arnoul of Champagne. Although Theobald was raised to be a warrior, he was inspired by reading the lives of the desert fathers to follow their way. With his father's reluctant consent, Theobald, in the company of another young nobleman named Walter, entered the abbey of Saint Remi at Reims. In their desire for the hermetic life, the pair left Reims to seek greater solitude—first in the forests of the Ardenne and later in the forest of Pettingen in present-day Luxembourg. Theobald and Walter supported themselves independently as day laborers on the neighboring farms, coming together again in the evening to chant and pray through the night. By their manner of life the hermits eventually became known. To escape their new fame, Theobald and Walter made a pilgrimage to Compostela in Spain, and then journeyed to Rome to venerate sites associated with the apostles and martyrs.

On their return from Rome, they found a wooded site at Salanigo near Vicenza suitable for a hermitage. Walter died within 2 years. By then Theobald had been ordained a priest by the bishop of Vicenza and had attracted several disciples who shared his way of life in the wilderness. Theobald's parents learned of his whereabouts, and, although quite old, they journeyed to Italy to see their long-departed son. With her husband's consent, Theobald's mother, Gisela, decided to end her years as a hermit in a cell near her son. Theobald eventually became very ill, perhaps with leprosy, and, in his final months, in 1066, made his profession as a Camaldolese monk.

REFERENCES 6, 36, 46

440

Theodard

MEMORIAL DAY **May 1**

PATRONAGE **Fever**

LIFE & LEGEND

Theodard was born at Montauriol, the site of which is now occupied by the city of Montauban. He studied law at Toulouse. According to Butler, "we first hear of him as the advocate retained by the cathedral authorities in a curious suit brought against them by the Jews of Toulouse, who, not unnaturally, objected to a sort of religious pageant in the course of which a Jew was publicly struck on the face before the cathedral doors." Archbishop Sigebold, who had come to Toulouse to hear the case, was so impressed by the young lawyer that he took him back with him to Narbonne. Sigebold ordained Theodard to the priesthood and made him his archdeacon. After Sigebold's death, Theodard succeeded him as archbishop of Narbonne. Theodard expended great energy and resources to ransom Christians taken captive by the Saracens during their raids on the coast, rebuilt the cathedral that had nearly been destroyed during a Saracen attack, and fed the hungry during a famine that lasted 3 years. The rigors and cares of his episcopal duties eventually affected Theodard's health, and he fell into a continuous fever. Hoping, perhaps, that a change of climate would improve his health, Theodard returned to his native Montauriol, where he died at the monastery of Saint-Martin in 893.

REFERENCES 6, 16, 36

441

Theodoric of Mont d'Or

MEMORIAL DAY **July 1**

PATRONAGE **Fever, rheumatism**

LIFE & LEGEND

Theodoric was born near Rheims. Sources agree that he married unwillingly, but disagree whether he convinced his wife to separate or whether he abandoned her when she refused to live with him celibately. In either case, Theodoric presented himself to Saint Remigius, bishop of Reims, who ordained him to the priesthood and advised a monastic life. Theodoric subsequently founded a monastic community at Mont d'Or near Reims. He was known for converting many pagans and unbelievers in Reims, including his own father, a former brigand, who died a monk in his son's monastery. Theodoric died of natural causes in 533. He is said to have cured King Theodoric of Austrasia of an eye disease, but he does not seem to be a patron of those with ocular disorders. The waters of a well associated with him at Aumenancourt (Aisne) were long noted for their power to heal those afflicted with fever and rheumatism.

REFERENCES 14, 36, 46

442

Theodulph

MEMORIAL DAY **May 1**

PATRONAGE **Toothache**

LIFE & LEGEND

Born into a noble family of Aquitaine, Theodulph abandoned the world as a very young man and placed himself under the spiritual direction of Saint Theodoric, the first abbot of the monastery of Mont d'Or. For 22 years, Theodulph labored in the fields and cared for farm animals. After Theodoric's death, the monks of Mont d'Or unanimously chose Theodulph to succeed him as abbot. Only then was he ordained to the priesthood. Theodulph died ca. 590.

REFERENCES 16, 36

443

Thérèse de Lisieux

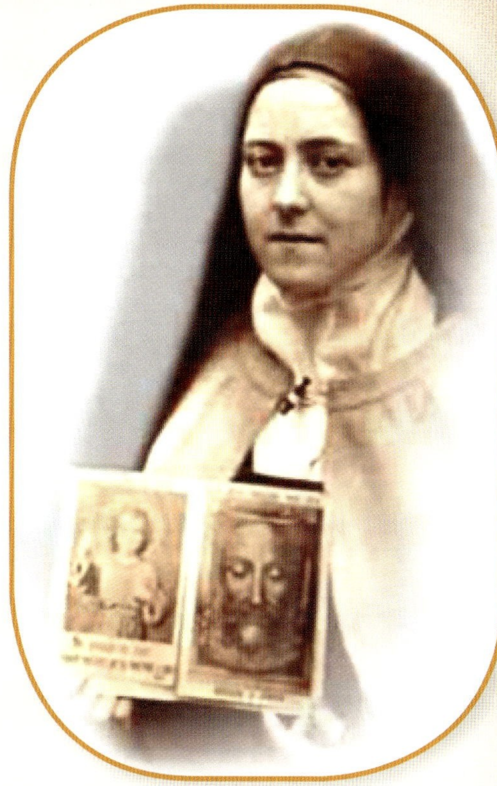

MEMORIAL DAY **October 1**

PATRONAGE **Tuberculosis, AIDS, France, Russia, several cities**

LIFE & LEGEND

Thérèse, whose name is derived from Greek, meaning "harvest," is also known as the Little Flower of Jesus. She was born in 1873 into a pious family in Alençon, France. In 2000, both her parents were approved by Pope Benedict XVI for beatification. The family moved to Lisieux when Thérèse was 4. She became a Carmelite postulant when she was 15 and took her final vows 2 years later. She died of tuberculosis in 1897 at age 24.

She was known for developing a simple approach to spiritual life that was understandable and imitable. She referred to it as The Little Way. It was the essence of her book, *Life of a Soul,* which was published posthumously and was the religious best seller of the twentieth century. Her major shrine is at the Basilique de Sainte-Thérèse in Lisieux, which remains a center for pilgrims and has been the site of many miracles. Pope Pius, during whose tenure her cause was initiated, referred to her as "the greatest of modern saints." She was beatified by Pope Pius XI in 1923 and canonized by him 2 years later. The 20 years between her death and canonization are a modern record for speed. In 1944, Pope Pius XII named her copatroness of France with Saint Joan of Arc. In 1997, Pope John Paul II named her as one of 33 Doctors of the Universal Church, one of only three women.

REFERENCES 6, 9, 45

444

Tiburtius

MEMORIAL DAY **August 11**

PATRONAGE **Fractures**

LIFE & LEGEND

Tiburtius is referred to in an epitaph of Pope Damasus. He was a subdeacon at Rome, and was betrayed to the authorities by an apostate during the persecution of the emperor Diocletian. Tiburtius walked barefoot unharmed over live coals and was then beheaded ca. 288 on the Via Labicana some 3 miles outside the walls of Rome. Tiburtius is noted for his healing of a workman who had broken one or more limbs after falling from a roof.

REFERENCES 6, 14, 36

445

Tillo

MEMORIAL DAY **January 7**

PATRONAGE **Fever**

LIFE & LEGEND

A Saxon by birth, Tillo was carried off by raiders to what is now the Low Countries, where he was held captive until ransomed by the charity of Saint Eligius. Tillo spent some time with Eligius at the abbey of Solignac. He was baptized there by the future saint and learned the art of goldsmithing. Before leaving to become bishop of Noyons in 640, Eligius ordained Tillo as a priest and charged him to become a missionary to the unconverted peoples of the Low Countries—especially around Tournai. Tillo did so, but eventually returned to the area around Solignac, where he lived as a recluse until his death of old age ca. 702.

REFERENCES 6, 16, 36

446

Timothy

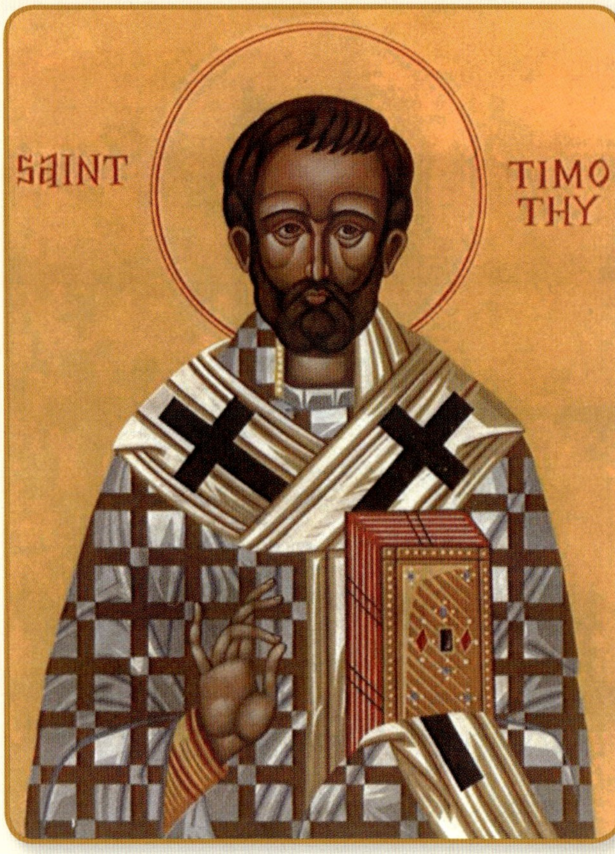

MEMORIAL DAY **January 24**

PATRONAGE **Stomach and intestinal disorders**

LIFE & LEGEND

Timothy, whose name is derived from Greek, meaning "honoring God," was born to a Greek gentile father and a Jewish mother ca. 17. He was converted to Christianity by Saint Paul the Apostle, whom he served as an assistant and comissionary. Paul either personally circumcised Timothy or had him circumcised so that he would be accepted by the Jews. Timothy accompanied Paul on many of his journeys. He initially joined Paul at Lystra, replacing Barnabas, and also traveled to Corinth, Macedonia, and Achaia. Timothy's report on the condition of the Christians in Thessalonica led to Paul's first letter to the Thessalonians.

Timothy was probably with Paul when the Apostle was imprisoned at Caesarea and then Rome. Timothy himself was imprisoned for a short period of time in Rome. He was the recipient of two canonical letters from Paul. Timothy served as the bishop of the Church in Ephesus for 15 years. At Ephesus, he was stoned to death ca. 80 (some indicate the date was ca. 90) when he tried to halt a pagan procession honoring Diana. In the fourth century, his relics were moved to the Church of the Holy Apostles in Constantinople.

REFERENCES 6, 9, 42

447

Trophimus of Arles

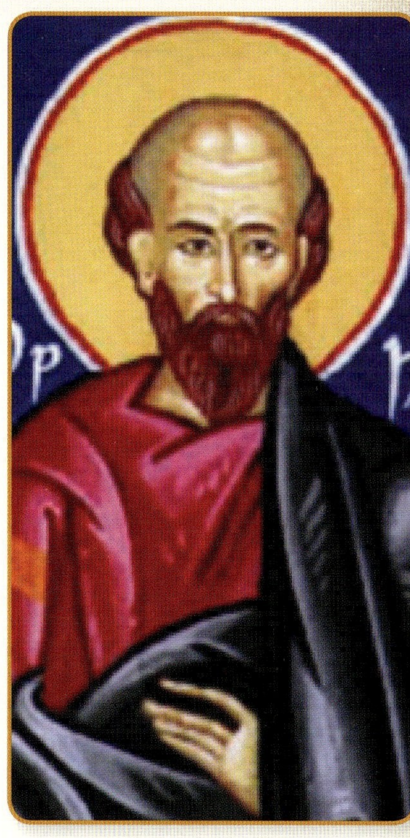

MEMORIAL DAY **December 29**

PATRONAGE **Gout**

LIFE & LEGEND

According to Saint Gregory of Tours, Trophimus was one of the six bishops sent from Rome with Saint Dionysius in the middle of the third century to evangelize Gaul. He became the first bishop of Arles and is mentioned in a letter of Pope Saint Zosimus to the bishops of Gaul in 417, which helped spread the Word at Arles. He is sometimes confused with Trophimus of the New Testament, whose feast day is also December 29. He is often represented without eyes or carrying his eyes.

REFERENCES 6, 14, 36

448

Turibius

MEMORIAL DAY **April 16**

PATRONAGE **Blindness**

LIFE & LEGEND

There were several saints named Turibius, and they are sometimes confused with one another. At least two of these saints share an April 16 feast day. This Turibius succeeded Saint Julian in the third century as bishop of Le Mans, and he is credited with healing several individuals of blindness and other eye diseases during his lifetime, accounting for his patronage.

REFERENCES 16, 36

U

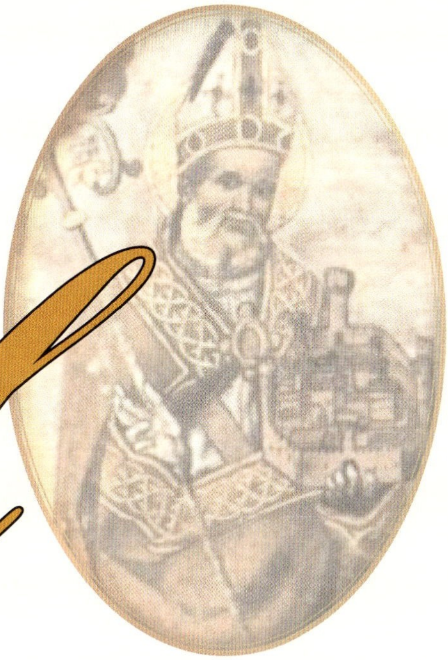

449
Ubaldo of Gubbio

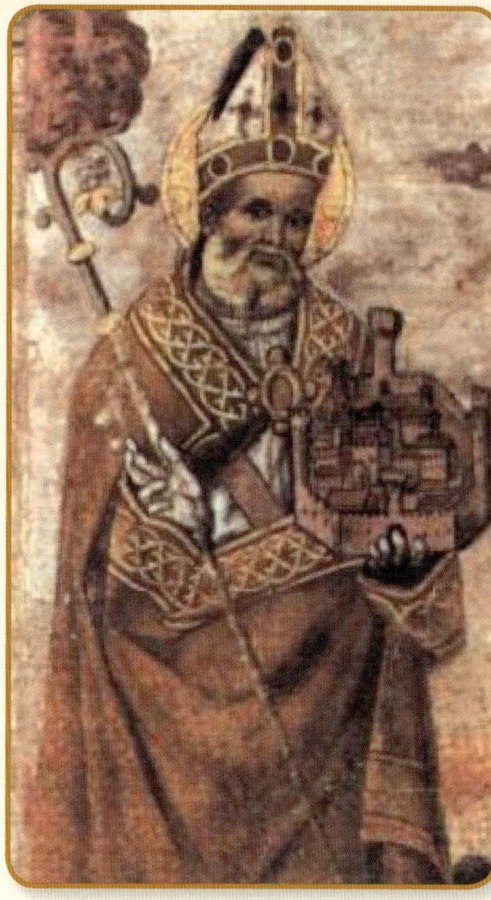

MEMORIAL DAY **May 16**

PATRONAGE **Migraine, neuralgia, autism, children's diseases, obsessive compulsive disorders, Gubbio (Italy)**

LIFE & LEGEND

Ubaldo, whose name has a Germanic derivation meaning "bold, brave," was born ca. 1084 at Gubbio, Italy, of noble parents named Baldassini. He was educated in the cathedral monastery of his native city and at the monastery of Saint Secondo. He returned to the cathedral monastery as prior. He divested himself of his family's riches by transferring them to the monasteries and to the care of the poor. He was noted for his humility and piety and was offered several bishoprics that he refused. He prevented Frederick Barbarossa from sacking Gubbio after Spoleto had been destroyed in 1155. Ubaldo died after a long and painful illness in 1160.

Many miracles were attributed to him during his life and after he died. Pope Celestine III canonized him in 1192. At the time of his canonization, his body was exhumed from the cathedral church in Gubbio at which time it was found to be incorrupt. The basilica of Sant Ubaldo is located on a hill overlooking the city. Its great windows depict episodes in the saint's life.

REFERENCES 6, 9

450
Udaut

MEMORIAL DAY **May 11**

PATRONAGE **Fever, labor, blindness**

LIFE & LEGEND

Udaut was born into a noble Italian family. While hunting one day, he gave chase to a hind that sought refuge in what turned out to be the hermitage of a holy man named Pancrace. Seeing the animal crouched at the holy man's feet seeking protection, Udaut was so moved that he asked Pancrace to give him instruction in the religious life. The two men left Italy together and settled in the central Pyrenees, where they evangelized the local people and where Udaut was ordained a priest. After Pancrace's death, Udaut went to Toulouse and from there to Rome with a party of Christians who wished to visit the tombs of the apostles, Peter and Paul. While in Rome, Udaut learned of the approach of Attila's Huns. He set out for the Danube, where he found the Huns and their allies. Udaut consoled those who had suffered greatly from the invaders and was able to mitigate to some extent the harshness of the Huns. Eventually Udaut was seized by Attila's brother and brutally flogged. Left for dead, Udaut recovered from the bloody beating and continued his work. Soon after, however, Udaut fell into the hands of Valamir, king of the Ostrogoths and one of Attila's allies, who ordered that Udaut be beaten to death. When he survived this, Valamir ordered Udaut to swallow molten lead. The saint blessed the liquid metal and swallowed it in a single draft without any ill effect. Udaut was released after this ordeal, and he returned to the Pyrenees. In 452, with Attila again threatening Italy, Valamir and his Ostrogoths followed a different route west toward the Pyrenees. At Ax, Valamir again encountered Udaut, who was evangelizing soldiers and discouraging them from sacrificing to Mars. This time, in 452, Valamir ordered Udaut to be rolled in a barrel lined with spikes on the inside, and finally he stabbed him through the heart.

REFERENCES 16, 36

451

Ulrich of Augsburg

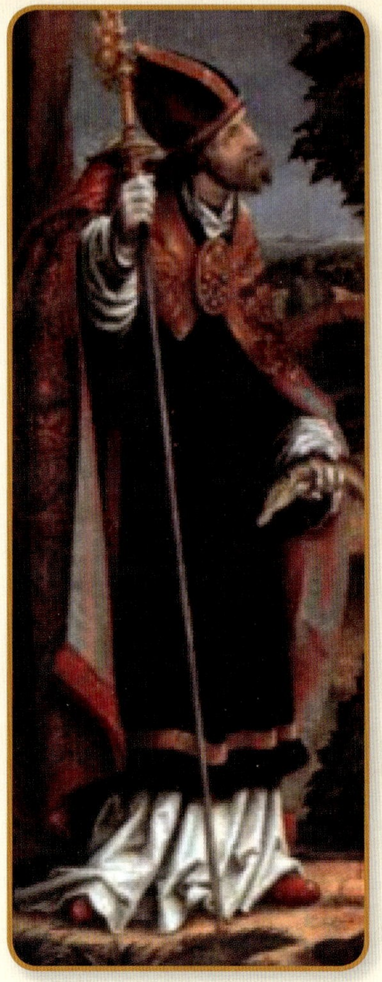

MEMORIAL DAY **July 4**

PATRONAGE **Fever, pregnancy, labor, fainting, rabies, physical frailty**

LIFE & LEGEND

Ulrich, whose name has a Germanic derivation, meaning "powerful through inheritance," was born in 890 in Zurich, Switzerland, the son of Count Hucpald and Thetbirga. Ulrich demonstrated himself to be an excellent student while being educated first at the abbey of Saint Gall and later under the care of his uncle Adalbero, bishop of Ausgburg. Ulrich himself became bishop of Augsburg in 923, and he led the effort to rebuild the city and its cathedral after it was sacked by the Magyars. Although he was a man of seemingly frail constitution, Ulrich was unstinting in his life of prayer, his administrative duties, and his charitable efforts on behalf of his flock.

He was noted for his work with the sick and built several churches within his bishopric region. When the Magyars again invaded Germany and laid siege to Augsburg, Ulrich organized the resistance, which held off the enemy until Emperor Otto arrived and defeated the invaders at the battle of Lechfeld in 955.

After 48 years as bishop, Ulrich retired to Saint Gall, naming his nephew (also named Adalbero) as his successor on the episcopal throne. This appointment caused some furor, and Ulrich had to answer to charges of nepotism for which he did penance shortly before he died in 973. He was buried in the church of

Saint Afra. During his life, women who drank from his chalice had easy births, and his pastoral cross was used to prevent or heal rabies in people bitten by rabid animals. Earth from his grave was used to repel rats. His canonization in 993 by Pope John XV is the first recorded canonization by a pope.

REFERENCES 6, 9, 16, 36, 45

452

Ursicinus

MEMORIAL DAY **June 19**

PATRONAGE **Physicians**

LIFE & LEGEND

Ursicinus was a physician who practiced in the city of Ravenna in the middle decades of the first century. After converting to Christianity, he became a victim of Nero's persecution of the new cult. Ursicinus was arrested in 67 by the consul, Gaius Suetonius Paulinus, former governor of Britain, and was condemned to death by decapitation. Trembling at the prospect of such a death, Ursicinus was encouraged in his resolve by no less a figure than Saint Vitale. In some accounts of his martyrdom, the body of Ursicinus rose from the ground, picked up its severed head, and carried it in both hands to its place of burial. There is disagreement whether Ursicinus was martyred at Ravenna or Mantua. The altar in the chapel of Saints Nazirius and Celsus in the church of Saint Vitale, Ravenna, is composed, in part, of fragments from the funeral monument of Ursicinus.

REFERENCES 16, 36, 50

453

Ursmar

MEMORIAL DAY **April 18 or April 19**

PATRONAGE **Fever, toothache, kidney diseases, bed wetting**

LIFE & LEGEND

Ursmar was born at Flogon near Avesmes. In 689, he was made abbot of the Lobbes monastery in Belgium, which had been founded 35 years earlier. He is credited with the foundation of other monasteries and is noted for the success of his missionary work in Flanders. He may have become a bishop. He died in 713.

REFERENCES 6, 14, 16, 36

454

Ursus (Orso) of Aosta

MEMORIAL DAY **February 1 or June 17**

PATRONAGE **Kidney diseases, back pain, rheumatism, labor**

LIFE & LEGEND

Ursus, whose name means "bear" in Latin, was an Irish monk who left his native island to carry the word of God to the people of Gaul and Italy during the sixth century. He first evangelized in the vicinity of Digne (Basses-Alpes), where he was active in refuting the Arian heresy. Ursus later crossed the Alps and settled in the city of Aosta, where he became archdeacon to its bishop, Jucundus. When the Gothic king, Theodoric, an Arian, expelled Jucundus from his episcopal throne, Ursus accompanied him into exile. After Jucundus' death, an Arian bishop assumed the episcopacy of Aosta, whereupon Ursus and some others founded a community outside the walls of Aosta at the site presently known as Sant'Orso.

REFERENCES 16, 36

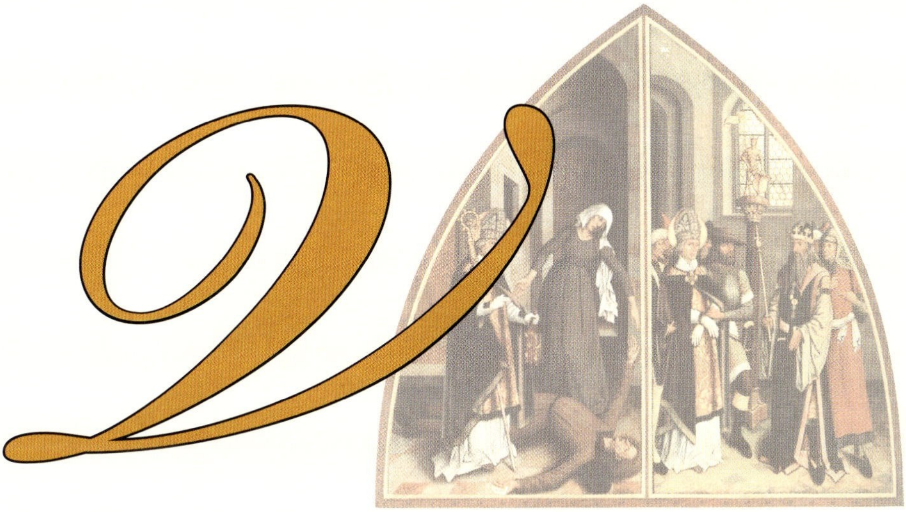

455

Valentine of Passau

MEMORIAL DAY **January 7**

PATRONAGE **Epilepsy**

LIFE & LEGEND

Valentine, whose name is derived from the same Latin root as "valor," meaning "healthy, strong," was an abbot who later became a missionary bishop in Rhaetia. He died ca. 440, and he was buried in the Tyrol. His remains were later transferred to Passau, where he was much venerated. Kerler suggests that Valentine's patronage of epilepsy stems from the similarity of the first syllable of his name (Val) with the term "fallende Sucht," or falling sickness, which is epilepsy.

REFERENCES 6, 36

456

Valentine of Rome

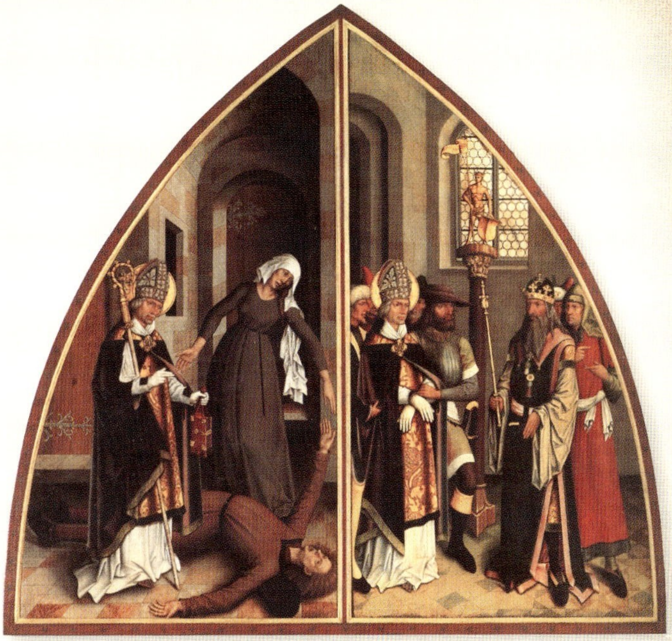

MEMORIAL DAY **February 14**

PATRONAGE **Fainting, epilepsy, plague, lovers, betrothed, beekeepers, greeting card makers, travelers**

LIFE & LEGEND

Valentine's name does not appear on an early list of Roman martyrs that was compiled in 354. He is said to have been a priest and physician in Rome. He was imprisoned for giving aid to martyrs, and, while in prison, he restored the sight of a jailer's daughter and subsequently converted the jailer. He is also depicted curing a crippled or epileptic child. He is said to have died ca. 269 after he was beaten and beheaded.

The *Legenda Aurae* of Jacobus de Voragine, written about 1260, indicates that Valentine was beheaded by Emperor Claudius, because he refused to deny Christ. He was buried on the Flaminian Way, and his relics were translated to the church of Saint Praxedes. Some of the relics were later donated by Pope Gregory XVI to the Whitefriar Street Carmelite Church in Dublin, Ireland.

A feast for the saint was decreed in 496 to commemorate him as a bishop and a martyr. The feast day was removed when the calendar was revised by the Church in 1969. The origin of Valentine's Day celebrations cannot be determined, but one interpretation relates to a Roman mid-February custom, in which boys drew girls' names in honor of the sex and fertility goddess, Februata Juno. Priests substituted Saint Valentine's name to supersede the pagan holiday.

REFERENCES 6, 9, 33

457
Vaury

MEMORIAL DAY **July 8**

PATRONAGE **Sick children**

LIFE & LEGEND

Born in the neighborhood of Reims, Vaury was recognized even by his contemporaries for the holiness of his life and the miracles that he worked. When Vaury made a pilgrimage to venerate the relics of Saint Martial at Limoges, the ecclesiastic authorities were able to keep Vaury near them by providing him a hermitage in the wilderness, called Bernage. Much later, the village of Saint-Vaury rose near this place. After his death, ca. 620, Vaury's tomb became a place of pilgrimage where miracles were often recorded. Pilgrims particularly invoked the saint to cure their sick children, carrying them in procession and placing their small bodies in the niche of the church in Saint-Julien, where Vaury's remains were interred.

REFERENCE 16

458

Vedastus (Vaast, Gaston)

MEMORIAL DAY **February 6**

PATRONAGE **Eye diseases, disabled people**

LIFE & LEGEND

A native of southwestern France, perhaps of Périgueux, Vedastus intended to lead a secluded monastic life, until he came to the notice of the bishop of Toul, who ordained him a priest. Vedastus was selected by the bishop to accompany Clovis I to Reims to instruct him in preparation for his baptism following his victory over the Alemanni. As Clovis and his party were about to cross the Aisne, Vedastus restored the sight of a blind beggar by making the sign of the cross on his eyes. Vedastus accompanied Saint Remigius on the latter's missionary tour to convert the Franks. It was Remigius who consecrated Vedastus as the first bishop of Arras in 500. When Vedastus first entered Arras, he found little evidence of Christianity except the ruins of a church and some elderly members of a shrunken community. For the next 40 years, Vedastus labored unceasingly to reestablish Christianity among his flock. He became bishop of Cambrai, France, ca. 510. When Vedastus died, ca. 540, the people of the town noted a luminous cloud ascend from his house.

REFERENCES 6, 16, 36, 46

459

Venantius of Camerino

MEMORIAL DAY **May 18**

PATRONAGE **Fractures, wounds, injuries**

LIFE & LEGEND

Born into a prominent pagan family of Camerino in central Italy, Venantius became a Christian at age 15. Although he was young, he was apprehended by the authorities and threatened with death if he did not abjure his faith and sacrifice to the traditional deities. Venantius refused, whereupon he was flagellated, had his bones broken on the cavaletto, was suspended upside-down over fire, and beaten so badly about the face that his teeth were knocked out and his jaw broken. Later, by order of the prefect, he was thrown into a ring with lions who did nothing more than lay about the boy's feet. Venantius was then cast off a cliff, only to pick himself up from the rocks beneath, uninjured. A number of those who had witnessed Venantius' ordeals were converted to Christianity by the example of his faith. These same people were beheaded with Venantius on May 18, 251. Butler maintains that this life of Venantius is a "fictitious history." Even if the official passio of the saint was elaborated much later than the third century, the historical existence of this adolescent martyr is evidenced by construction in the fifth century of a basilica named in his honor outside Camerino's eastern gate, where he was supposed to have been buried.

REFERENCES 3, 6, 46

460

Venantius of Tours

MEMORIAL DAY **October 13**

PATRONAGE **Fever**

LIFE & LEGEND

Venantius was a native of Bourges in the sixth century and was engaged to marry a young woman of that city. While in Tours, he visited the monastery of Saint-Martin. He was so taken by the life of the monks there that he decided to join them. In time, Venantius became abbot. Numerous healings of fever were recorded at his tomb.

REFERENCES 16, 36

461

Ventura of Castello

MEMORIAL DAY **September 7**

PATRONAGE **Hernia**

LIFE & LEGEND

Ventura was parish priest of the church of San Bartolomeo near Valdipetrina in the vicinity of Città di Castello (Umbria). One day, ca. 1250, Ventura encountered a muleteer in the woods who was cursing and blaspheming terribly. When the priest gently corrected the muleteer, the man became so enraged that he killed Ventura with an axe and hid the body under a pile of stones. Shortly thereafter, it was observed that a dove kept striking the bell of San Bartolomeo with his beak and then flying off toward the woods. After this happened several times, a party followed the dove and discovered the priest's martyred body. The priest was buried in the church of San Bartolomeo, which not long afterward became known as San Ventura. One of the men who had carried Ventura's body back from the woods was immediately cured of his hernia—thus Ventura's patronage of those suffering from this disorder. On the saint's feast day, it used to be the custom to place children on Ventura's tomb to preserve them from hernia.

REFERENCES 16, 36, 46

462

Veranus

MEMORIAL DAYS **October 19, November 11**

PATRONAGE **Plague, rabies, mental disorders**

LIFE & LEGEND

Veranus began his religious life during the sixth century as a recluse in the wilderness of the Vaucluse. He built a sanctuary dedicated to the Virgin in the region that was maintained into modern times. When this region came to be ravaged by a dragon, Veranus cornered the beast in its cave, chained it, and led it into the mountains far from human habitation. When it became impossible for him to avoid the attention and praises of men, he traveled through Provence and northern Italy, preaching and working miracles, including the subjugation of another dragon in Liguria. On his return to Gaul, Veranus was made bishop of Cavaillon near Avignon. He also served as an ambassador for King Gontran and was godfather to a son of Childbert II, king of Austrasia. His presence was recorded at several regional Church councils. Veranus was successively invoked for the cessation of plague in the city of Nivers, where his remains were transferred from Cavaillon.

REFERENCES 16, 36

463

Veronus

MEMORIAL DAY **March 31**

PATRONAGE **Fever, headache**

LIFE & LEGEND

Little more is known of Veronus than he lived during ninth century at the time of the Norman depredation of present-day Belgium, and that he died at Lembeek, near Hal, on the border of Hainault and Brabant.

REFERENCES 16, 36

464

Victor of Campbon

MEMORIAL DAY **August 31**

PATRONAGE **Fever**

LIFE & LEGEND

Victor built an oratory in his native village of Campbon in the diocese of Nantes during the sixth or seventh century and lived there as a recluse. Du Broc de Segange maintains that Victor attained "perfect tranquility of soul, rivaling in his purity the state of the angels." The holy man was buried in his oratory, where his remains lay until dispersed during the Norman invasions in the ninth century. A shrine to the saint remains in the church of Saint Victor at Campbon, where Victor was invoked for the cure of fever.

REFERENCES 16, 36

465

Victurnianus

MEMORIAL DAY **September 30**

PATRONAGE **Mental disorders**

LIFE & LEGEND

Victurnianus was born into a noble family of Scotland in the seventh century. Early in life he made the decision to dedicate himself wholly to God. Turning his back on the world and his patrimony, Victurnianus secretly made his way to Gaul, where he built a hermitage on the banks of the Vienne near the city of Limoges. He was disappointed in his hopes for a life of solitude, however, because his reputation spread throughout the neighboring territory, a place remote enough to be known as "the shadowy valley." Today this area is occupied by the village of Saint-Victurnien. Many people came to Victurnianus to be healed of their maladies, especially mental disorders. After his death, Victurnianus was buried in the place where he had built his hermitage, and a sanctuary was erected in his honor. Behind the principal altar are two circular openings where the insane and those afflicted with mental disorders place their heads when they invoke the saint.

REFERENCES 16, 36

466

Vincent de Paul

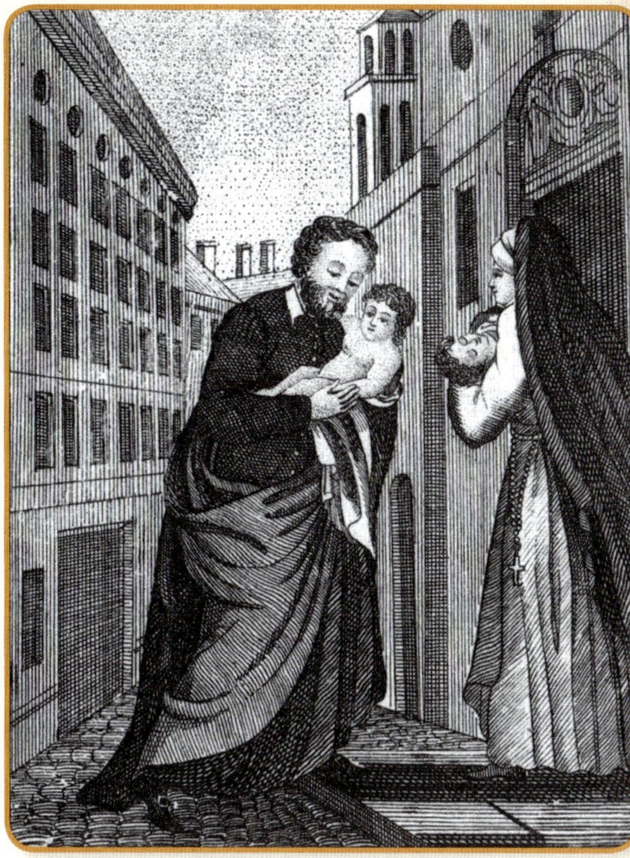

MEMORIAL DAY **September 27**

PATRONAGE **Hospital workers, lepers, charities, horses, prisoners**

LIFE & LEGEND

Vincent, whose name is derived from Latin, meaning "conquering," was born in Gascony, France, in 1581 into a peasant family. He was educated by Franciscan friars before undertaking divinity studies at the University of Toulouse. Shortly after he was ordained at age 20, he was captured by Turks while returning to Toulouse from Marseilles by sea, taken to Tunis, and sold into slavery. He was freed in 1607 by his master, whom he had converted to Christianity. Vincent returned to France, where he served as a parish priest near Paris, and he became almoner to Queen Marguerite of Valois and took charge of the parish at Clichy.

He entered the services of the influential Gondi family but left to concentrate on his prime mission of charity. He founded the first conference on charity for assisting the poor. Some of his initial efforts were directed toward convicts in the galleys, and he converted many of these men. He founded the Congregation of the

Daughters of Charity and the Congregation of Priests of the Mission (Lazarists), which was dedicated to the evangelization of country people. The Daughters, consisting of as many as 200 women of high rank, nursed the sick-poor at the Hotel-Dieu and in the prisons, and provided care for foundlings.

Vincent established ecclesiastic conferences and seminaries throughout France and was chaplain at the court of Henry IV. His charitable activities extended throughout France and beyond to Italy, Ireland, Scotland, Poland, Madagascar, and Barbary. He died in 1660 and was canonized by Pope Clement XII in 1737. His name is attached to an island nation in the Caribbean Sea and a Catholic health care system in New York City.

REFERENCES 6, 9

467

Vincent Ferrer

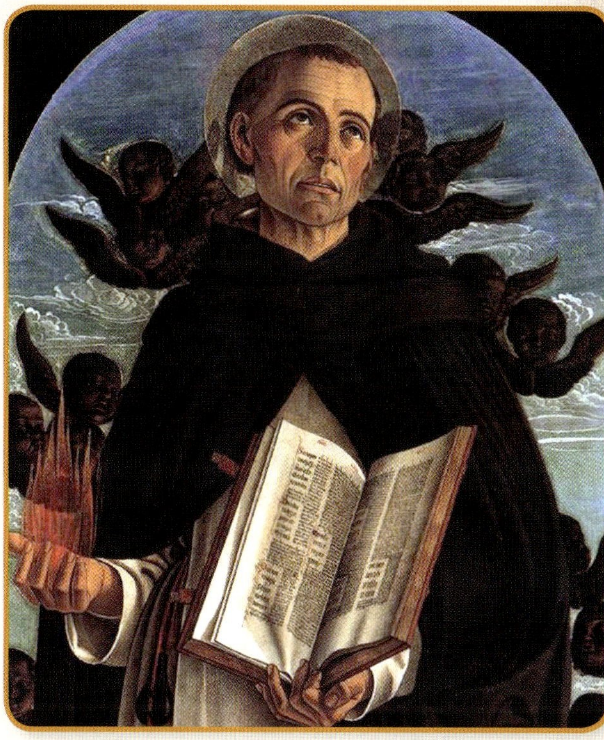

MEMORIAL DAY **April 5**

PATRONAGE **Fever, headache, epilepsy**

LIFE & LEGEND

Vincent was born in Valencia in 1350, the fourth child of the Anglo-Scottish nobleman, William Stewart Ferrer, and his Spanish wife, Constantia Miguel. Vincent joined the Dominican Order in 1367. He studied in Barcelona and then received a doctorate of theology from the University of Lleida, where he became professor of philosophy at the age of 21. Vincent returned to Barcelona in 1373. He was transferred to Toulouse by his nervous superiors, however, after he correctly prophesied the arrival of corn-laden ships during a famine afflicting Barcelona. He returned to Barcelona the following year and was ordained to the priesthood.

In 1379, Vincent entered the service of Pedro Cardinal de Luna, who was elected as the antipope known as Benedict XIII in 1394, the second in the Avignon line of popes during the Great Schism. Benedict was supported by Vincent, who at the time maintained the legitimacy of the popes at Avignon. Between 1385 and 1390, Vincent taught in Valencia and served as confessor to Yolanda, queen of Aragon. He was cited for heresy by the Inquisition for maintaining that Judas had done penance. The charge was dismissed, however, by the antipope. Vincent then joined Benedict in Avignon and was appointed his confessor. Vincent refused a cardinal's hat from Benedict following a serious illness during which he had a vision of Christ accompanied by Saint Dominic de Guzman and Saint Francis of Assisi. The saintly pair directed Vincent to henceforth devote himself to preaching, and then they restored him to health. Vincent began his preaching career in 1399, and over the next two decades traveled the length and breadth of Europe, from northern Italy to the Netherlands, and from Switzerland to Moorish Spain. He attracted great crowds everywhere he went, converted many, and motivated numerous others to repent. Many believed he had the gift of tongues, because he was understood wherever he appeared, although he spoke only his own language.

By 1408, Vincent had changed his stance on the papacy and tried to convince Benedict XIII to renounce his claim to the papal throne so that the schism dividing the Church might be closed. Benedict refused, and Vincent returned to Spain, where he continued his preaching mission. During this stay, Vincent was influential in the election of Ferdinand to the throne of Castile and convinced Ferdinand to renounce his loyalty to the pope in Avignon and recognize the pope in Rome. The Great Schism ended when Ferdinand agreed to do so.

Vincent spent the final 3 years of his life preaching in France. He died at Vannes, Brittany, on April 5, 1419, and was interred at the cathedral of Vannes. Vincent was canonized by Pope Callistus III in 1455. During the celebration, 800 of his miracles were read aloud.

REFERENCES 6, 9, 14, 16, 36, 45, 46

468
Vitalis of Salzburg

MEMORIAL DAY **October 20**

PATRONAGE **Pregnancy, delivery**

LIFE & LEGEND

Vitalis was a disciple of Saint Rupert and succeeded his mentor as bishop of Salzburg. He died ca. 730, and numerous miracles were reported to have taken place at his tomb.

REFERENCES 16, 36, 46

469
Vitus

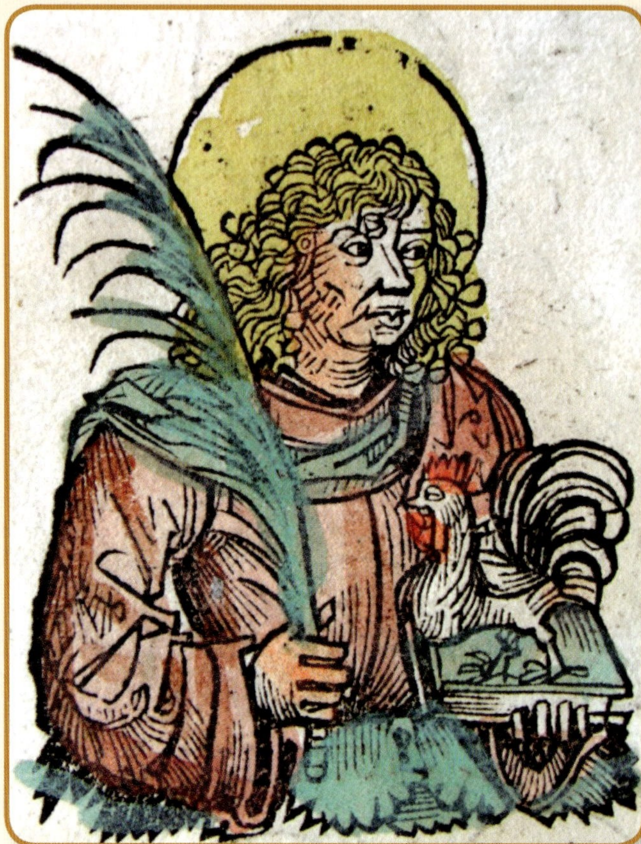

MEMORIAL DAY **June 15**

PATRONAGE **Animal bites, epilepsy, lethargy, lightning, storms, actors**

LIFE & LEGEND

Vitus, whose name means "life" in Latin, was the son of a pagan Sicilian senator. He was converted to Christianity when he was 12 years old by his nurse, Saint Crescentia, and his tutor, Saint Modestus. The threesome was arrested at the request of Vitus' father and imprisoned. They were freed by angels and fled to Luciana and later Rome, where Vitus exorcised Emperor Diocletian's son. This miracle was attributed to sorcery, and, along with Crescentia and Modestus, Vitus was arrested, tortured, and thrown to the lions, which refused to attack them. The prisoners were then executed ca. 303 by immersion into a cauldron of boiling oil. A rooster was thrown into the pot with Vitus and became his symbol, which accounts for his patronage against oversleeping. As Vitus was dying, a storm broke out in the region and destroyed several pagan temples, thereby accounting for his patronage against storms and lightning.

In the fourteenth century, in France and Germany, Saint Vitus was included on the roster of the Fourteen Holy Helpers. In the sixteenth century, Germans danced before Saint Vitus' statue on his memorial day to ensure a year of good health. The word chorea, meaning "dance" in Greek, was first applied by the sixteenth-century physician, Paracelsus, to the frenzied movements. The dancing resembled the movements associated with Sydenham's chorea, which later became known as Saint Vitus' dance. This explains his patronage for dancers, entertainers, and epileptics.

Sydenham's chorea took its name from the seventeenth-century English physician, Thomas Sydenham, who gave the name "chorea" to the facial twitching and convulsive movements, usually a consequence of rheumatic fever, occurring mainly in female children and generally self-limiting.

As patron saint of Czechoslovakia, Saint Vitus' name is attached to the cathedral at Prague. In 1969, his memorial day was restricted to local calendars and removed from the Roman Catholic Calendar.

REFERENCES 6, 9, 45

470

Vulganius

MEMORIAL DAY **November 3**

PATRONAGE **Colic, calculi, hernia**

LIFE & LEGEND

Vulganius was an Englishman by birth. He left home to pursue a religious life in Gaul during the seventh century. He landed at Wissant (Pas-de-Calais), evangelized in the vicinity of Boulogne and Thérouanne, and settled as a hermit in the abbey of Saint-Waast-d'Arras. He died ca. 704 in Arras and was purportedly buried at Christ Church, Canterbury, in a chest on the beam beyond the altar of Saint Stephen. At some undetermined period, his body was transferred to Lens, in Artois, which chose this saint for its patron and has preserved his relics.

REFERENCES 16, 36

W

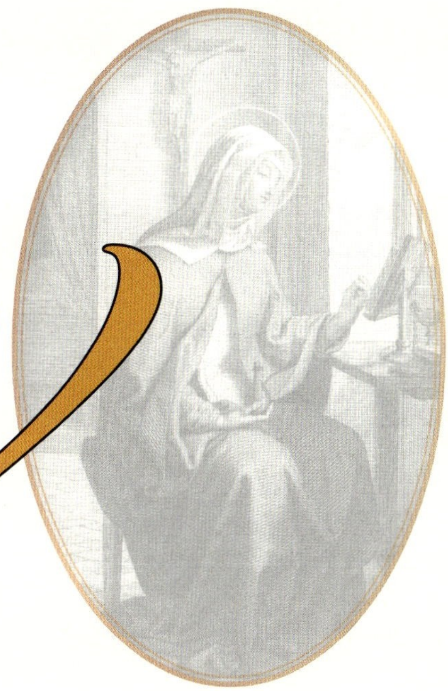

471 Walaricus (Valéry)

MEMORIAL DAY **April 1**

PATRONAGE **Hernia, insanity**

LIFE & LEGEND

Walaricus was born in the Auvergne. He committed the entire psalter to memory while tending sheep. While still a boy, he was taken by his uncle for a visit to the monastery at Antoingt near Issoire, and Walaricus opted to remain there. He later entered the abbey of Saint-Germain-d'Auxerre, and then moved to the monastery at Luxeuil to be under the spiritual direction of Saint Columban. It was there that Walaricus professed his monastic vows. When Columban was expelled from Luxeuil by King Theodoric, Walaricus and a monk named Waldolanus became missionaries in Neustria, the northwestern part of modern France. Longing for a secluded life, Walaricus built a hermitage near the sea at the mouth of the Somme. Even in seclusion, however, he attracted disciples, whom he organized into the community later known as Leucone ca. 614. From here Abbot Walaricus evangelized the Pas-de-Calais and eastern length of the English Channel. He died ca. 620.

REFERENCES 6, 14, 16, 36

472
Walburga

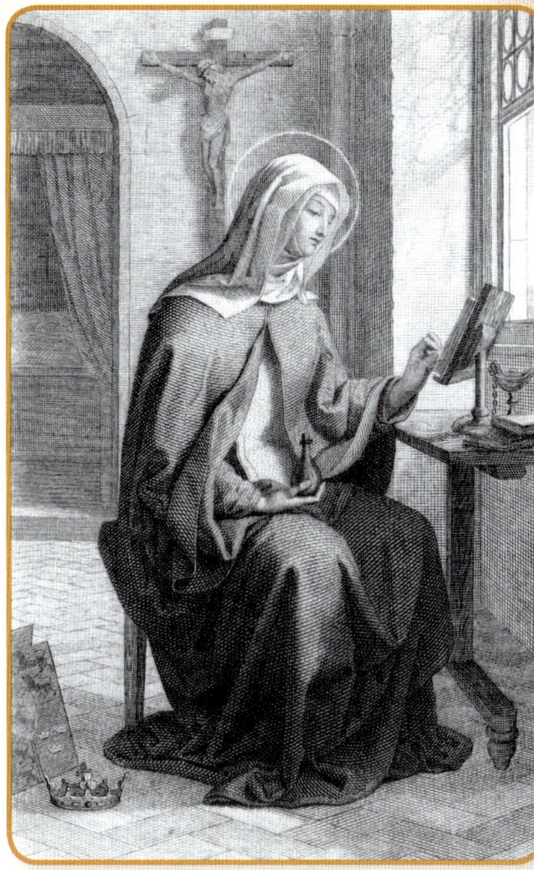

MEMORIAL DAYS **February 25, May 1**

PATRONAGE **Coughs, plague, dog bites and rabies, lung diseases, harvest, sailors and storms**

LIFE & LEGEND

The name of Walburga is derived from Old German, meaning "strong protection." Walburga was born in Devonshire, England, ca. 710, the daughter of Saint Richard the King, and the sister of Saint Willibald and Saint Winebald. She studied and became a nun at Wimborne monastery in Dorset, England. Her education prepared her for writing about the life of Saint Winebald and the travels of Saint Willibald to Palestine. As a consequence of these productions, she is regarded as the first woman author of England and Germany.

Saint Boniface, Walburga's mother's brother, was one of the first missionaries to call on women for assistance. Walburga responded to the call and initially went to Antwerp, where a church bearing the name of Saint Walburga exists. She moved on to Heidenheim, where she served as abbess near her brother, Winebald, who was in charge of the monastery. When Winebald died, Walburga added the charge of the monastery to her own duties. She evangelized and cured illnesses of pagans during her life.

She died in Swabia, Germany, in 779. She was laid to rest next to Winebald, and many miracles took place at the tomb. A rock where her relics were placed exuded an oil that effected miraculous cures, particularly of the plague and rabies. Her remains were translocated to Eichstadt, Germany, and placed in the Church of the Holy Cross, which is now called Saint Walburga's. She was canonized by Pope Adrian II ca. 872.

REFERENCES 6, 9

473
Walfroy

MEMORIAL DAY **July 7**

PATRONAGE **Gout, foot disorders, paralysis**

LIFE & LEGEND

Born in Lombardy, Walfroy crossed the Alps to pursue a monastic life at the monastery of Atane (Limousin), then under the direction of the future Saint Yriez. Once on a journey with Saint Yriez, the holy man showed Walfroy a mountain dedicated to Diana and surmounted by a colossal statue of the goddess. To counter the pagan association of the mountain, Walfroy became a stylite (ascetic) at its highest point. Atop the column he erected, Walfroy was able to stand or kneel, but unable to lie down. Saint Gregory of Tours visited Walfroy atop his column and relates the austerities and hardships the monk endured in all seasons. His example moved many in the surrounding villages to convert to Christianity and to pull down the statue of Diana. At the behest of local bishops, Walfroy eventually descended from his column to live in a monastery he founded in honor of Saint Martin. When this monastery burned down in 598, Walfroy moved to Yvois, where he was ordained a priest by Magneric, archbishop of Treves.

REFERENCES 16, 36

474

Walstan

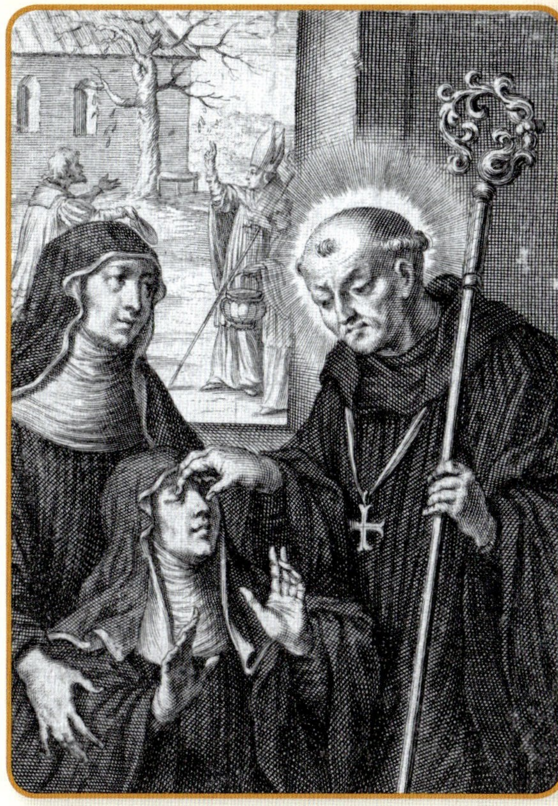

MEMORIAL DAY **May 30**

PATRONAGE **Fever, blindness, lameness, paralysis**

LIFE & LEGEND

Born into a noble and wealthy family of Bawburgh, near Norfolk in England, Walstan left his family at age 12 to live as a medicant pilgrim. To this end he became a farmhand in nearby Taverham. Walstan lived in poverty, giving most of his wages, his clothes, and even his shoes to the poor. He was known for austerity and the gift of miracles. One of his employers wanted to make him an heir, but Walstan asked only for a pregnant cow. Walstan died suddenly one day in 1016 while working in a field. The cow's twin calves carried his body to Bawburgh church where they passed through the solid walls and left Walstan's body at the altar. He was buried at Bawburgh, where his grave became a site of pilgrimage by those seeking a miraculous cure for their infirmities.

REFERENCES 6, 16, 36

475

Walter of Poitiers (Gauthier)

MEMORIAL DAY **January 22**

PATRONAGE **Fever, paralysis, epilepsy**

LIFE & LEGEND

Walter, whose name has a Germanic derivation, meaning "leader of the army," was born into a noble family in Brabant. He became a monk at the abbey at Citeaux and a teacher of theology. He was made bishop of Poitiers in 1279, in spite of his reluctance to assume the office. He was deposed from the episcopal seat of Poitiers by Pope Clement V, who had had difficulties with Walter when serving as archbishop of Bordeaux. Walter returned to his monastery, where he died in 1307.

REFERENCES 16, 36

476
Walter of Pontoise

MEMORIAL DAY **April 8**

PATRONAGE **Fever, eye diseases, rheumatism**

LIFE & LEGEND

Walter was a native of Andainville in Picardy. Trained in the liberal arts, he taught philosophy and rhetoric before entering the Benedictine abbey of Rebois-en-Bris. Later, against his own will, he was chosen by King Philip I to become abbot of the new monastery founded at Pontoise by the Count of Amiens. Although he had hoped for a life of seclusion and prayer on entering the monastic life, Walter obeyed. He was never comfortable in his responsibilities and eventually fled Pontoise to take refuge in Cluny, where he hoped to resume the life of a simple monk. He was discovered there, however, by monks from Pontoise and compelled to return to his abbey. Some time later, Walter again fled Pontoise, settling this time in a hermitage on an island in the Loire near Tours. Once again he was discovered and forced to return to Pontoise. Finally, on a journey to Rome, Walter petitioned Pope Gregory VII to be relieved of his office as abbot of Pontoise. The pope refused and admonished him to accept the burden of his abbacy, though contrary to his own spiritual aspirations. Walter obeyed, carried on the duties of his office, and founded a convent for women at Bertaucourt. In 1095, Walter died suddenly of a fever, which accounts for that patronage.

REFERENCES 6, 16, 36

477

Werenfrid (Guerfroy)

MEMORIAL DAY **August 27**

PATRONAGE **Gout, joint diseases**

LIFE & LEGEND

Werenfrid was one of the 12 apostles sent from England by Saint Willibrord to evangelize the Frisians and to preach the Holy Gospel in Germany. He converted a great number of idolators in the village of Elste in Holland, and he enjoyed the same success at Westerwoert, where he died ca. 780 after having accompanied Saint Swithbert on several of his missions. His death roused great emotion throughout Holland. When the villages of Elste and Westerwoert disputed over Werenfrid's remains, it was agreed to harness a wagon bearing the saint's relics and let it go wherever God might direct. According to one legend, the oxen that pulled the wagon went to Elste, where great miracles have been worked at Werenfrid's tomb ever since. According to others, the coffin was placed in the river and it floated down to settle in Elste. This interpretation is commemorated on the Overbetuwe coat of arms.

REFERENCES 16, 36, 45

478

William Firmatus

MEMORIAL DAY **April 24**

PATRONAGE **Headache**

LIFE & LEGEND

Born into a noble family of Tours, William served as a soldier before commencing the study of medicine in 1026. He enjoyed a successful medical practice, acquiring both fame and some degree of wealth. Du Broc de Segange relates that William one day encountered a demon in the form of an ape seated on the chest where he kept his money. When asked why he was seated on William's property, the demon responded, "It is my property that I am guarding and not yours." Perceiving his own avarice, William renounced the world and gave all he had to the poor. With his mother, he retired to a secluded spot near Tours into a life of solitude and poverty.

After the death of his mother, he withdrew even further into the forest of Concise, near Laval. He made two pilgrimages to the Holy Land. During one of these he was imprisoned by the Saracens, but released. Following both pilgrimages, William returned to a hermetic life near Mantilly. During a drought, he struck the ground with his staff and caused a spring of water to appear. After his death in 1103, William's holiness continued to be revealed by miraculous cures attributed to his intercession.

REFERENCES 6, 16, 50

479

William Tempier

MEMORIAL DAY **March 27**

PATRONAGE **Hemorrhage**

LIFE & LEGEND

William Tempier was a native of Poitiers. He entered the monastery of Saint-Helaire-de-la-Celle, of which he became a canon regular and eventually abbot. In 1184, he was chosen bishop of Poitiers, and he devoted himself to eradicating simony within his diocese and countering secular interference in Church affairs. William was buried in 1197 behind the high altar of the church of Saint Cyprien in Poitiers. His tomb became a place of pilgrimage and the site of healing miracles, in particular for those afflicted with hemorrhage.

REFERENCES 6, 16, 36

480 Willibrord

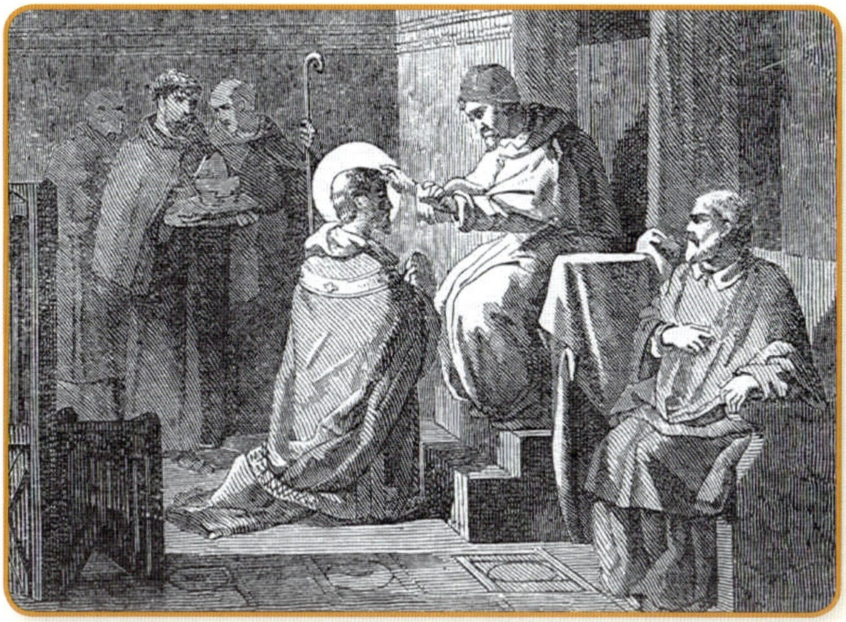

MEMORIAL DAY **November 7**

PATRONAGE **Epilepsy, convulsions**

LIFE & LEGEND

Willibrord, the son of Saint Hilgis, was born in Northumbria, England, in 658, and was sent at age 7 to study in the monastery at Ripon. At age 20 he went to Ireland, where he spent 12 years in Irish monastic schools. Willibrord was ordained at age 30. The following year (690), he was sent with 11 other monks to Friesland to serve as a missionaries. Landing at the mouth of the Rhine, the English missionaries preached in Lower Friesland under the protection of Pepin of Herstal, who had recently conquered the region from the pagan ruler, Radbod. Willibrord traveled to Rome to receive the pope's blessing for his mission. He was sent to Rome a second time by Pepin, who wanted Willibrord to be consecrated a bishop. In 695, Willibrord was made bishop of the Frisians, the founding bishop of Utrecht, by Pope Sergius I, who also gave him the name Clement.

On his return to Friesland, he established his see at Utrecht. Willibrord founded Echternach monastery in Luxembourg, which quickly became a center of ecclesiastic influence in the region. He extended his missionary activities to Upper Friesland and, with less success, into Denmark. In 714, he baptized Charles Martel's son, Pepin the Short, who later became king of the Franks. A year later, Pepin of Herstal's holdings in Friesland were reconquered by Radbod, who burned Willibrord's churches, murdered some of his clergy, and caused many to apostatize. After Radbod's death in 719, Willibrord resumed preaching among the Frisians, now with the assistance of Saint Boniface.

Willibrord, known as the Apostle of the Frisians, died in 739 at Echternach at age 81. His relics are at Echternach and in the Cathedral of Saint Catherine in Utrecht. Butler describes a dance performed by hundreds or even thousands at Willibrord's shrine each Whitsunday: "The participants, four or five abreast and hand-fasted or arm-in-arm, proceed with a hopping or dancing motion, in which for every three steps forward they take two back, in time to a traditional tune played by bands." Du Broc de Segange maintains that this dance commemorates Willibrord's deliverance of his diocese from "an epidemic of Saint Guy's dance," a choreiform movement disorder otherwise known as "Sydenham's chorea" or "Saint Vitus' dance."

REFERENCES 6, 16, 36, 46

481

Wolfgang

MEMORIAL DAY **October 31**

PATRONAGE **Stroke, paralysis, stomach diseases, apoplexy**

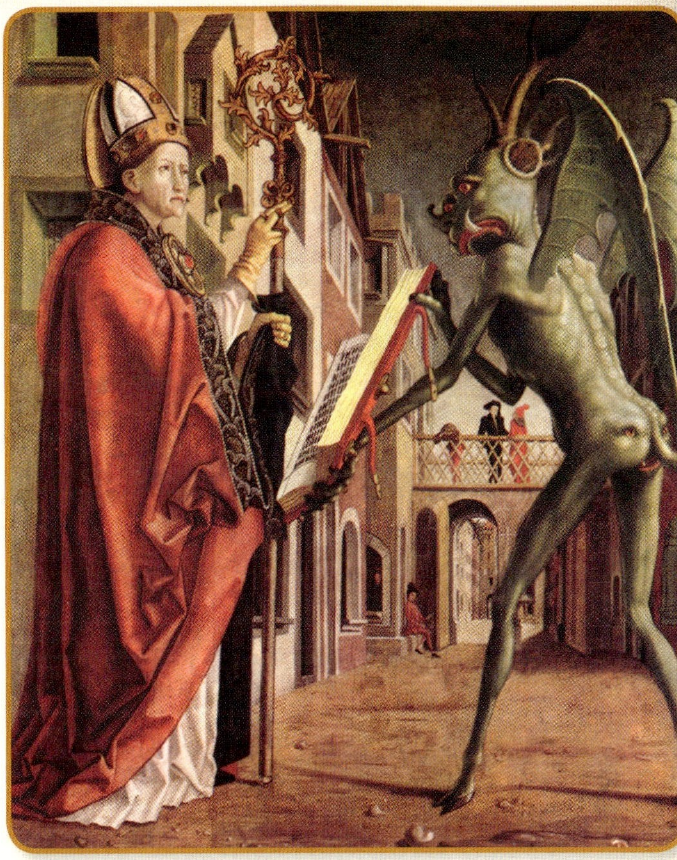

LIFE & LEGEND

Wolfgang, whose name means "wolf going," was one of the three great German saints of the tenth century; the other two were Saint Ulrich and Saint Conrad of Constance. Wolfgang was born ca. 934 into a Swabian noble family, and he began his ecclesiastic studies at home before entering the monastic school at Reichenau Abbey. He studied at Würzburg and Trier and then entered the Benedictine Order at the Abbey of Maria Einsiedelm in Switzerland, where he was ordained in 968. Two years later he was made director of the abbey school. In 972, he evangelized the hostile Magyars in what is now Hungary. That same year he was made bishop of Regensberg, Germany. In that capacity, he was the tutor of Emperor Henry II, the German King and Holy Roman Emperor, who was later canonized as Saint Henry II. Wolfgang was noted for reforming the convents in his bishopric, his preaching, his teaching ability, and his care of the needy. The latter earned him the designation of The Great Almoner.

Toward the end of his life he became a hermit. He died while traveling in 994. He was buried in the crypt of Saint Emmeram church in Regensburg. Many miracles were ascribed to his relics, and he was canonized in 1052 by Pope Leo IX.

REFERENCES 9, 45

Z

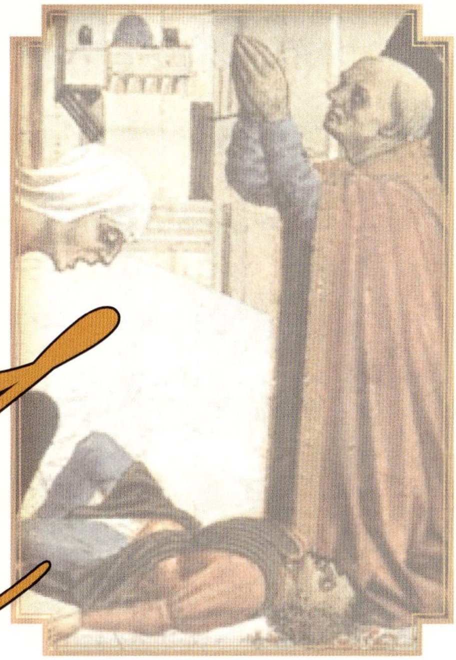

482
Zenaide

MEMORIAL DAY **Not known**

PATRONAGE **Physicians, disease in general**

LIFE & LEGEND

Zenaide was a relative of the Apostle Paul, and, like the Apostle, hailed from Tarsus, where he practiced as a physician. After his conversion to Christianity, Zenaide retired to a cave near the city of Demetriade, together with his sister Saint Filonilla, where he continued to practice the healing art and perform other good works. He died a hermit, and, because he treated every sort of malady, is regarded as the patron saint of diseases in general.

REFERENCE 50

483

Zenobius

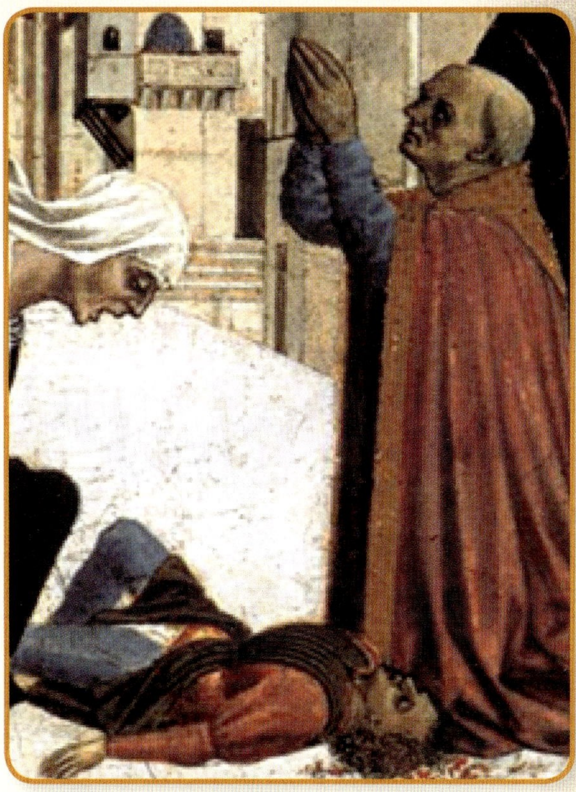

MEMORIAL DAY **May 25**

PATRONAGE **Headache, Florence**

LIFE & LEGEND

Zenobius was born in Florence in the middle of the fourth century. He was baptized at 21 by Bishop Theodore, who also ordained Zenobius and made him an archdeacon. On the advice of Saint Ambrose of Milan, Zenobius was sent by Pope Damasus on a diplomatic mission to the imperial court at Constantinople. On the death of Theodore, Zenobius was made bishop of Florence. He evangelized Florence and the surrounding countryside, combatted the Arian heresy, led a life of exemplary holiness, and performed miracles, including bringing the dead back to life. Zenobius died ca. 417.

REFERENCES 6, 9, 16, 36, 45, 46

484
Zoilus

MEMORIAL DAY **June 27**

PATRONAGE **Pain**

LIFE & LEGEND

Zoilus was one of 20 Christians martyred together at Cordova during the persecution of the emperor Diocletian, ca. 304. He was born into a patrician family of Cordova, and he was a Christian from infancy. Du Broc de Segange relates that one of Zoilus' torturers "wanted to make him suffer a torment that was entirely new, so he struck him repeatedly on the lower vertebrae of the spine, until by this means he forced out his entrails. Without a doubt, this is what gave Spaniards the idea of invoking the holy martyr against pains in the side."

REFERENCES 6, 16, 36

485

Zosimus

MEMORIAL DAY **March 30**

PATRONAGE **Plague**

LIFE & LEGEND

Zosimus was born to prosperous landowners near the city of Syracuse in Sicily. At age 7, he was placed in the monastery of Santa Lucia, where he was assigned the task of tending the saint's tomb. He was displeased with the monastic life until he had a vision from Saint Lucia, who indicated that she was angry with him. The Holy Mother assuaged Saint Lucia's anger, and, in turn, Zosimus became more accepting of the monastic life.

Zosimus became a monk in the community of Santa Lucia, where he was inconspicuous and little regarded by the other brothers. When the abbot Faustus died, the monks asked the bishop of Syracuse to appoint his successor. The bishop came to the monastery, convened the monks, and asked whether all the brotherhood was present. When told that only Zosimus was absent, because he was ordered to watch the front gate, the bishop sent for him. When Zosimus entered the room, the bishop is said to have exclaimed, "Ecco il vostro abbate!" (Here is your abbot!) A few days later Zosimus was ordained to the priesthood. The humble Zosimus surprised many with the zeal and wisdom he displayed in managing the abbey. In 649, Zosimus was made bishop of Syracuse, an office he held until he died, ca. 660.

REFERENCES 6, 16, 36

References

1. Badouin M. Origine et signification thérapeutique des clés des saints dans le traitement de la rage. Bull Soc Française Hist Méd 9:32-43, 1910.
2. Baring-Gould S. The Lives of the Saints, 2 vols. London: John C. Nimmo, 1897-1898.
3. Bocchi L. Sul culto di San Venanzio matire come protettore dei traumatizzati. Chir Organi Mov 46:162-165, 1958.
4. Brewer EC. A Dictionary of Miracles. Philadelphia: Lippincott, 1894.
5. Briggs CV. The Encyclopedia of Angels. New York: Plume, 1997.
6. Butler A. Butler's Lives of the Saints, 12 vols. Allen, TX: Christian Classics, 1996.
7. Butler A. Vies des Pères, des Martyrs et des Autres Principaux Saints, 22 vols. Louvain, Belgium: Vanlinthout & Vandenzande, 1835.
8. Caracci P. Il culto dei santi taumaturghi in Friuli. Pagine Stor Med 14:34-38, 1970.
9. Catholic encyclopedia. Available at *www.catholic.org/encyclopedia.*
10. The Catholic University of America Press. Saint Gregory the Great: Dialogues. New York: Fathers of the Church, 1959.
11. Chaudon LM, ed. Nouveau Dictionnaire Historique, 13 vols, 8th ed. Lyon, France: Bruyset Ainé, 1804.
12. Clendening L. The plague saints. Bull Soc Med History Chic 4:133-141, 1930.
13. Cunningham LS. The Meaning of Saints. San Francisco: Harper and Row, 1980.
14. Delaney JL. Dictionary of Saints. Garden City, NY: Doubleday, 1980.
15. Donaghy TJ. Lives of the Saints II. New York: Catholic Book Publishing, 1992.
16. Du Broc de Segange L. Les Saints Patrons des Corporations et Protecteurs, 2 vols. Paris: Bloud et Barral, 1887.
17. Duffin J. Medical miracle. Sat Night 112:29-42, 1997.
18. Dunbar A. A Dictionary of Saintly Women, 2 vols. London: George Bell & Sons, 1904.
19. Encyclopedia Britannica. Available at *www.britannica.com.*
20. Encyclopaedia Judaica, 2nd ed. Detroit: Macmillan, 2007.
21. Farmer DH. The Oxford Dictionary of Saints. Oxford: Oxford University, 2004.

22. Fatovic-Ferencic S, Dürrigl MA, Repanic-Braun M. Two unconventional testimonies of urolithiasis in the 18th century on the 1600th anniversary of St. Liborius' death. Scand J Urol Nephrol 32:245-249, 1998.
23. Fay HM. Quelques saints guérisseurs de la lèpre dans le sud-ouest de la France. Bull Soc Française Hist Méd 6:32-38, 1907.
24. Fletcher R. On some diseases bearing names of saints. Bristol Med Chir J 30:295-315, 1912.
25. Fosseyeux M. Les saints protecteurs contre la 'male' mort ay moyen-âge et la renaissance. Bull Soc Française Hist Méd 29:339-449, 1935.
26. Giussano GP. The Life of St. Charles Borromeo, 2 vols. London: Burns & Oates, 1884.
27. Glaire JB. Dictionnaire Universel des Sciences Ecclésiastiques, 2 vols. Paris: Poussielgue Frères, 1868.
28. Goodier A. Saints for Sinners. Garden City, NY: Image Books, 1959.
29. Gray A, Brittain F. A History of Jesus College, Cambridge. Cambridge: Silent Books, 1988.
30. Gregory of Tours. History of the Franks. London: Penguin, 1977.
31. Guérin P, Giry F, eds. Les Petits Bollandistes, 17 vols, 7th ed. Bar-le-Duc, France: Typographie Des Celestins, 1872-1874.
32. Guyotjeannin C. Notes sur quelques saints guérisseurs bretons. Rev Hist Pharm 20:479-483, 1971.
33. Jacobus de Voragine. The Golden Legend: Readings on the Saints. Princeton: Princeton University, 1993.
34. Jewish virtual library. Available at *www.jewishvirtuallibrary.org.*
35. Jogues I. René Goupil, 1608-1642: Jogue's Narrative. Available at *www.wyandot.org/goupil.htm.*
36. Kerler DH. Die Patronate der Heiligen. Ulm: Heinrich Kerler, 1905.
37. McBrien R. Lives of Saints. San Francisco: Harper, 2001.
38. Meige H. Deux saints guérisseurs des foux: Saint Menoux et Saint Dizier. Bull Soc Française Hist Méd 3:471-475, 1904.
39. Merritt HS. The legend of St. Achatius. Art Bull 45:258, 1963.
40. Miller MJ. Joseph Moscati: saint, doctor, miracle-worker, 2004. Available at *www.catholiceducation.org/articles/catholic-stories/cs0067.html.*
41. Moule L. Saint-Eloi guérisseur et la legende du pied-coupé. Bull Soc Française Hist Méd 9:103-147, 1910.
42. New Catholic Dictionary. New York: Universal Knowledge Foundation, 1929.
43. One Hundred Saints: Their Lives and Likenesses Drawn from Butler's "Lives of the Saints" and Great Works of Western Art. Boston: Little Brown, 1993.

44. Oxford Dictionary of National Biography, 22 vols. London: Oxford University, 1963-1990.
45. Saint Augustine's Abbey, Ramsgate. The Book of Saints: A Dictionary of Servants of God Canonized by the Catholic Church, 5th ed. London: A & C Black, 1966.
46. Santi beati e testimoni. Available at *www.santiebeati.it.*
46a. Severus S. On the Life of St. Martin. Roberts A, tr. New York: Christian Literature, 1890.
47. Shewsbury JFD. The saints and epidemic disease. Birm Med Rev 19:209-224, 1956.
48. Stephens SDG. St. Cadoc and the healing of the deaf. J Largyng Otol 104:1-3, 1990.
49. Teresa of Avila. The Life of Teresa of Jesus: The Autobiography of Teresa of Avila. New York: Doubleday, 1991.
50. Vitiello M. Evoluzione del concetto di 'medico' e medici santi. Minerv Med 60:1271-1300, 1969.
51. Ward B. Harlots of the Desert. Kalamazoo: Cistercian, 1987.
52. Woodward KL. Making Saints. New York: Touchstone, 1996.

Calendar of Saints

January

1 Basil the Great Félix of Bourges Thaumast	*2* Adelard Defendens	*3* Daniel of Padua Genevieve	*4* Pharaildis Rigobert	*5*	*6* Peter Thomas	*7* Tillo Valetine of Passau
8 Lucian of Beauvais Severinus of Noricum	*9* Marciana	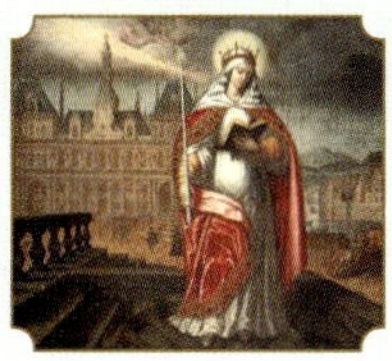	*11*	*12*	*13*	*14* Felix of Nola Nomadia
15 Bonitus Maurus	*16* Fursey Roland of Chèzery	*17* Anthony the Great Sulpicius Pius	*18*	*19*	*20* Molagga Sebastian	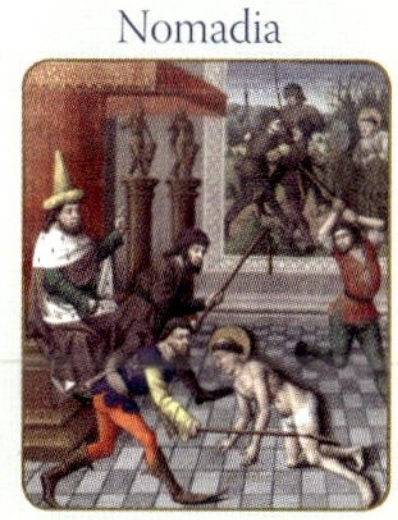
22 Anastasius the Persian Dominic of Sora Inventus Walter of Poitiers	*23* Emerentiana	*24* Francis de Sales Timothy 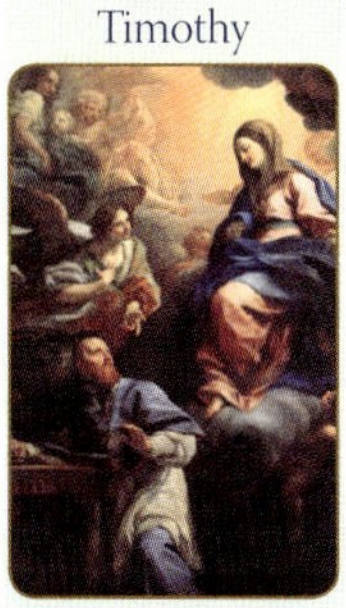	*25* Praejectus of Clermont	*26* Marus	*27*	*28*
29 Arnould Gildas Sulpicius Severus	*30* Aldegonde Haberilla					

February

1 Leontius Ursus of Aosta	2 Hadeloga	3 Blase	4	5 Agatha	6 Alderic Hildegund Vedastus	7 Chrysolius
8	9 Ansbert Apollonia	10 Charalampos Scholastica	11	12 Eulalia of Barcelona Julian the Hospitaler Ludan	13 Gilbert of Meaux Guimerra Licinius	14 Valentine of Rome
	16 Juliana of Nicomedia	17	18	19 Conrad of Piacenza Loup of Chalon	20	21 Peter Damian
	23 Polycarp	24 Mathias the Apostle	25 Avertan Caesarius of Nazianzen Walburga	26	27 Honorina of Conflans Julian of Alexandria Leander	28

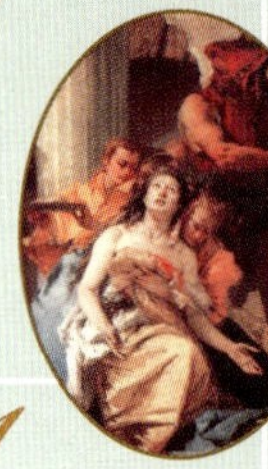

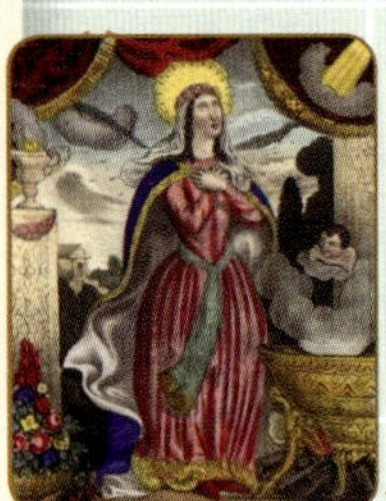

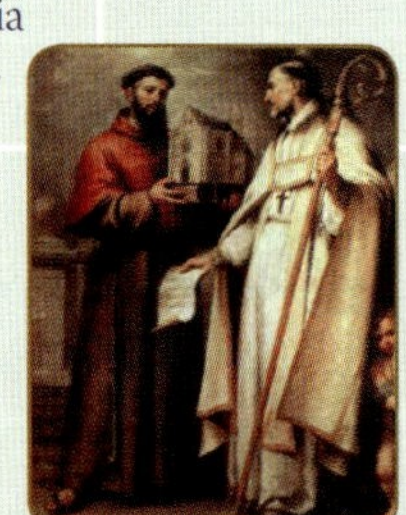

March

1 Albinus of Angers Leo of Rouen Swithbert	2 Charles the Good	3 Cunégonde Guenole	4 Casimir	5	6 Colette Senan of Saint-Pol-de-Léon	7
8 John of God	9		11	12	13 Gerald of Mayo	14 Lubin of Chartres
15 Matrona of Capua	16 Gregory of Armenia	17 Gertrude of Nivelles	18 Salvator of Horta	19 Joseph	20 Cuthbert of Lindisfarne	
22 Paul of Narbonne	23	24 Catherine of Vadstena	25		27 William Tempier	28
29	30 Quirinus Regulus Zosimus	31 Albana Balbina Veronus				

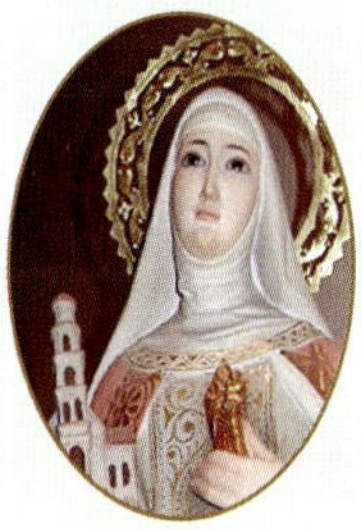

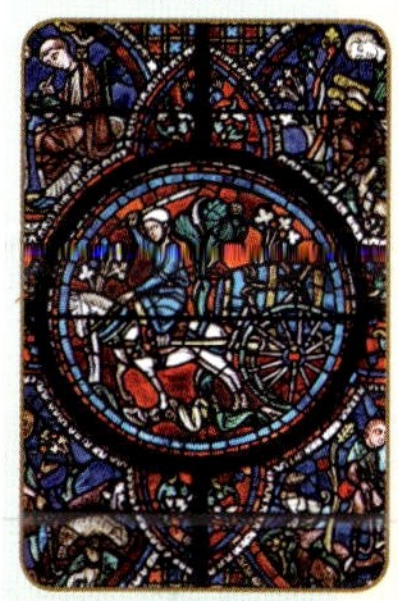

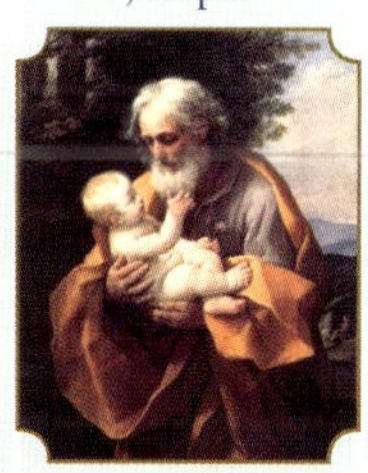

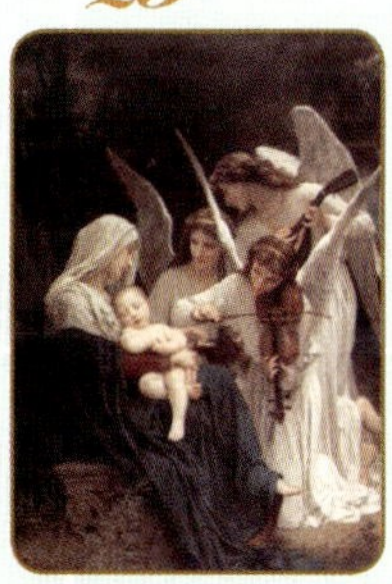

April

1 Hugh of Grenoble; Walaricus	2 Francis of Paola	3 Mary of Egypt	4 Benedict the Moor	5 Vincent Ferrer	6	7 Aybert
8 Walter of Pontoise	9 Casilda of Toledo; Gaucherius	10 Macarius of Antioch	11 Godeberta		13	14
15 César de Bus	16 Drogo; Engratia; Joachim of Siena; Turibius	17 Donanus; Gebuinus of Lyon	18 Agapitus; Ursmar	19	20	21
	23 George	24 Beuve; William Firmatus	25 Fidelis of Spello; Franca of Piacenza	26 Berthilon; Richarius	27	28 Aphrodisius
29 Catherine of Siena; Hugh of Cluny; Peter of Verona	30 Desideratus; Eutropius; Forannan; Onenna					

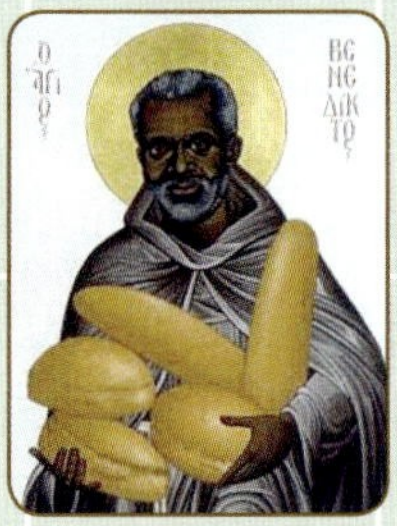

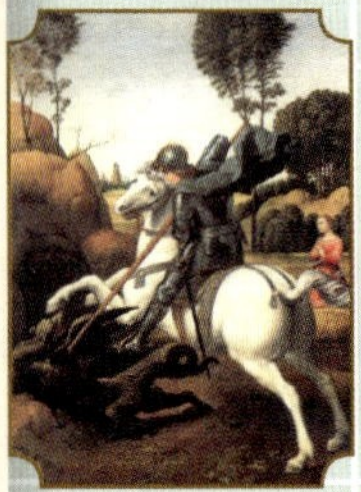

May

1 Bertha ■ Joseph Marculf ■ Peregrine Laziosi Sigismund of Burgundy Theodard ■ Theodulph Walburga	**2** Anthony della Chiesa Athanasius Flamina Germanus of Scotland	**3**	**4** Godehard	**5** Avertinus Lando	**6**	**7** Domitian of Maestricht Gibrian Serenicus and Serenus
8 Achatius Aurelianus of Limoges	**9** Beatus	**10** Catald of Taranto Job	**11** Gengulf Udaut	**12** Danio Pancras of Rome	**13** Mucius Rolande Servatius	**14**
15 Dymphna Guimerra	**16** Adamo of Fermo Gens Ubaldo of Gubbio	**17** Framechildis Ratho	**18** Felix of Split Venantius of Camerino	**19**	**20** Baudelius Bernardino of Siena	**21** Isberga Ortarius
22 Boetianus Loup of Limoges Quiteria Rita of Cascia	**23** Desiderius of Langres Desiderius of Vienne Guibert	**24** Gerard of Lunel	**25** Philip Neri Zenobius	**26** Godo Priscus	**27** Hildevert	**28** Germanus of Paris
29 Maximinus of Besançon	**30** Walstan	**31** Petronilla Simplicianus				

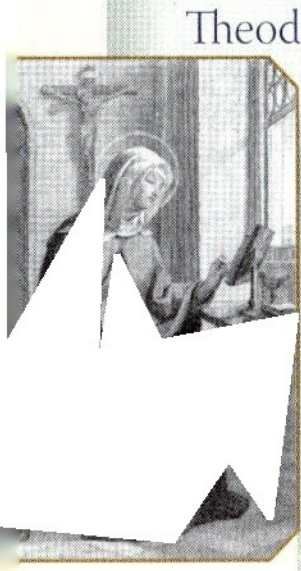

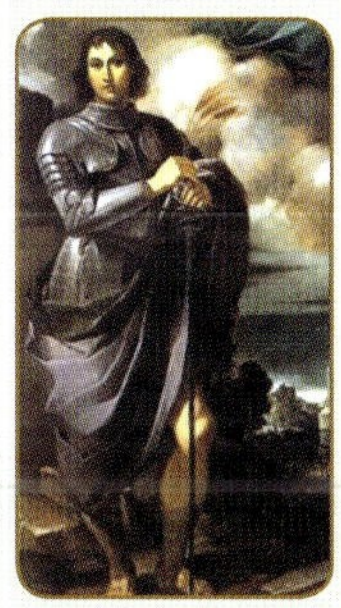

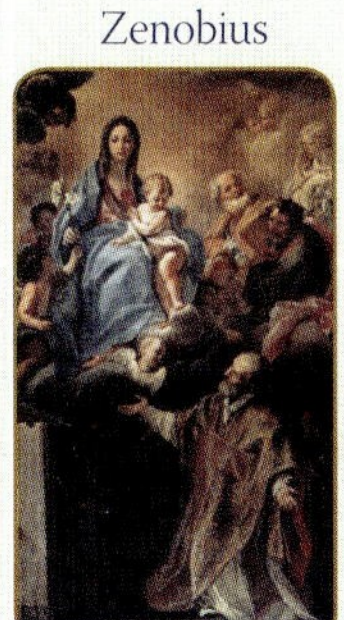

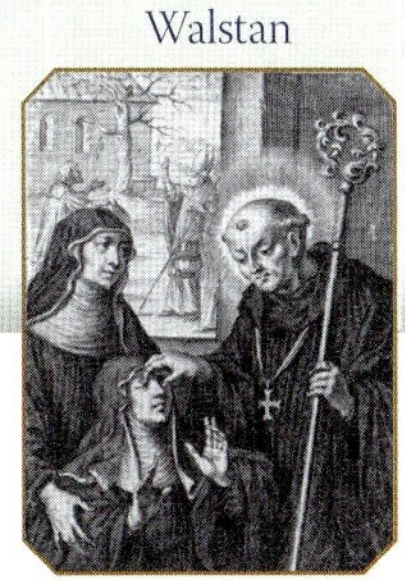

June

1 Caprasius; Clarus of Albi; Florentius	2 Erasmus 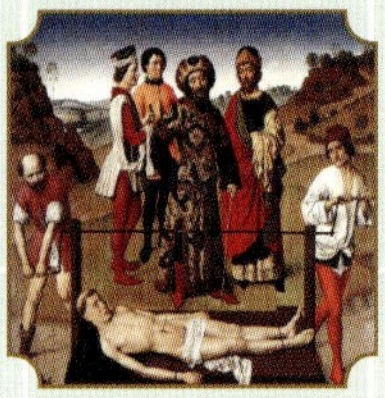	3 Clotilda; John the Great Sinner; John of Ortica	4	5 Placido of Recanati	6 Claude of Besançon; Jean François Régis; Norbert	7 Eugenia; Gilbert of Neufontaines; Meriadoc
8 Fortunatus of Fano; Medard; Syre		10 Landericus	11 Amable; Macra	12 Cunera	13 Anthony of Padua	14
15 Abraham of Saint Cirgues; Crescentia; Psalmodius; Vitus	16 Berthaldus of Reims; Lutgardis	17 Alena; Hervé; Teresa and Sanchia of Portugal	18 Calogeros	19 Deodatus; Gervasius of Milan; Juliana Falconieri; Ursicinus	20	21 Alban of Mainz; Aloysius Gonzaga; Engelmund; Lazarus the Poor Man; Leutfridus ■ Méen
22 Consortia	23 Agrippina of Mineo; Etheldreda; Mary of Oignies	24 Frisius; John of Arras	25 Emilien	26 Dizaint; Medicus	27 Zoilus	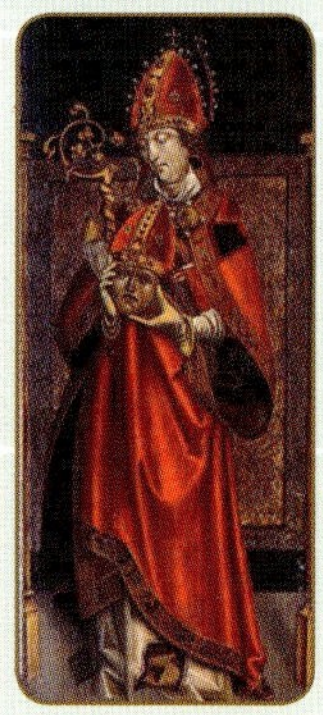
29 Peter the Apostle 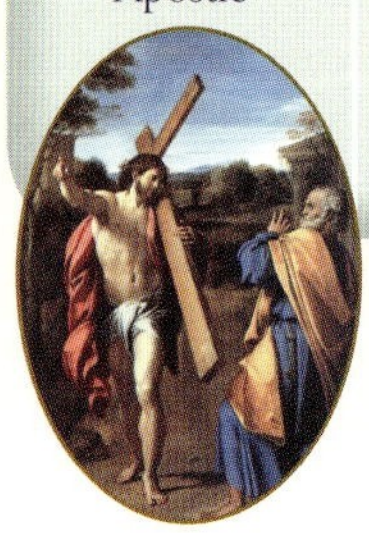	30 Donatus; Martial of Limoges; Theobald of Provence					

July

1 Gall of Clermont Theodoric of Mont d'Or	2 Otto of Bamberg	3 Raymond of Toulouse	4 Ulrich of Augsburg	5	6 Godeleva	7 Ethelburga Félix of Nantes Walfroy
8 Kilian Vaury	9 Paulina do Coração Agonizante de Jesus	10 Amalburga of Maubeuge Amalburga of Munsterbilzsen Pacificus	11 Alexander Benedict of Nursia Hidulf	12 Lucius of Cavargna Menoux	13 Henry II	14 Camillus of Lellis
15 Apronia Bonosa	16 Reineldis	17 Fredegand	18 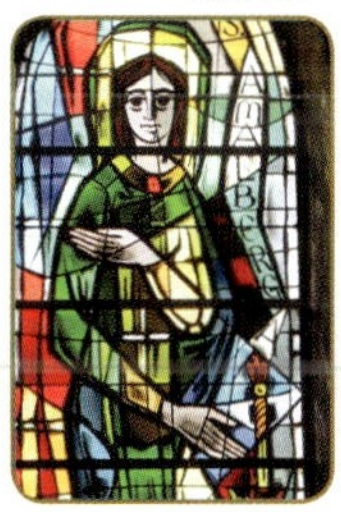	19 Bernulph of Utrecht	20 Margaret of Antioch	21 Julia of Troyes
22 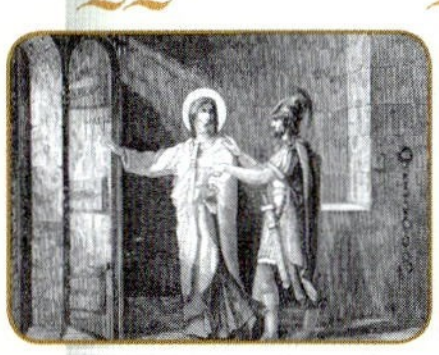	23 Apollinaris of Ravenna Balthasar Liborius of Le Mans	24 Christine of Saint Trond	25 Christopher James the Greater	26 Anne 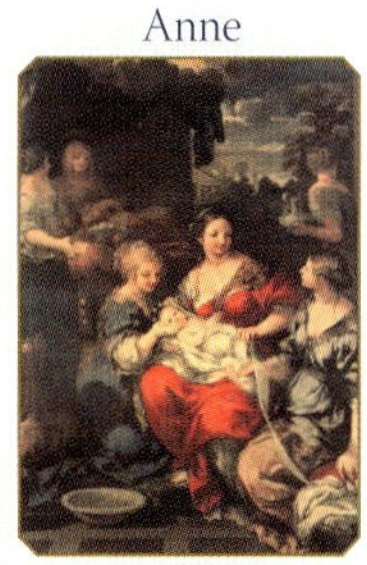	27 Pantaleon	28
29 Lazarus of Bethany Loup of Troyes Martha of Bethany	30 Peter Chrysologus	31 Germanus of Auxerre				

August

1 Alphonsus Maria de Liguori Friard	2	3 Asperenus Godfrey of Le Mans	4	5 Oswald of Northumbria	6 Stapinus	7 Albert of Trapani
8 Cyriacus	9 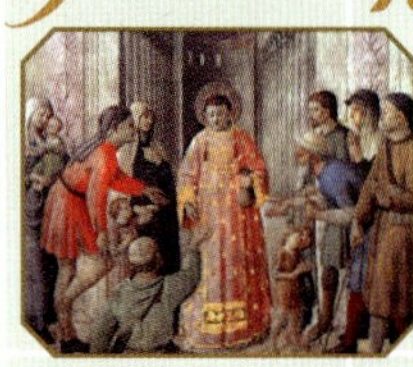	10 Lawrence	11 Clare of Assisi Dinoaldus Philomena Tiburtius	12 Porcarius	13 Radegunde 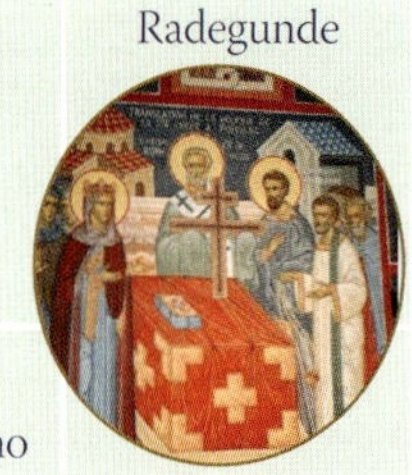	14 Maximilian Kolbe
15 Arnulf of Soissons Stanislaus Kostka	16 Fraimbaud Roch	17 Hyacinth Mamas	18 Fiacre	19 Ezekiel Moreno y Diaz Marianus		21 Jeanne Françoise de Chantal Severus of Agde
22 Symphorian	23 Philip Benizi	24 Bartholomew Ouen of Rouen Rose of Lima	25 Gregory of Utrecht Maginus of Tarragona	26	27 Gebhard of Konstanz Werenfrid	28 Julian of Brioude
29 John the Baptist Sabina	30 Fiacre	31 Albertinus Raymond Nonnatus Victor of Campbon	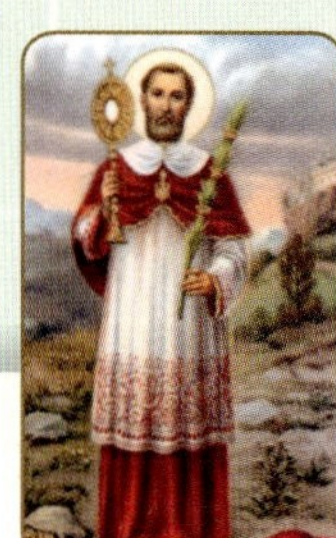			

September

1 Fiacre Giles Juliana of Collalto Loup of Sens	2	3 Gregory the Great Remaclus	4 Rosalia	5	6 Magnus of Füssen	7 Clodoald Eustace Madelbertha Regina of Alise Ventura of Castello
8 Adrian of Nicomedia	9 Omer	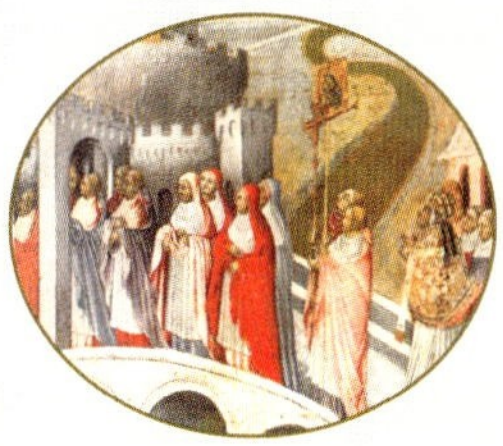		12 Guy of Anderlecht	13 John Chrysostom	14 Notburga
15 Baldus Orana Roland de'Medici	16 Cornelius	17 Lambert of Maastricht Reginald	18 Ferreolus	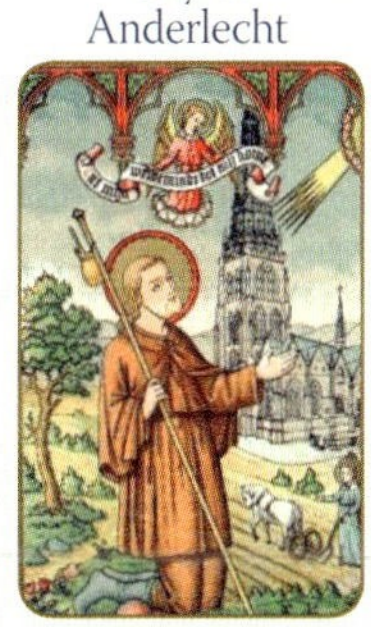	20	21
22 Maurice	23	24 Cadoc of Llancarfan Dalmatius Moner Germer	25 Firminus Loup of Lyon	26 Cosmas and Damian	27 Ceranus Hiltrude Vincent de Paul	28 Annemund Exsuperius
29 Michael the Archangel Raphael	30 Victurnianus				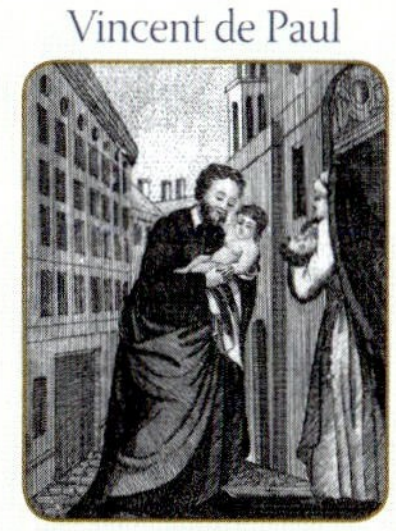	

October

1 Bavo Piat Remigius Thérèse de Lisieux	2 Leodegar	3 Gerard of Brogne Leudomer	4 Teresa of Ávila	5 Charitina Enimia	6 Bruno of Cologne Faith	7
8	9 Bernard of Rodez Denis Gislenus	10 Gereon Tanche	11 Gummarus Taracus	12 Libaria	13 Colman of Stockerau Edward the Confessor Leobonus Venantius of Tours	14 Burchard Manechildis
15 Austriclinianus Leonard of Vandoeuvre	16 Dulcidius of Agen Gerard Majella Gratus Magnobodus Mommolinus	17 Ignatius of Antioch Margaret Mary Alacoque	18 Luke the Evangelist	19 Peter of Alcántara Rene Goupil Veranus	20 Vitalis of Salzburg	21
22 Candida Nepotianus	23 Amo Léothade Luglius and Luglianus Romanus of Rouen		25 Balsamia	26	27	28
29 Baldus Germanus of Montfort Mazerand	30	31 Quintinus Wolfgang				

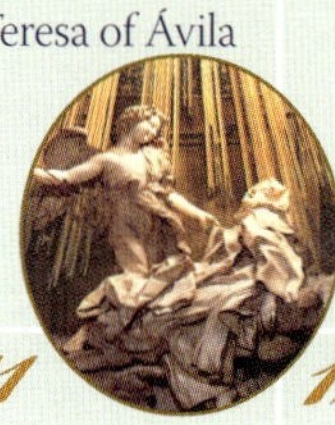

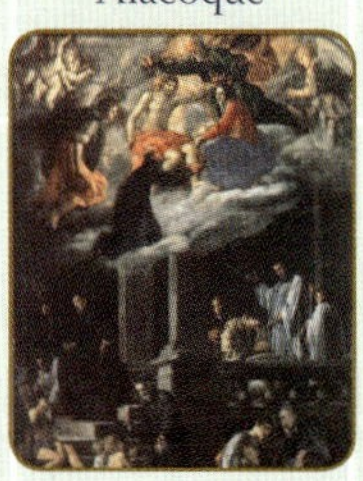

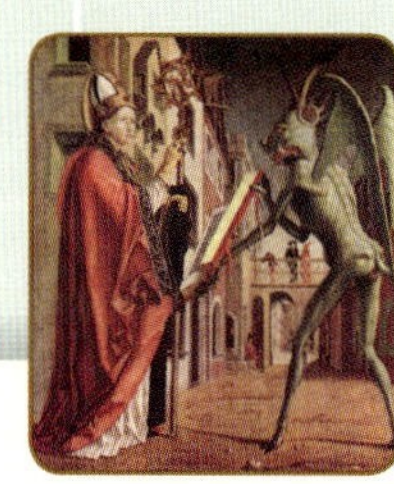

November

1 Maturinus	2	3 Gobrianus, Hubert of Liège, Pirminus, Vulganius	4 Charles Borromeo, Clarus of Vexin	5 Bertilia, Gunsaldus, Millefort	6 Leonard of Noblac	7 Willibrord 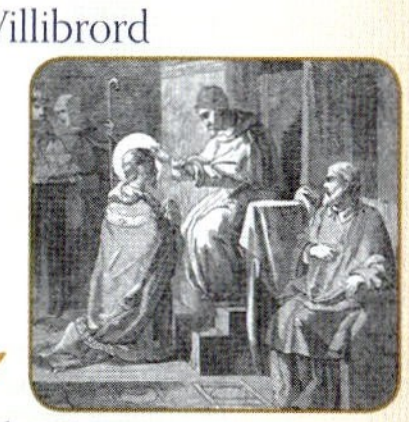
8 Castorius	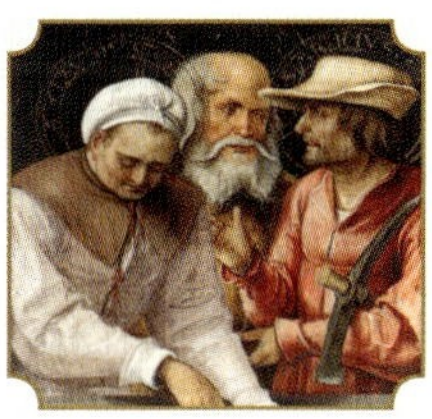	10 Aedh Mac Bricc, Andrew Avellino	11 Martin of Tours, Mennas, Veranus	12	13 Quintianus	14 John Licci
15 Cessator, Malo	16 Balsamia, Giuseppe Moscati, Namphanius	17 Anianus	18 Maudez	19 Elizabeth of Hungary, Patroclus	20 Edmund the Martyr 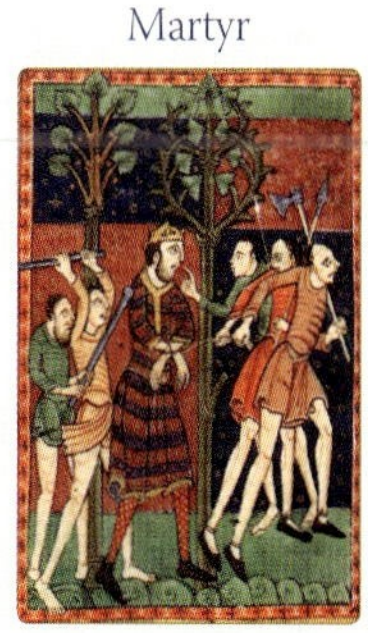	21 Columban
22	23 Phaletrus	24 Portianus	25 Catherine of Alexandria	26		28
29 Saturninus of Toulouse	30 Andrew the Apostle 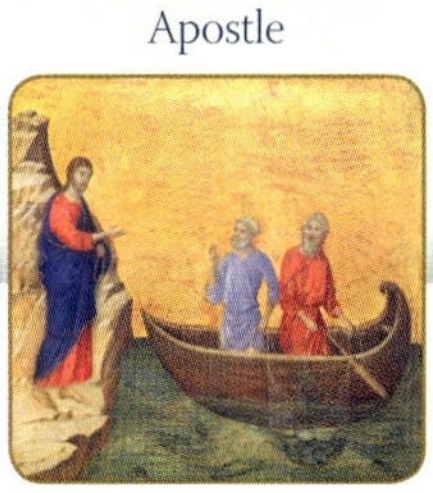					

December

1 Eligius	2 Bibiana	3 Francis Xavier	4 Anno Barbara Osmund	5	6 Aemilianus Nicholas of Bari	7 Fara
8	9 Leocadia		11 Damasus	12	13 Josse Lucy of Syracuse Odile	14 Nicasius
15	16 Ida of Nivelle	17	18 Flavitus	19	20 Dominic of Silos	21 Honoratus of Toulouse
22	23 Asclepius of Limoges Hartman of Brixen Marguerite d'Youville Servulus	24	25	26		28
29 Ebrulf Trophimus of Arles	30	31 Columba of Sens				

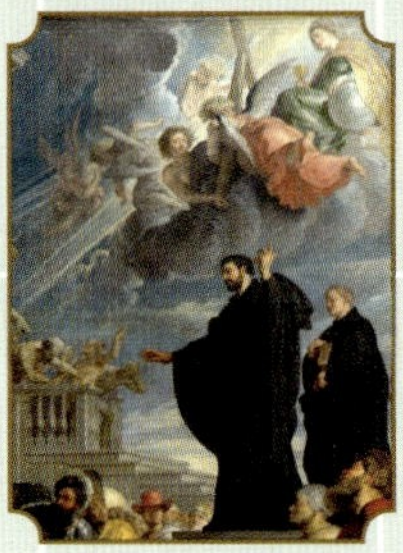

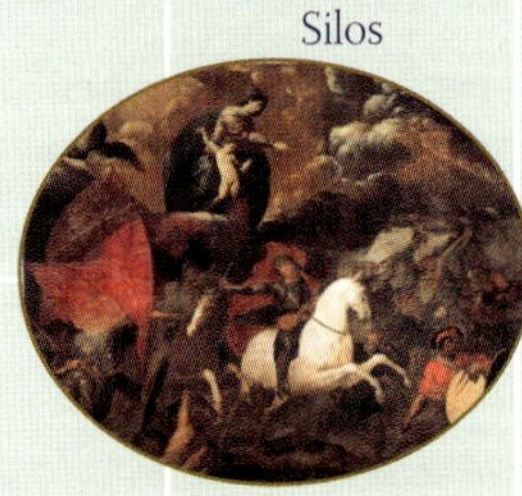

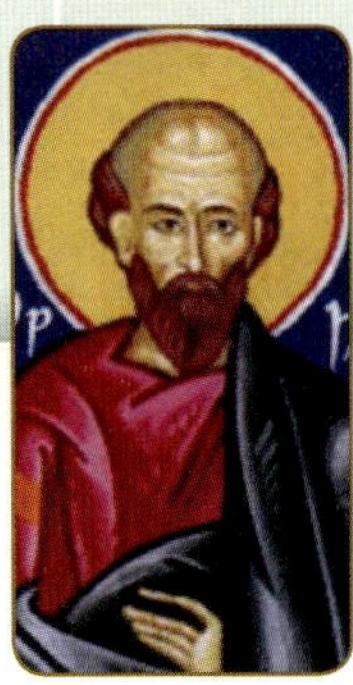

Index of Medical Conditions

A

ABORTION Catherine of Vadstena
AIDS Aloysius Gonzaga, Peregrine Laziosi, Thérèse de Lisieux
ALCOHOLISM John of God, Martin of Tours
AMPUTATION Anthony the Great
ANGINA (*See also* HEART DISEASES) Blase, Swithbert
APOPLEXY Andrew Avellino, Wolfgang
APPENDICITIS Erasmus
ARM PAIN AND FRACTURES Amalburga of Maubeuge
ARTHRITIS Alphonsus Maria de Liguori, James the Greater, Ortarius
ASTHMA Alderic, Gunsaldus

B

BACK PAIN Marguerite d'Youville, Ursus of Aosta
BLINDNESS (*See also* EYE DISEASES) Catald of Taranto, Clarus of Vexin, Cosmas and Damian, Fara Godeleva, Leodegar, Leudomer, Lucy of Syracuse, Lutgardis, Mucius, Odile, Omer, Paul of Narbonne, Porcarius, Portianus, Psalmodius, Raphael, Rolande, Turibius, Udaut, Walstan
BOILS Clodoald, Magnobodus
BREAST DISEASES Agatha, Aldegonde, Giles, Macra, Peregrine Laziosi
BREASTFEEDING - *See* LACTATION
BRUISES Amalburga of Maubeuge

C

CALCULI Apollinaris of Ravenna, Benedict of Nursia, Burchard, Drogo, Emilien, Fiacre, Fursey, Gebuinus of Lyon, Godehard, Lambert of Maastricht, Liborius of Le Mans, Ratho, Rolande, Syre, Vulganius

CANCER Aldegonde, Beatus, Bertilia, Eutropius, Ezekiel Moreno y Diaz, Fiacre, Giles, Peregrine Laziosi, Philomena

CEREBRAL DISORDERS Méen

CHILDBIRTH Alexander, Anne, Anthony of Padua, Apronia, Balsamia, Baudelius, Benedict the Moor, Beuve, Colette, Cunégonde, Daniel of Padua, Desiderius of Langres, Dominic of Silos, Drogo, Erasmus, Eulalia of Barcelona, Gebhard of Konstanz, Gerard Majella, Gislenus, Hildegund, Honoratus of Toulouse, Hyacinth, Jeanne Françoise de Chantal, Juliana of Nicomedia, Leo of Rouen, Leonard of Noblac, Licinius, Lutgardis, Margaret of Antioch, Marguerite d'Youville, Marianus, Mary of Oignies, Norbert, Notburga, Peregrine Laziosi, Peter of Verona, Pirminus, Psalmodius, Raymond Nonnatus, Rita of Cascia, Rose of Lima, Sulpicius Severus, Udaut, Ulrich of Augsburg, Ursus of Aosta, Vitalis of Salzburg

CHILDREN'S DISEASES Abraham of Saint Cirgues, Albinus of Angers, Aldegonde, Anianus, Boetianus, Clotilda, Cunégonde, Eustace, Eutropius, Felix of Split, Fidelis of Spello, Gengulf, Germanus of Montfort, Gibrian, Gislenus, Haberilla, John the Baptist, Leonard of Noblac, Leutfridus, Loup of Lyon, Maurice, Pharaildis, Priscus, Psalmodius, Ubaldo of Gubbio, Vaury

CHOLERA Charalampos, Defendens, Luglius and Luglianus, Nicasius, Roch

COLDS Maurus

COLIC Agapitus, Baldus, Charles Borromeo, Emerentiana, Erasmus, Fiacre, Fursey, Gens, Gervasius of Milan, Liborius of Le Mans, Mamas, Psalmodius, Serenicus and Serenus, Thaumast, Vulganius

CONTAGIOUS DISEASES Adelard, Christine of Saint Trond, Godeberta, Hidulf, Juliana of Nicomedia, Leobonus, Lucy of Syracuse, Martial of Limoges, Peter Thomas, Roch

CONVULSIVE DISORDERS (*See also* EPILEPSY) Bibiana, Claude of Besançon, Cornelius, Firminus, Gislenus, John the Baptist, Loup of Sens, Scholastica, Willibrord

COUGH Blase, Quintinus, Walburga

CRAMPS Cadoc of Llancarfan, Maurice, Pancras of Rome

CROUP Guibert

D

DEAFNESS Adelard, Aurelianus of Limoges, Cadoc of Llancarfan, Christopher, Drogo, Eugenia, Francis de Sales, Leonard of Vandoeuvre, Meriadoc, Orana, Ouen of Rouen

DEFORMITIES Eutropius, Gervasius of Milan, Isberga

DENTITION, INFANT Agapitus, Dalmatius Moner

DIABETES Paulina do Coração Agonizante de Jesus
DIARRHEA Germanus of Auxerre, Loup of Limoges
DISABILITY Claude of Besançon, Dizaint, Eutropius, Gibrian, Giles, Henry II, Lutgardis, Malo, Maximinus of Besançon, Servulus, Ulrich of Augsburg, Vedastus, Walstan
DISEASE (IN GENERAL) Camillus of Lellis, Catherine of Siena, Medicus, Zenaide
DROPSY - *See* **HYDROPS**
DRUG ADDICITION Maximilian Kolbe
DYSENTERY Eulalia of Barcelona, Fiacre, Guy of Anderlecht, Loup of Sens, Lucy of Syracuse, Matrona of Capua, Polycarp, Roch

E

EAR DISEASES Aurelianus of Limoges, Cornelius, Eugenia, Polycarp, Quirinus
ECZEMA Anthony the Great
EDEMA Onenna
EPIDEMIC DISEASES Cosmas and Damian, Eligius, Godeberta, Godo, Hidulf, Julian of Brioude, Leobonus, Macarius of Antioch, Martial of Limoges, Placido of Recanati, Remigius, Roch, Sebastian
EPILEPSY Adamo of Fermo, Alban of Mainz, Albana, Annemund, Anthony the Great, Aphrodisius, Avertinus, Balthasar, Bibiana, Catald of Taranto, Christopher, Cornelius, Defendens, Dinoaldus, Dymphna, Ebrulf, Frisius, Gerard of Lunel, Gervasius of Milan, Giles, Gislenus, Guy of Anderlecht, Hildevert, Joachim of Siena, John the Baptist, John Chrysostom, John the Great Sinner, Lambert of Maastricht, Leobonus, Léothade, Loup of Sens, Maturinus, Millefort, Namphanius, Nomadia, Philip Benizi, Quirinus, Valentine of Passau, Valentine of Rome, Vincent Ferrer, Vitus, Walter of Poitiers, Willibrord
ERGOTISM Anthony the Great, Genevieve
ERYSIPELAS Anthony the Great, Benedict of Nursia, Firminus
EYE DISEASES AND INJURY (*See also* BLINDNESS) Aldegonde, Alena, Aloysius Gonzaga, César de Bus, Clare of Assisi, Clarus of Albi, Clarus of Vexin, Colette, Columba of Sens, Cyriacus, Etheldreda, Eustace, Fara, Félix of Bourges, Felix of Nola, Flamina, Franca of Piacenza, Fursey, Guimerra, Hervé, Joseph, Leodegar, Leudomer, Libaria, Lubin of Chartres, Lucius of Cavargna, Lucy of Syracuse, Magnus of Füssen, Odile, Omer, Porcarius, Portianus, Raphael, Reineldis, Roland of Chèzery, Stanislaus Kostka, Symphorian, Vedastus, Walter of Pontoise

F

FAINTING Ulrich of Augsburg, Valentine of Rome
FEVER Abraham of Saint Cirgues, Adelard, Albert of Trapani, Aldegonde, Alderic, Amalburga of Maubeuge, Amalburga of Munsterbilzsen, Amo, Ansbert, Anthony della Chiesa, Anthony of Padua, Arnould, Austriclinianus, Aybert, Barbara,

Benedict of Nursia, Berthilon, Castorius, Charles the Good, Chrysolius, Claude of Besançon, Clotilda, Colette, Cornelius, Damasus, Desiderius of Vienne, Dominic of Sora, Domitian of Maestricht, Donanus, Donatus, Dulcidius of Agen, Ebrulf, Eustace, Exsuperius, Félix of Bourges, Firminus, Flavitus, Friard, Fursey, Gall of Clermont, Gaucherius, Genevieve, Gens, Gerard of Brogne, Germanus of Paris, Germanus of Scotland, Germer, Gertrude of Nivelles, Godeleva, Godfrey of Le Mans, Hadeloga, Hiltrude, Hugh of Cluny, Inventus, Isberga, Josse, Julia of Troyes, Julian of Brioude, Leobonus, Leontius, Loup of Chalon, Loup of Limoges, Luglius and Luglianus, Mary of Egypt, Mary of Oignies, Mazerand, Medard, Millefort, Nepotianus, Otto of Bamberg, Pacificus, Patroclus, Peter of Alcántara, Peter the Apostle, Peter Chrysologus, Petronilla, Piat, Placido of Recanati, Praejectus of Clermont, Quintianus, Radegunde, Raymond Nonnatus, Reginald, Regulus, Remigius, Richarius, Rigobert, Salvator of Horta, Serenicus and Serenus, Severus of Agde, Sigismund of Burgundy, Stanislaus Kostka, Teresa and Sanchia of Portugal, Thaumast, Theobald of Provence, Theodard, Theodoric of Mont d'Or, Tillo, Udaut, Ulrich of Augsburg, Ursmar, Venantius of Tours, Veronus, Victor of Campbon, Vincent Ferrer, Walstan, Walter of Poitiers, Walter of Pontoise

FISTULA Fiacre

FOOT DISORDERS Gervasius of Milan, Ludan, Maximinus of Besançon, Peter the Apostle, Servatius, Walfroy

FRACTURES AND DISLOCATIONS Amalburga of Munsterbilzsen, Drogo, Félix of Nantes, Gummarus, Jean François Régis, Sigismund of Burgundy, Stanislaus Kostka, Symphorian, Syre, Tiburtius, Venantius of Camerino

G

GALLSTONES Benedict of Nursia, Drogo

GANGRENE Fiacre

GLANDULAR DISORDERS Cadoc of Llancarfan

GOITER Balbina, Blase, Gunsaldus

GOUT Andrew the Apostle, Anno, Austriclinianus, Baldus, Bonitus, Gebuinus of Lyon, Gobrianus, Gregory the Great, Julian of Alexandria, Kilian, Leander, Leontius, Marus, Maurice, Maurus, Maximinus of Besançon, Ortarius, Quirinus, Stapinus, Sulpicius Pius, Trophimus of Arles, Walfroy, Werenfrid

H

HEADACHE Achatius, Aedh Mac Bricc, Aldegonde, Alexander, Anastasius the Persian, Asperenus, Athanasius, Avertinus, Bibiana, Colette, Denis, Emilien, Engratia, Eutropius, Fiacre, Fraimbaud, Framechildis, Gerard of Lunel, Gereon, Gratus, Gurloes, Hildegund, Hugh of Grenoble, Juliana of Collalto, Lando, Leonard of Noblac, Maurus, Menoux, Meriadoc, Odile, Pancras of Rome, Peter Damian,

Peter of Verona, Roland of Chèzery, Roland de'Medici, Saturninus of Toulouse, Severinus of Noricum, Severus of Agde, Simplicianus, Taracus, Teresa of Ávila, Ubaldo of Gubbio, Veronus, Vincent Ferrer, William Firmatus, Zenobius

HEAD INJURIES John Licci

HEART DISEASES Dulcidius of Agen, Fursey, John of God, Philip Neri, Philomena, Piat, Quiteria, Stanislaus Kostka, Swithbert, Teresa of Ávila

HEMORRHAGE Alexander, Asclepius of Limoges, Casilda of Toledo, Consortia, Fiacre, Gervasius of Milan, Lucy of Syracuse, Martha of Bethany, Matrona of Capua, Sabina, Tanche, William Tempier

HEMORRHOIDS Alexander, Fiacre

HERNIA Alban of Mainz, Albertinus, Baudelius, Bertilia, Calogeros, Catald of Taranto, Conrad of Piacenza, Danio, Drogo, Emilien, Fursey, Gummarus, John of Arras, Lambert of Maastricht, Osmund, Ratho, Rolande, Syre, Ventura of Castello, Vulganius, Walaricus

HERPES Anthony the Great, George, Psalmodius

HYDROPS Albana, Eutropius, Firminus, Fursey, Gilbert of Meaux, Lubin of Chartres, Malo, Onenna, Quintinus

I

IMBECILITY Columban

IMPOTENCE Gummarus

INCONTINENCE Gervasius of Milan

INCURABLE DISEASES Christine of Saint Trond, Joseph, Landericus, Praejectus of Clermont

INFECTIONS Agrippina of Mineo

INFERTILITY Adrian of Nicomedia, Agatha, Albert of Trapani, Alexander, Andrew the Apostle, Anne, Anthony of Padua, Bernulph of Utrecht, Casilda of Toledo, Colette, Faith, Fiacre, Francis of Paola, Gilbert of Neufontaines, Guenole, Hyacinth, Jean François Régis, John of Ortica, Maginus of Tarragona, Margaret of Antioch, Mathias the Apostle, Medard, Nicholas of Bari, Phaletrus, Philip Neri, Philomena, Reginald, Remaclus, Sulpicius Severus, Theobald of Alba

INFLAMMATORY DISEASES Benedict of Nursia

INTESTINAL DISORDERS Charles Borromeo, Erasmus, Loup of Limoges, Rolande, Timothy

J

JAUNDICE Albert of Trapani, Gerard of Brogne

JOINT DISEASES Burchard, Gebuinus of Lyon, James the Greater, Kilian, Leander, Ortarius, Philip Neri, Werenfrid

K

KIDNEY DISEASES Albinus of Angers, Benedict of Nursia, Burchard, Friard, Gurloes, Lambert of Maastricht, Margaret of Antioch, Sulpicius Pius, Ursmar, Ursus of Aosta

KIDNEY STONES Alban of Mainz

KNEE DISORDERS Roch

L

LABOR - ***See*** **CHILDBIRTH**

LACTATION Gilbert of Neufontaines, Giles

LAMENESS - ***See*** **DISABILITY**

LEG DISORDERS AND INJURIES Jean François Régis, Ludan, Maximinus of Besançon, Peregrine Laziosi, Philip Neri, Quirinus, Servatius, Stapinus

LEPROSY Agrippina of Mineo, Cessator, Edward the Confessor, Enimia, Francis Xavier, George, Giles, Job, Julian the Hospitaler, Lazarus of Bethany, Lazarus the Poor Man, Loup of Troyes, Lucian of Beauvais, Magnobodus, Méen, Philip Benizi, Quiteria, Radegunde, Vincent de Paul

LEUKEMIA Giuseppe Moscati, Marguerite d'Youville

LIMB REPLANTATION Anthony of Padua

LUMBAGO Lawrence, Sulpicius Pius

LUNG DISEASES Bernardino of Siena, Cunera, Walburga

M

MEASLES Adelard, Maginus of Tarragona

MENTAL ILLNESS Amable, Avertinus, Bertha, Berthaldus of Reims, Columban, Drogo, Dymphna, Ebrulf, Eugenia, Germanus of Auxerre, Giles, Gratus, Hervé, Hidulf, Hildevert, Job, John the Great Sinner, Maturinus, Medard, Menoux, Osmund, Patroclus, Quiteria, Raphael, Romanus of Rouen, Ubaldo of Gubbio, Veranus, Victurnianus, Walaricus

MISCARRIAGE Catherine of Siena, Catherine of Vadstena

MOTION SICKNESS Erasmus

MUTENESS - ***See*** **SPEECH IMPEDIMENTS**

N

NAUSEA Juliana Falconieri

NECK DISORDERS Arnould

NEUROLOGIC DISORDERS Bartholomew, Caprasius, Dymphna, Firminus, Menoux

NEURALGIA Ubaldo of Gubbio

NURSING - ***See*** **LACTATION**

O

OBESITY Leonard of Noblac

P

PAIN Loup of Chalon, Zoilus

PARALYSIS Adelard, Bonitus, Catald of Taranto, Christopher, Clotilda, Dizaint, Fursey, Gregory of Utrecht, John Licci, Marus, Maurus, Ortarius, Osmund, Paul of Narbonne, Quirinus, Servulus, Walfroy, Walstan, Walter of Poitiers, Wolfgang

PLAGUE Adrian of Nicomedia, Aedh Mac Bricc, Aloysius Gonzaga, Avertan, Barbara, Bernardino of Siena, Bruno of Cologne, Calogeros, Casimir, Catald of Taranto, Catherine of Siena, Charalampos, Charles Borromeo, Christopher, Colman of Stockerau, Cuthbert of Lindisfarne, Deodatus, Edmund the Martyr, Félix of Nantes, Florentius, Fortunatus of Fano, Francis of Paola, Francis Xavier, Fredegand, Gall of Clermont, Genevieve, George, Gerald of Mayo, Giles, Godeberta, Godo, Gregory the Great, Hidulf, Job, John the Great Sinner, Julia of Troyes, Leocadia, Luglius and Luglianus, Macarius of Antioch, Manechildis, Martha of Bethany, Martial of Limoges, Michael the Archangel, Molagga, Nicasius, Oswald of Northumbria, Peter Thomas, Pirminus, Quirinus, Quiteria, Raymond of Toulouse, Remigius, Roch, Rosalia, Saturninus of Toulouse, Sebastian, Senan of Saint-Pol-de-Léon, Serenicus and Serenus, Valentine of Rome, Veranus, Walburga, Zosimus

POISON Benedict of Nursia, Pirminus

POLIO Margaret Mary Alacoque

PREGNANCY Agapitus, Anne, Anthony of Padua, Arnulf of Soissons, Balsamia, Baudelius, Bernard of Rodez, Beuve, Drogo, Emerentiana, Ethelburga, Eulalia of Barcelona, Faith, Gerard Majella, Gislenus, Hartman of Brixen, Honoratus of Toulouse, Honorina of Conflans, Joseph, Leo of Rouen, Madelbertha, Maginus of Tarragona, Margaret of Antioch, Peregrine Laziosi, Pirminus, Raymond Nonnatus, Ulrich of Augsburg, Vitalis of Salzburg

PREMATURE BIRTH Catherine of Vadstena

R

RABIES Denis, Dominic of Silos, Dominic of Sora, Forannan, Germanus of Auxerre, Gildas, Guy of Anderlecht, Hubert of Liège, Otto of Bamberg, Peter Chrysologus, Quiteria, Ulrich of Augsburg, Veranus, Walburga

RACHITIS Méen, Millefort

RAPE VICTIMS Dymphna

RECTAL DISEASES Fiacre

RESPIRATORY PROBLEMS - *See* **LUNG DISEASES**

RHEUMATISM Burchard, Caprasius, Ethelburga, Ferreolus, Firminus, James the Greater, Kilian, Leander, Lubin of Chartres, Maurus, Méen, Nicholas of Bari, Servatius, Stapinus, Theodoric of Mont d'Or, Ursus of Aosta, Walter of Pontoise

S

SCABIES Aldegonde, Cessator, Fursey, Job, Julian the Hospitaler, Magnobodus, Méen, Mennas, Radegunde, Regina of Alise

SCROFULA Balbina, Cadoc of Llancarfan, Candida, Clodoald, Donanus, Edward the Confessor, Eligius, Gerard of Brogne, Hildevert, Leontius, Marculf, Maurus, Méen, Quirinus

SCURVY Firminus

SEA SICKNESS Erasmus

SEXUALLY TRANSMITTED DISEASES Fiacre, George, Job, Leonard of Noblac, Psalmodius, Symphorian

SICKNESS - *See* **DISEASE (IN GENERAL)**

SKIN DISEASES Anthony the Great, Bartholomew, Bonosa, Enimia, Fursey, George, Isberga, Job, Julian the Hospitaler, Magnobodus, Marculf, Martin of Tours, Méen, Patroclus, Peregrine Laziosi, Regina of Alise, Reineldis, Roch

SLEEPWALKING Dymphna

SMALLPOX Bonosa, Maginus of Tarragona, Mathias the Apostle, Nicasius, Rita of Cascia, Rose of Lima, Saturninus of Toulouse

SNAKEBITES - *See* **VENOM**

SPEECH IMPEDIMENTS Adelard, Drogo, Mommolinus, Mucius, Syre

SPLENIC DISEASES Phaletrus

SPRAINS Drogo

STARVATION Anthony of Padua

STERILITY - *See* **INFERTILITY**

STOMACH DISORDERS Charles Borromeo, Dulcidius of Agen, Emerentiana, Gregory the Great, Juliana Falconieri, Roland of Chèzery, Timothy, Wolfgang

STROKE Andrew Avellino, Wolfgang

SUDDEN DEATH Andrew Avellino, Barbara, Catherine of Alexandria

T

THROAT DISORDERS Alban of Mainz, Albert of Trapani, Andrew the Apostle, Arnould, Bertilia, Blase, Cunera, Godeleva, Gunsaldus, Ignatius of Antioch, Lucy of Syracuse, Peter Damian, Quirinus, Remigius, Swithbert

TINEA Enimia, Ignatius of Antioch, Méen, Radegunde

TONGUE DISEASES Catherine of Alexandria

TOOTH DISORDERS Agapitus, Alena, Apollonia, Baldus, Blase, Ceranus, Charitina, Christopher, Crescentia, Dalmatius Moner, Desideratus, Dominic of Sora, Elizabeth of Hungary, Engelmund, Forannan, Gregory of Armenia, Ida of Nivelle, Medard, Osmund, Rigobert, Thaumast, Theodulph, Ursmar

TRANSPLANTATION Cosmas and Damian
TUBERCULOSIS Bernulph of Utrecht, Pantaleon, Thérèse de Lisieux
TYPHOID Adelard
TYPHUS Adelard

U

ULCERS Aldegonde, Charles Borromeo, Fiacre, Job, Maudez, Quirinus, Radegunde, Reineldis
URINARY STONES Apollinaris of Ravenna, Burchard, Emilien, Godehard, Liborius of Le Mans
URINARY TRACT DISORDERS Alban of Mainz, Rolande

V

VENOM Amable, Dominic of Sora, Josse, Pirminus, Vitus
VERTIGO Avertinus, John the Baptist, Orana, Saturninus of Toulouse
VOMITING Juliana Falconieri

W

WHOOPING COUGH Bavo, Blase, Nicasius
WORMS Hildevert, Millefort, Psalmodius
WOUNDS AND INJURIES Aldegonde, Amalburga of Maubeuge, Edmund the Martyr, Marciana, Maudez, Maximinus of Besançon, Peregrine Laziosi, Quiteria, Reineldis, Rita of Cascia, Rose of Lima, Sebastian, Venantius of Camerino

Y

YELLOW FEVER Albert of Trapani

Index of Medical Specialties

AMBULANCE DRIVERS
Michael the Archangel

ANESTHESIOLOGISTS
Rene Goupil

BREASTFEEDING
Gilbert of Neufontaines, Giles

CARDIOLOGISTS
Philip Neri

DENTISTS
Apollonia, Cosmas and Damian, Lambert of Maastricht

DERMATOLOGISTS
Bartholomew

DIETICIANS
Martha of Bethany

EMERGENCY MEDICAL TECHNICIANS
Michael the Archangel

HOSPICE
Elizabeth of Hungary

HOSPITAL ADMINISTRATORS
Basil the Great, Francis Xavier, Martha of Bethany

HOSPITAL WORKERS
Camillus of Lellis, Job, Vincent de Paul

HOSPITALS
Camillus of Lellis, Elizabeth of Hungary, John of God, Joseph

MEDICAL SOCIAL WORKERS
Jean François Régis

MEDICINE
Luke the Evangelist

MIDWIVES
Cosmas and Damian, Pantaleon, Raymond Nonnatus

NURSES
Agatha, Camillus of Lellis, Catherine of Alexandria, Catherine of Siena, John of God, Margaret of Antioch, Raphael

OBSTETRICIANS
Raymond Nonnatus

OPHTHALMOLOGY
Lucy of Syracuse

OPTICIANS
Hubert of Liège

OTORHINOLARYNGOLOGISTS
Blase

PHARMACISTS
Aemilianus, Cosmas and Damian, James the Greater, Nicholas of Bari, Roch

PHYSICIANS
Caesarius of Nazianzen, Cosmas and Damian, Giuseppe Moscati, Luke the Evangelist, Pantaleon, Raphael, Roch, Ursicinus, Zenaide

PLASTIC SURGEONS
Bartholomew

PODIATRISTS
Peter the Apostle

PROCTOLOGISTS
Fiacre

PSYCHIATRISTS
Dymphna

RADIOLOGISTS
Michael the Archangel

SURGEONS
Cosmas and Damian, Lambert of Maastricht, Luke the Evangelist, Quintinus, Roch

TELEMEDICINE
Clare of Assisi

UROLOGY
Liborius of Le Mans

WET NURSES
Agatha, Lambert of Maastricht, Mamas

Illustrations

A

ACHATIUS *Martyrdom of San Acacio,* Anonymous. Museo National del Prado, Madrid, Spain.

ADELARD *Saint Adelard Distributing Alms,* Hans the elder Burgkamair, ca. 1500.

ADRIAN OF NICOMEDIA

AEDH MAC BRICC

AGAPITUS Artist unknown, from a painting on the wall of the Cathedral at Palestrina, Italy.

AGATHA *The Martyrdom of Saint Agatha,* Giovanni Battista Tiepolo, ca. 1750. Gemäldegalerie, Berlin, Germany.

AGRIPPINA OF MINEO

ALBAN OF MAINZ Anonymous Tyrolean painter, sixteenth century. National Gallery of Art, Washington, DC.

ALDEGONDE

ALOYSIUS GONZAGA Unknown Italian painter, ca. 1790.

ALPHONSUS MARIA DE LIGUORI

AMALBURGA OF MAUBEUGE

ANASTASIUS THE PERSIAN

ANDREW THE APOSTLE *The Calling of the Apostles Peter and Andrew,* Duccio di Buoninsegna, 1308-1311. National Gallery of Art, Washington, DC.

ANDREW AVELLINO Unknown artist, nineteenth century.

ANIANUS *Saint Mark Healing the Cobbler Anianus,* Giovanni Battistada da Conegliano, 1499. Gemäldegalerie, Berlin, Germany.

ANNE *The Nativity of the Virgin,* Pietro de Cortona. Musée du Louvre, Paris.

ANTHONY THE GREAT *Christ Appearing to Saint Anthony Abbot During His Temptation,* Annibale Carracci. National Gallery, London, UK.

ANTHONY OF PADUA *Anthony of Padua With the Infant Jesus,* Antonio de Pereda, seventeenth century.

APOLLINARIS OF RAVENNA

APOLLONIA *Saint Apollonia,* Francisco de Zurbarán. Musée du Louvre, Paris.

ARNOULD

ARNULF OF SOISSONS *Saint Arnold of Soissons,* ca. 1490-1500. Museum voor Schone Kunsten, Ghent, Belgium. Photo by Roel Renmans.

ATHANASIUS

B

BARBARA

BARTHOLOMEW Michelangelo Buonarroti, ca. 1510. Sistine Chapel, The Vatican.

BASIL THE GREAT *Saint Basil Dictating His Doctrine,* Francisco de Herrera the Elder. Musée du Louvre, Paris.

BAVO Geertgen tot Sint Jans, late fifteenth century.

BENEDICT THE MOOR

BENEDICT OF NURSIA *Saint Benedict in Prayer,* Master of Messkrich, 1538 or later. Staatsgalerie, Stuttgart, Germany.

BERNARDINO OF SIENA *Saint Bernardino of Siena,* Domenikos Theotocopoulos (El Greco). Museo del Greco, Toledo, Spain.

BLASE Predella panel from stories in *Life of Saint Blaise: The Wolf Returning the Pig to the Poor Widow,* Sano di Pietro. Pinacoteca, Spain.

C

CADOC OF LLANCARFAN

CAMILLUS OF LELLIS

CASILDA OF TOLEDO *Saint Casilda,* Francisco de Zuberón, ca. 1640. Museo Nacional del Prado, Madrid, Spain.

CASIMIR

CASTORIUS *The Roman Martyr Saints Claudius, Castorius, and Simplicius,* Hans Suess Kulmbach, 1520.

CATALD OF TARANTO Statue of Saint Catald in the Cathedral of Saint Cataldo, Taranto, Italy.

CATHERINE OF ALEXANDRIA *Catherine of Alexandria,* Caravaggio, ca. 1598. Thyssen-Bormenisza Collection, Madrid, Spain.

CATHERINE OF SIENA *Saint Catherine of Siena Dictating Her Dialogues to Raymond of Capua,* Giovanni de Paolo, fifteenth century. Detroit Institute of Arts, Detroit, Michigan.

CATHERINE OF VADSTENA

CHARLES BORROMEO *Saint Carlo Borromeo,* Orazio Borgianni, 1610-1616. The Hermitage, Saint Petersburg, Russia.

CHRISTOPHER *Saint Christopher,* Master of the Embroidered Foliage. Gemäldegalerie, Dresden, Germany.

CLARE OF ASSISI *Saint Clare Driving Saracens Out of San Damiano by the Force of Her Prayers* (detail), Follower of Guido de Siena, fourteenth century. Pinacoteca Comunale, Spain.

CORNELIUS Stained glass. National Gallery of Art, Washington, DC.

COSMAS AND DAMIAN *Limb Transplantation Miracle by Saints Cosmos and Damian,* Swabian wood-panel painting, ca. 1500. Württembergische Landesmuseum, Stuttgart, Germany.

CUNÉGONDE

CUTHBERT OF LINDISFARNE Aidan Hart.

CYRIACUS From a stain glass window. Pfarrkirche Saint Pelagus, Weitnau, Germany.

D

DENIS *Saint Denis,* Boucicant Master. Musée Jacquemart, André, Paris.

DOMINIC OF SILOS *The Madonna Guiding Saint Dominic to Victory Over the Albigensians,* Giovanni Battista Crespi, ca. 1632. Museo Civico, Cremona, Italy.

DROGO *Saint Isidore,* Bartolomé Estéban Murillo, 1655.

DYMPHNA

E

EDMUND THE MARTYR *Life of Saint Edmund,* unknown artist, mid-twelfth century. Pierpont Morgan Library, New York, NY.

EDWARD THE CONFESSOR *Richard II Presented to the Virgin Child by His Patron Saints* (the Wilton Diptych), French School, ca. 1394-1399. National Gallery, London, UK. (Left panel, from left to right: Edmund, Edward the Confessor, John the Baptist.)

ELIGIUS *Saint Eligius,* Petrus Christus, 1449. Metropolitan Museum of Art, New York, NY.

ELIZABETH OF HUNGARY

ERASMUS *Martyrdom of Saint Erasmus,* Bouts the Elder, 1458. Sankt Peterskerk, Louvain, Belgium. (Detail of triptych.)

ETHELDREDA

EUSTACE *The Vision of Saint Eustace,* Pisanello, 1438-1442. National Gallery, London, UK.

EZEKIEL MORENO Y DIAZ

F

FELIX OF NOLA *The flogging of Felix of Nola.*

FIACRE

FRANCIS OF PAOLA *The Vision of Saint Francis of Paola,* Bartolomé Estebán Murillo, 1670. J. Paul Getty Museum, Los Angeles, California.

FRANCIS DE SALES *The Virgin Appears to Saint Francis de Sales,* Carlo Maratta. Pinacoteca e Musei Comunali, Forli, Italy.

FRANCIS XAVIER *Miracles of Saint Francis Xavier,* Peter Paul Rubens. Jesuit Church, Antwerp, Blegium.

G

GENEVIEVE Unknown artist, seventeenth century. Musée Carnavelet, Paris.

GEORGE *Saint George and the Dragon,* Raffaello Sanzio da Urbino (Raphael), ca. 1506. National Gallery of Art, Washington, DC.

GERARD MAJELLA

GERTRUDE OF NIVELLES Saint Gertrude of Nivelles statue. Nivelles, Belgium.

GILES *Saint Giles and the Hind,* Master of Saint Giles, sixteenth century. National Gallery, London, UK.

GISLENIUS

GIUSEPPE MOSCATI

GODELEVA *Strangulation of Godelina.* Procession Chapel, Gistel, Belgium.

GREGORY THE GREAT *The Procession of Saint Gregory to Saint Angelo,* Giovanni di Paolo. Musée du Louvre, Paris.

GUY OF ANDERLECHT

H

HENRY II *Emperor Henry II,* fifteenth century painting. Tafelbild Brünn, Mährische, Moravia.

HUBERT OF LIÈGE *The Conversion of Saint Hubert,* Studio of the Master of the Life of the Virgin. National Gallery, London, UK.

HYACINTH *Three Dominican Saints,* Giovanni Battista Piazzetti, 1738. Santa Maria del Gesuati, Venice. (Detail.)

I

IGNATIUS OF ANTIOCH *Saint Ignatius in Glory and the Works of the Jesuit Fathers,* Giovanni Battista Caracciolo, ca. 1629. Museo Correale di Terranova, Sorrento, Italy.

J

JAMES THE GREATER *Saint James Major,* Master Boucieant. Musée Jacquemart, Andrés, Paris.

JEANNE FRANÇOISE DE CHANTAL

JOB *Illustrations to the Book of Job,* engraved prints by William Blake, published 1826.

JOHN THE BAPTIST *The Baptism of Christ,* Bartolomé Estéban Murillo, ca. 1655. Gemäldagalerie, Berlin, Germany.

JOHN CHRYSOSTOM *Saint John Chrysostom Altar,* Sebastiano del Piombo, 1509. San Giovanni Cristostomo, Venice, Italy.

JOHN OF GOD *Saint John of God,* Bartolomé Estéban Murillo, 1647-1682. Museo Municipal de Játiva, Spain.

JOHN THE GREAT SINNER

JOSEPH *Saint Joseph With the Christ Child in His Arms,* Guido Reni, 1620s. The Hermitage, Saint Petersburg, Russia.

JULIANA OF NICOMEDIA

L

LAMBERT OF MAASTRICHT *Martyrdom of Saint Lambert,* fifteenth century. Maastricht, the Netherlands.

LAWRENCE *The Martyrdom of Saint Laurence,* Agnolo Bronzino, 1571. Church of Saint Lorenzo, Florence, Italy.

LAZARUS OF BETHANY *The Raising of Lazarus,* Sebastiano del Piombo, 1517-1519. National Gallery, London, UK.

LEANDER *Saint Leander,* Bartolomé Estéban Murillo, 1655. Seville Cathedral, Seville, Spain.

LEODEGAR

LEONARD OF NOBLAC *The Resurrection of Christ With SS. Leonard of Noblac and Lucia,* Giovanni Antonio Boltraffio, 1491. Gemäldegalerie, Berlin, Germany.

LIBORIUS OF LE MANS Relief in the Trinity Chapel of the Paderborn Cathedral, Germany.

LUBIN OF CHARTRES Stained glass window at Chartres Cathedral of Notre Dame.

LUCY OF SYRACUSE *Saint Lucie,* Beccafumi Domenico di Pace. National Portrait Gallery, Washington, DC.

LUKE THE EVANGELIST *Saint Luke Painting the Virgin's Portrait,* Marten de Vos, 1602. Koninklijk Museum voor Shone Kunsten, Antwerp, Belgium.

LUTGARDIS *Santa Lutgarde,* Francisco de Goya, 1787. Monasterio de San Joaquín y Santa Ana, Valladolid, Spain.

M

MAMAS *Fresco of Saint Mamas,* sixteenth century. Chapel of Saint Mamas, village of Sotira, Cyprus.

MARGARET OF ANTIOCH

MARGARET MARY ALACOQUE *Alacoque Contemplating the Sacred Heart of Jesus,* Corrado Giaquinto, ca. 1765.

MARGUERITE D'YOUVILLE

MARTHA OF BETHANY *Christ in the House of Mary and Martha,* Tintoretto, ca. 1580. Alte Pinakothek, Munich, Germany.

MARTIN OF TOURS *Saint Martin and the Beggar,* Domenikos Theotocopoulos (El Greco), 1597-1599. National Gallery of Art, Washington, DC.

MARY OF EGYPT

MAURICE *Martyrdom of Saint Maurice and His Legions,* Domenikos Theotocopoulos (El Greco), 1580-1581. Chapter House, Monastery of El Escorial, Spain.

MAXIMILIAN KOLBE

N

NORBERT *Saint Norbert,* Marten Pepijn, 1637. O.-L. Vrouwekathedraal, Antwerp, Belgium.

NOTBURGA

O

ODILE

OSMUND

P

PANCRAS OF ROME *San Pancrazio,* Giovan Battista Barbieri (Guercino), ca. 1616.

PANTALEON

PAULINA DO CORAÇÃO AGONIZANTE DE JESUS

PEREGRINE LAZIOSI

PETER OF ALCÁNTARA *Ecstacy of Saint Peter of Alcantara,* Melchior Perez Holguin, eighteenth century. National Museum of Art, La Paz, Bolivia.

PETER THE APOSTLE *Christ Appearing to Saint Peter on the Appian Way (Domine, Quo Vadis?),* Annibale Carracci, 1601-1602. National Gallery, London, UK.

PETER DAMIAN
PETRONILLA
PHILIP BENIZI *Saint Phillip,* Peter Paul Rubens, ca. 1610-1612. Museo del Prado, Madrid, Spain.
PHILIP NERI *The Appearance of the Virgin to Philip Neri,* Carlo Maratta, ca. 1675.
PHILOMENA
POLYCARP

R

RADEGUNDE *Redegund With Bishop Euphronisus and Venatius Fortunatus, Receiving the Cross and Gospel Book.* Abbaye de Saint Antoine in Isère, France.
RAPHAEL
RAYMOND NONNATUS
REMIGIUS *The Baptism of Clovis,* Master of Saint Giles, ca. 1500. National Gallery of Art, Washington, DC.
RENE GOUPIL Jesuit Singapore Website, *www.jesuit.org.sg.*
RITA OF CASCIA
ROCH Minor Library, University of Rochester Medical Center, Rochester, NY.
ROSALIA *Rosalina With Angels,* Miguel Cabrera, ca. 1740.
ROSE OF LIMA *The Virgin Mary and Child With Three Dominican Saints,* Giovanni Battista Tiepolo. Santa Maria del Rosario (Gesuati), Venice. (Panel foreground from left to right: Rose of Lima, Catherine of Sienna, and Agnes of Mentepulciano.)

S

SCHOLASTICA Scholastica and her twin brother, Saint Benedict, at the foot of the cross. Fresco from Sacro Speco (Holy Grotto), Subiaco, Italy.
SEBASTIAN *Saint Sebastian,* Tiziano Vecellio (Titian), ca. 1570. The Hermitage, Saint Petersburg, Russia.
SERVATIUS
SEVERINUS OF NORICUM by Albrecht Dürer.
SIGISMUND OF BURGUNDY *Sigismondo Malatesta (d. 1468) Kneeling Before His Patron, Saint Sigismund of Burgundy,* Piero della Francesca, 1451. Tempio Malatestiano, Rimini, Italy.
STANISLAUS KOSTKA *Stanislaus Kostka Beaten by His Brother,* Andrea Pozzo, late sixteenth century. Church of Saint Ignazio, Rome, Italy.
SWITHBERT
SYMPHORIAN *Martyrdom of Saint Symphorian,* Jean Auguste Dominique Ingres, 1480-1481.

T

TERESA OF ÁVILA *The Ecstasy of Saint Teresa,* Gianlorenzo Bernini, 1645-1652. Santa Maria della Vittoria, Rome, Italy.

THÉRÈSE DE LISIEUX Saint Thérèse of Lisieux, nineteenth century. Private collection.

TIMOTHY

TROPHIMUS OF ARLES

U

UBALDO OF GUBBIO

ULRICH OF AUGSBURG

V

VALENTINE OF ROME *Saint Valentine Heals the Epileptics and Rebukes the Worshippers of False Gods,* Bartholomeus Zeitblom. Bayerische Staatsgemäldesammlungen, Munich, Germany.

VINCENT DE PAUL

VINCENT FERRER

VITUS

W

WALBURGA

WALSTAN

WILLIBRORD *Consecration of Saint Willibrord,* eighteenth century.

WOLFGANG *Saint Wolfgang and the Devil,* panel of Pacher's Fathers of the Church altarpiece, ca. 1483. Alte Pinakothek, Munich, Germany.

Z

ZENOBIUS